The Placebo Effect in Manual Therapy

Improving Clinical Outcomes in your Practice

T0187142

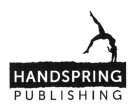

HANDSPRING
PUBLISHING

The Placebo Effect in Manual Therapy

Improving Clinical Outcomes in your Practice

Brian Fulton RMT
Registered Massage Therapist, Ontario, Canada

Forewords by **Leon Chaitow ND DO**
State Registered Osteopathic Practitioner (UK), Honorary Fellow
and formerly Senior Lecturer, University of Westminster, London, UK;
Editor in Chief *Journal of Bodywork and Movement Therapies*; Director,
Ida P Rolf Research Foundation (USA); Member Standing Committees,
Fascia Research Congress & Fascia Research Society (USA)

and

Ruth Werner BCTMB
Board Certified in Therapeutic Massage and Bodywork
Past President, Massage Therapy Foundation
Trustee, Massage Therapy Foundation
Author of *A Massage Therapist's Guide to Pathology*

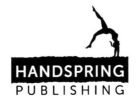

HANDSPRING
PUBLISHING

Edinburgh

HANDSPRING PUBLISHING LIMITED
The Old Manse, Fountainhall,
Pencaitland, East Lothian
EH34 5EY, United Kingdom
Tel: +44 1875 341 859
Website: www.handspringpublishing.com

First published 2015 in the United Kingdom by Handspring Publishing

ISBN 978-1-909141-29-2

British Library Cataloguing in Publication Data
A catalogue record for this book is available from the British Library

Important notice
It is the responsibility of the practitioner, employing a range of sources of information, their personal experience, and their understanding of the particular needs of the patient, to determine the best approach to treatment.
Neither the publishers nor the authors will be liable for any loss or damage of any nature occasioned to or suffered by any person or property in regard to product liability, negligence or otherwise, or through acting or refraining from acting as a result of adherence to the material contained in this book.

Commissioning Editor, Mary Law
Design by Pete Wilder, Designers Collective
Cover design by Bruce Hogarth, KinesisCreative
Cartoons by Wesley Donkers
Photographs 2.6 and 2.10 by Divino Mucciante
Copyediting by Lynn Watt
Typeset by DSM Soft
Printed Bell & Bain Limited

Contents

Foreword

Leon Chaitow ND DO

This important book explains, in appropriate and easily digestible detail, the potency and power of ways in which self-regulating potentials can be harnessed – by means of that much mentioned, but little understood factor – placebo.

Manual therapy involves a multitude of interactions between the person receiving and the person providing the treatment. On a physical level there will be contact that most commonly involves hands being placed on the tissues being addressed. Apart from the particular tissues involved, this contact involves such variables as the size of the area being contacted, the degree of force being applied (ranging from minimal to forceful), for seconds or minutes, in a sustained or variable manner, static or moving, with the process being passive or with active participation by the recipient.

The intent of the provider adds further variants – to stimulate, to mobilize, to calm, to stretch, to compress or distract and more – possibly involving objectives to enhance functionality, or to remove obstacles to recovery.

And, depending on the overall age, condition and resilience of the individual, as well as the status of the local tissues being addressed (for example tense, congested, inflamed, hypertonic, flaccid, painful or pain-free), the ideal outcome may be measured by the degree of improvement – how much more functional, less painful, is the condition or situation, compared with pre-treatment?

When a patient reports marked benefit following a previous treatment, it is likely that both you and the patient will credit the particular treatment protocol – and your skill in delivering it – as the reason for the improvement.

Such processes might be seen as a simple matter of cause and effect – resulting from predictable biomechanical and psychosocial influences. However, such an assumption would not necessarily be accurate. For one thing, the condition may be one that would have improved on its own, since self-regulation is the norm rather than the exception.

In reality the 'effect' of manual treatment is only partly dependent on the efficiency of the delivery of appropriate techniques and methods. The other half of the equation involves the self-regulating potentials of the individual. And some of that response is not tissue-related.

Self-regulating, self-repairing, self-healing influences emerge from a variety of deep pools of homeostatic potential that reside both in the recesses of the brain as well as in the systems of the body.

Broken bones mend, cuts heal, infections are overcome – with and without therapeutic interventions – and sometimes despite these. *If only we could tap into that deep pool of homeostatic potential!*

Vincent and Lewith (1995) have described placebo as a term that incorporates *'a set of disparate phenomena.'* But what might these *disparate phenomena* be? Lougee and colleagues (2013) include the following as possible components of placebo:

> *The natural history of the illness; the patient's (and practitioner's) expectations and beliefs; the degree of suggestibility or persuasion of the patient; the all-important patient–practitioner relationship and interaction; any conditioning influences; as well as reasons for seeking care – and of course the healing environment.*

The author of this book, Brian Fulton, has delved deeply into the topic of placebo to deliver a text that can help you learn how to harness and work with placebo – as well as how to avoid the pitfalls of the nocebo effect.

The many chapters, written in a satisfyingly accessible way, take you through definitions and historical aspects of the subject, before going into biological, psychological, ethical and practical operational aspects in which you should be able to absorb the essence of what is required to utilize this powerful innate force for good, on a daily basis.

This does not mean that the manual treatments that you offer become superfluous, but that their potential can be vastly enhanced by using simple methods that encourage well-being – with the aid of placebo.

Corfu, Greece
February 2015

REFERENCES

1. Lougee H et al (2013) The suitability of sham treatments for use as placebo controls in trials of spinal manipulative therapy: a pilot study. *J Bodyw Mov Ther* 17(1):59–68.
2. Vincent C, Lewith G (1995) Placebo controls for acupuncture studies. *J R Soc Med* 88(4):199–204.

Foreword

Ruth Werner BCTMB

We already know that touch feels good; why ask why?

I once had a chiropractor who came very highly recommended. His understanding of the principles of his science was flawless. But he treated me dismissively, he seldom made eye contact, and when a neck adjustment sent an electric jolt down my arm and I flinched, he shrugged and said, 'Well, chiropractic isn't for everybody'. Here was someone who understood his technique perfectly, but his ability to convey his skill into a positive outcome was impaired by his inability to make a useful personal connection. (I promptly fired him, and found someone else.)

The use of touch to promote well-being is as ancient as the first caress a mother ever gave to her baby, but the field of touch research is still in its early days. We continue to struggle with questions such as if manual therapies work, and for whom, in what circumstances, under what conditions and done by what level of professional. Then come questions of how well manual therapies compare with other interventions for effectiveness, safety, and cost. Dosing studies attempt to define the sweet spot where manual therapies find their peak usefulness, balanced with pragmatic considerations like cost and convenience.

All these inquiries can be framed as yes-or-no questions to help develop our knowledge of how to get the best from manual therapy, as we understand it.

But the research examined here by Brian Fulton goes beyond yes-or-no questions. It takes a brave researcher to undertake the question not of **if**, but of **how** touch affects function. We see that it appears to improve our sense of well-being and ability to cope with everyday life stressors – but how? We see that people with anxiety disorders and depression report improved symptoms when they receive welcomed touch, but why? In the best of all possible worlds the answers to these questions allow us to hone our skills so that we can achieve positive outcomes on purpose instead of by accident. To the frustration of some traditional scientists, it can be difficult to untangle how much of a positive outcome is due to the skin-to-skin intervention, and how much is due to the subjective and complex interactions that happen between a practitioner and a patient. And ultimately, the solution is not one or the other; it is both.

In this book the author has focused on a phenomenon that is sometimes considered to be statistical 'noise' that comes up between a research question and its results – the placebo effect. He has made a compelling argument that this noise can be as interesting and elucidating as any typical result. In the world of manual therapies, as in any relationship that relies heavily on a level of trust and positive expectations between practitioners and their patients, that relationship itself turns out to be as important for the patient as any exchange of skills or advice. In other words, if we like our clinician, and we know that s/he has our best interest at heart, and we expect his or her work to be effective, then – voila! We are more likely to have a positive outcome than if we didn't have that sense of warmth and unconditional positive regard that is the basis of the therapeutic relationship. This leads to the larger question: how can we harness that power?

So, yes, it's important to know what happens in a session of manual therapy, from the molecular changes in the tissues up through lines of force that stretch fascia or stimulate nerve endings. But at an even more fundamental level, understanding how to maximize the power of a good therapeutic relationship is just as vital, much more subtle, and usually under-addressed. Most manual therapists are not taught to embrace the power of the therapeutic relationship, and to use it to its fullest. This book will help to fill some of that vacuum, and I look forward to seeing how it influences new generations of hands-on health care providers.

Waldport, OR, USA
February 2015

Preface

When my career as a massage therapist began, I had a large number of techniques at my disposal from the 2-year training that massage therapists receive in Ontario, Canada. As each year went by, my techniques improved and I continued with my postgraduate education, taking many courses with most of them being technique-based. Five years into my career I encountered Stuart Taws, who taught a course called Soft Tissue Release©, a system based on an osteopathic technique that works on the nervous system and soft tissue jointly by starting with point pressure on a muscle in the shortened position, then quickly lengthening it. However, instead of introducing us to his technique, Stuart spent the first few hours of this 2-day course talking about 'you'. By you, of course he meant the first person singular... 'me'. He made it very personal, talking about your attitudes, your approach, your ego, your preconceived notions as a health professional, and how any of these could be barriers to the therapeutic relationship. He also talked about the doctor within all of us, about deep consciousness, quantum physics, and other esoteric topics, tying them all into the therapeutic relationship that exists between the practitioner and the patient. Finally, he linked all of these topics to the science of his therapy. This approach impressed me deeply. I was finally taking an evidence-based techniques course with a holistic approach; an approach that looks at the 'big picture'.

Meeting Stuart was kismet in that I had just completed a magazine article on the placebo effect and, while he was not using that particular word, further investigation and research in the placebo effect would reveal that this was largely a matter of semantics. What we both knew was that the patient already has an amazing internal healing system. The question was: what techniques and approaches could you use to re-start this healing system in areas of the body where it seems stalled?

So then... as a practitioner, how do you augment your patients' internal healing systems? Clearly, knowledge, assessment skills, competency and technique are essential elements in manual therapy... full stop! I do not wish to suggest that these are not essential tools in manual therapy; they are unquestionably essential if you are going to know what and whom you are treating, and how you are going to treat any given condition. However, understanding how to maximize the healing response in your patient is also an essential piece of the puzzle. Jerome D. Frank MD, PhD, in his seminal work on this topic entitled *Persuasion and healing* (Frank 1991), states:

> *My position is that technique is not irrelevant to outcome. Rather, I maintain that the success of all techniques depends on the patient's sense of alliance with an actual or symbolic healer.*

Before completing this book, I read dozens of books on mind/body medicine and the placebo effect, and perused hundreds of clinical trials. Information was gathered from many sources for the purposes of creating an assemblage of facts, theories and methods for manual practitioners to employ, to the end of improving therapeutic outcomes for their patients. Admittedly, I have relied on conclusions and insights from experts in this area of healing, based on information gathered from clinical trials and systematic reviews that they have either performed or examined.

Before proceeding further, I would like to speak to the limits of my abilities in tackling the daunting task of this book. There are currently 5096 medical journals indexed at National Institutes of Health/US National Library of Medicine that are accessible via through PubMed/MEDLINE. A recent search on PubMed for 'placebo' generated just under 170 300 results. This number changes not so much by the day as by the hour. Typing 'placebo effect' into PubMed's search engine in June 2014 returned 66 792 results. Currently, approximately 10 peer-reviewed papers are added to PubMed's database per day containing the term 'placebo effect'. I make no claim to have combed over all of the journals and studies, nor do I put myself forth as an expert on this subject. Rather, just like you, I am a manual practitioner on a journey to improve himself, the lot of his patients, and the knowledge base of other practitioners.

What is clear is that scientific interest in studying this phenomenon has reached critical mass. Look at these year-specific results for the search term 'placebo effect' in PubMed's database (i.e. this number represents the number of studies that were published in that specific year on this topic.)

'Placebo effect' in PubMed	
Year	Year-specific Results
1972	13
1982	563
1992	1491
2002	2331
2013	3865

I think that these results speak for themselves. Interest has continued to grow dramatically in this topic and, as yet, shows no sign of letting up. In 2011 Harvard Medical School instituted the Program in Placebo Studies and the Therapeutic Encounter (PiPS) at Beth Israel Deaconess Medical Center. All of this points to just how important this topic has become. This is no longer something that is only of interest to fringe groups outside of the mainstream medical paradigm. The medical establishment has definitely stood up and taken notice of this very real phenomenon.

It would seem that the time is right for a book such as this, especially one tailored to the manual therapy professions. As you read through this book, you will see both older and newer reference sources. This is because I am attempting to give the reader a retrospective of how we got to where we are now with this fascinating healing phenomenon, as well as providing recent research on the placebo effect.

I hope that this book helps to re-inspire you in your role as a health care provider, just as researching and writing it has done for me.

Brian Fulton RMT
Ontario, Canada
March 2015

Acknowledgements

I want to thank Stuart Taws for practicing what I have always believed in theory and for teaching me confidence in what I do, by showing a deep confidence in his methods and outcomes.

I want to thank Dr Howard Brody MD for researching and writing so competently on this topic. His book, *The Placebo Response*, impressed me so deeply that it started me on a journey that eventually led to this book.

Brian Fulton RMT

Introduction to the Book

Why write about the placebo effect?

If you think that this topic is not terribly important because your patients are responding only to your treatment modality and not to a placebo effect, then perhaps you might want to look at the 2011 peer-reviewed paper published by the *Journal of Manual and Manipulative Therapy,* 'Placebo response to manual therapy: something out of nothing?' The authors look at 94 different research papers on manual therapy and on the placebo effect and draw some relevant inferences about the placebo effect in manual therapy. Some of the papers reviewed clearly suggest that what you and I think may be happening is not exactly what **is** happening. The evidence points to a strong placebo component in what we do in our collective professions, as the conclusions of this study suggest (Bialosky et al. 2011):

> *We suggest that manual therapists conceptualize placebo not only as a comparative intervention, but also as a potential active mechanism to partially account for treatment effects associated with manual therapy. We are not suggesting manual therapists include known sham or ineffective interventions in their clinical practice, but take steps to maximize placebo responses to reduce pain.*

The evidence-based model is not affecting many practitioners' mindsets quite as quickly as was assumed. There are several reasons for this, but certainly one is that many of us in the field of manual therapy operate from instinct and our own practice logic. We are not easily swayed by one study that says our model is deficient in some manner. However, when multiple studies say the same thing, it is definitely time to change our ways and adopt a different approach, or even a new paradigm.

Another interesting review of evidence is a 2010 paper, 'Effectiveness of manual therapies: the UK evidence report'. The authors looked at 49 recent relevant systematic reviews, 16 evidence-based clinical guidelines, plus an additional 46 randomized controlled trials (RCT) that had not yet been included in systematic reviews and guidelines. The authors reviewed 26 categories of conditions containing RCT evidence for the use of manual therapy: 13 musculoskeletal conditions, four types of chronic headache and nine non-musculoskeletal conditions. This report (Bronfort et al. 2010), published in *Chiropractic and Manual Therapies* (the official journal of the Chiropractic & Osteopathic College of Australasia, the European Academy of Chiropractic and The Royal College of Chiropractors), recognizes the important role that manual therapy plays in treating a wide variety of ailments, but even in this the authors state:

> *Additionally, there is substantial evidence to show that the ritual of the patient practitioner interaction has a therapeutic effect in itself separate from any specific effects of the treatment applied. This phenomenon is termed contextual effects. The contextual or, as it is often called, non-specific effect of the therapeutic encounter can be quite different depending on the type of provider, the explanation or diagnosis given, the provider's enthusiasm, and the patient's expectations.*

Evidence supporting the placebo response

The goal of this book is to help you improve your clinical outcomes by applying the lessons learned from placebo trials and other studies. As mentioned, placebos are used in most drug trials and in most of these studies, the control (placebo) group's health improves. This is rather fascinating when you consider that these individuals were typically given an inert substance. Clearly, something is going on with the patient's own healing system. This book largely cites placebo trials but there are lessons to be gleaned from other comparative studies as well. My desire is to present evidence of any non-manual component of the practitioner–patient relationship that will augment healing and consider ways that we, as practitioners, can apply these concepts in our practice to improve therapeutic outcomes. While accessing and engaging the patient's inner healer is a deeply complex matter that is only partly understood, some very important lessons have been learned about this topic. We have Henry Beecher MD, who had to get by without anesthetic in a combat area during WWII and, interestingly, the pharmaceutical industry to thank for some fascinating insights into the placebo effect. Tens of thousands of studies have been conducted around the placebo. I say 'around' because the placebo wasn't initially studied per se by the pharmaceutical industry but studied by default as a baseline against which to compare drugs in clinical trials. However, concurrently, some researchers, physicians, anthropologists, and others with a deep scientific interest in the body's ability to heal itself, have examined and analyzed many of these studies and drawn some interesting conclusions. In addition, this same group have also designed some fascinating studies that have specifically examined the placebo effect in more recent decades, providing several illuminating discoveries. The pharmaceutical industry eventually stood up and took notice of the placebo effect because they had too many drugs that could not outperform placebos. As a result, they have a deep vested interest in minimizing this effect in drug trials.

This book is largely, but not entirely, about the lessons from those studies. In this book we will look at any factor that improves the health outcome of a patient outside of the obvious skills that we hold as health practitioners; in other words anything outside of assessment, treatment, remedial exercises and homecare.

As you look at the literature, it is fascinating to discover that the placebo effect is not just some statistical anomaly. Participants' healing systems are turned on in almost every study that includes being given an inert substance such as a sugar pill. Furthermore, it is not always a pill that acts as a placebo. Sometimes it is a phrase, a presence or a sham procedure that elicits a placebo response. Sometimes it is one in 100 participants that respond, and other times it's 100 people out of 100. Typically, it is a notable percentage of participants who see both subjective and objective improvement. The goal of this book is to tease out why this healing response happens so that you might be able to reproduce these results in a more predictable manner in a clinical setting, not by actually using placebo pills but rather by 'being' the placebo. In other words, our offices, our treatment rooms, our words, our actions and we ourselves are the actual symbols that elicit the placebo response from the patient.

The placebo effect is still part of the Wild, Wild West of medicine, and as such, there is a lot of exploration to be done. We don't know the names of many of the towns that we are passing through, and haven't yet learned all of the laws of the land. In this world, it appears that belief, conditioning and meaning are powerful triggers for release of neurotransmitters in the brain. The guns are components of the immune and endocrine system that become enhanced or suppressed. There are several models that attempt to explain the mechanisms of action, but what is not known far outweighs what is known. Researchers will keep on searching for workable theories and definite pathways and mechanisms, but for the purposes of this book, we will largely confine ourselves to studies that find repeatability of results.

Semantics

At the beginning of this project, I was torn as to whether or not to use the phrase 'placebo' in this book at all, since this word does arrive with a fair bit of baggage. For example, the existence of the word 'placate' suggests a historical perspective of hollowness surrounding the root word placebo. The literal translation of the word placebo, from Latin, 'I will please'* seems woefully inadequate to describe a way to activate healing systems within the patient. Phrases such as 'the healer within' or 'healing power of the mind' more aptly describe what is going on, but these words are largely owned by an alternative health community that takes much on faith and tends not to be as concerned with whether or not an approach has passed the test of scientific scrutiny. As a result these terms carry baggage that is not helpful to an 'evidence-based' discussion. In the end, I returned to the term 'placebo effect/response', but even the medical community is aware that it is

---

*The word placebo ('I will please' in Latin) entered the English language by way of a peculiar mistranslation of the 116th Psalm that read, 'I will please the Lord' rather than 'I will walk before the Lord'. In the medieval Catholic liturgy this verse opened the Vespers for the Dead. Because professional mourners were sometimes hired to sing vespers, 'to sing placebos' came to be a derogatory phrase describing a servile flatterer. By the early 19th century, 'placebo' had come to mean a medicine given 'more to please than to benefit the patient'.

now time for a new or broader term. Dr Fabrizio Benedetti concluded in his 2008 review of current literature entitled 'Mechanisms of placebo and placebo-related effects across diseases and treatments', *'It is now clear that the term placebo effect is too restrictive'* (Benedetti 2008). However, for the time being, until our collective understanding of the topic improves, we will continue with the use of this accepted MeSH (US National Library of Medicine's Medical Subject Headings MeSH®) term.

Just to give you an idea of how inadequate the term 'placebo effect' is, here is a partial list of labels for this phenomenon that I encountered while researching this book. Many people had their own favorite term that they wanted to use instead. As mentioned, the most common MeSH term is placebo; however, this term can be combined with other MeSH terms to generate searches such as 'placebo effect', 'placebo response', 'placebo analgesia' etc. However, even researchers find this term confining and some make alternative suggestions. The fact that so many people seem to be inventing new terms suggests perhaps that 'placebo effect' falls short of the mark.

Perhaps if you put all of the following concepts together, you would have a good term to describe just what is going on. The order of terms below is simply aesthetic – phrases with more letters ended up at the bottom of the list:

- The hope effect
- The belief effect
- Placebo response
- The healer within
- The placebo effect
- Contextual healing
- Meaning response
- Non-specific effects
- Remembered wellness
- Our deep unconscious
- The body's own wisdom
- Healing power of the mind
- Meaning and context effect
- The endogenous health care system
- Releasing the body's inner pharmacy
- Our natural health care management system.

The hope effect touches on the idea that hope of healing is relevant. It is well recognized in the psychiatric community that hopelessness inpatients can retard recovery or even hasten death. The first person that I found using this phrase was Jerome D. Frank in his seminal work *Persuasion and Healing* (Frank & Frank 1991). As a psychiatrist, Frank was fascinated with this component of the therapeutic relationship and was an early writer on this topic.

The belief effect, coined by Dylan Evans in his book *Placebo: Mind Over Matter in Modern Medicine* (Evans 2004), aptly describes much of what is going on. However, there are studies where participants were specifically told that they were being given an inert placebo, and subjects still improved. Also, conditioning studies in animals have yielded powerful placebo effects, but belief, as we know it, is not at play in animal populations.

Placebo response is typically used interchangeably with 'placebo effect'. Response is often the more correct way of labelling the body's reaction to a placebo that has been administered. Both are accepted Medical Subject heading (MeSH) terms and have been since 1990 and these terms are used in the bulk of the research papers. It is a well-understood term, and while it contains baggage, it has a universal currency in the research world (similar to 'ATP' in the body).

Contextual healing is a term coined by Ted Kaptchuk, the director of The Program in Placebo Studies and the Therapeutic Encounter (PiPS) at Harvard Medical School. Kaptchuk has one of the most prominent positions in this field and has led a number of illuminating studies on this topic. Kaptchuk co-authored a paper in 2008 with Franklin Miller, 'The power of context: reconceptualizing the placebo effect'. The authors propose an alternative expression to 'placebo effect' since a placebo is not even used in many studies that attempt to understand this phenomenon (Miller & Kaptchuk 2008):

> *The placebo is a methodological tool for understanding contextual healing but is not itself responsible for clinical effects that emanate from the clinician–patient relationship. Conceptualizing the placebo effect as contextual healing suggests that theoretical understanding and scientific experimentation related to this phenomenon should aim at isolating and elucidating those factors in the clinician-patient encounter that contribute causally to improvement in outcomes for patients.*

The concept of the **body's own wisdom** involves the important idea that our body does an amazing job of carrying out all its complex functions (including healing), without conscious intervention.

Meaning response is Daniel Moerman's attempt at a fresh term. Moerman is a professor of Anthropology at University of Michigan-Dearborn and is author of *Meaning, Medicine and the Placebo Effect*. As an anthropologist, he approaches this subject from a different angle but there is ample defense for this term. As we will see later there are many explanations of, or components to, the placebo effect but the leading three that are recognized in literature are: 1) expectation; 2) conditioning; and 3) meaning. The gist of his argument is that everything could be lumped into meaning.

Both **the healer within** and **our natural health care management system** could also be viewed as ways of describing the body's own wisdom and ability to heal itself.

'**Non-specific effects**' is a term you will encounter in the literature and it is often followed by an explainer such as placebo effect or contextual effects. As a term, non-specific effects is about as illuminating as a match in a cave. It strikes me that this term is actually misleading. Is reduced blood pressure, pain reduction or improved function non-specific? Are changes in brain activity observed in PET scans or tissue changes viewed by sigmoidoscope non-specific? No, they are quite specific and highly measurable. What is not specific is the cause. The *effect* of this phenomenon can actually be wonderfully specific.

Remembered wellness is Herbert Benson's figurative 'hat in the ring'. Benson, author of *The Relaxation Response,* is an American cardiologist and founder of the Mind/Body Medical Institute at Massachusetts General Hospital in Boston. His contention is that our bodies know how to fix themselves, but they become stuck for one reason or another, and these studies demonstrate ways to get the body to 'remember' again.

Our deep unconscious is a term used by Stuart Taws referring to that part of our patient that we need to give messages to when we are treating them. Sigmund Freud and Carl Jung originally developed and explored the concept of the deep unconscious. Some modern thinkers, such as Robert Langs, see the deep unconscious as an innate mechanism, which is able to heal emotional wounds and point to adaptive solutions in the face of environmental challenges and trauma.

The healing power of the mind from Deepak Choprah tends, at first glance, to be a bit Cartesian-minded. However, once you see the mind (and neural tissue) as being present everywhere in the body, the term sounds more holistic.

Meaning and context effect (MAC) is a term spearheaded by Dr Wayne Jonas of the Samueli Institute in Alexandria, Virginia. As you can see, it combines two terms discussed previously. Jonas points out that the clinical encounter itself is the therapeutic agent and that meaning and context are the filters through which the patient determines the value of the encounter, which then creates a healing effect.

Fabrizio Benedetti, who has pretty much spent his life devoted to researching this phenomenon, uses the term **endogenous health care system**. This phrase uses a mixture of scientific and holistic words to describe what he sees as an innate system that has evolved in social species where members can put their care in the trust of other members. This allows individuals to spend precious physical resources on healing, instead of on immediate threats or concerns. The thinking is that this gave an evolutionary advantage to groups that cared for its members.

Finally, **releasing the body's inner pharmacy** is Howard Brody's addition to this list. He suggests visualization exercises to aid in turning on this healing system or pharmacy. Visualization helps with many other human endeavours, so it would make sense that it would also help in this arena as well.

If you prefer one of these terms, or another one of your own, then please feel free to mentally substitute your term whenever you see *'placebo effect'*. I am personally not married to any term and admittedly only adopt placebo effect/response as a convention for the purpose of exploring and understanding the phenomenon. I will leave it to the experts to battle over what term is most appropriate. In the end, however, most of us in health care are not looking for new labels as much as we are looking for ways to improve therapeutic/clinical outcomes.

Manual therapy and the placebo response

Although there is a sincere effort to make a science of this topic, you already know as a practitioner that what works for patient 'A' may or may not work for patient 'B'. This applies to your manual technique, your language and your approach. Likewise, healing techniques based on the placebo effect need to be tailored to the individual patient. In the end you will see, and hopefully be enthused about the fact, that improving therapeutic outcomes involves not only the development of a new set of psychosocial techniques, but also the re-examination of your own beliefs and assumptions in order to consider what conscious and unconscious ideas you are passing on to your patients about their health and healing. Manual therapy is, in my opinion, a wonderful blend of science and art. Improving clinical outcomes by applying the concepts in this book is exactly the same. There are principles, concepts and methods but eventually you will have to 'make them your own' and tailor these concepts to each and every patient.

The practical examples suggested in Part 2 of this book are geared toward any-one working in the manual therapy professions such as (but not limited to) physi-cal medicine and rehabilitation (physiatry) osteopathy, chiropractic, physical therapy, massage therapy, athletic therapy, kinesiology, occupational therapy or any other type of manual therapy. On the other hand, the concepts presented in this book are universal. They are applicable to anyone who has the sacred honor and privilege of helping someone on their journey out of illness, injury or pain, to a state of improved health. As health care providers, we are truly in a sacred and honoured position. Patients put us at a higher level and come to us hoping or expecting to be healed. This belief, hope or expectation is the beginning point of the placebo effect, and there is a lot that we as practitioners can do to support the dynamic that creates this phenomenon, or to undermine it, as you will see in the sections ahead.

The intent of this book is not for you develop ways to 'trick' your patient. Cer-tainly, your professional code of conduct as a health professional would keep you from going down this path. However, the placebo effect clearly does exist and if, along with proper assessment, knowledge and techniques (already in your pos-session), you apply the concepts presented here in your practice, you will not only be acting ethically… you will, in fact, be acting in the patient's best interest. How-ever, ethical questions are almost never black and white. Therefore, there is a sec-tion devoted exclusively to the matter of ethics and informed consent around this issue at the end of Part 1.

The three parts of this book

The first part of the book, Understanding the placebo effect, gives the background to many aspects of the placebo and paints a historical picture of its use. It also contains some conceptual topics, such as the nature of belief and body-mind medicine. If these seem too fluffy, perhaps you could pass over them and move on to the 'meat and potato' sections. Overall, I believe that Part 1 will convince you that the placebo effect is in fact real, measurable and that its effects can sometimes last for years. We will also look at the dark side of this phenomenon, known as the nocebo effect. We will see what the critics have to say about this, and then finally we will, as mentioned, examine ethical issues around your decision to employ techniques in this book.

The second part, Concepts and application, presents a separate concept in each section, and then helps you employ the theory with examples that can immediately be applied in practice. Do not feel that you have to read this section from beginning to end, or in any order at all. As you read each of these sections, you will see that you are already using the placebo effect in your practice but now you will have more knowledge about how it works. By the very nature of your personality, you will recognize that you will be more competent in execution of some of these concepts than in others. You can choose to use the areas where you are weak as an opportunity for personal growth or you can simply say 'that's not for me' and go with your strong suit, enhancing areas where you are already comfortable.

Finally, Part 3 is a short section that takes a much broader look at healing and medicine. It brings in alternative models from some conceptual thinkers in the world of biology and health. Part 3 is not as much about the placebo effect as it is about our notions concerning healing. It paints a slightly different picture and may influence you to look at the body in a different way when treating people. If nothing else, I hope that it opens your mind a bit, and this is always a good thing.

Part 1

Understanding the Placebo Effect

There is no 'choice' about whether or not to 'use' the placebo (and nocebo) effects. Those effects are going on in every medical encounter between patient and physician. They exist whether we want them to or not; whether we are consciously exploiting them or not. The 'choice' is about how we go about using them: well or poorly, blindly or thoughtfully.

Dr Howard Brody,
Director of the Institute for Medical Humanities
of the University of Texas (Brody 2012, p. 15).

I regard the placebo response as a pure example of healing elicited by the mind: far from being a nuisance, it is, potentially, the greatest therapeutic ally doctors can find in their efforts to mitigate disease. I believe further that the art of medicine is the selection of treatments and their presentation to patients in ways that increase their effectiveness through the activation of placebo responses.

Dr Andrew Weil,
Director of the Arizona Center for Integrative Medicine
at the University of Arizona (Weil 1995, p. 52)

DEFINITION OF A PLACEBO

As always, the best place to start is at the beginning. To begin down this road we need to have a common definition of a placebo. Webster's Dictionary online (Merriam Webster 2013) has a very 'safe' definition of the placebo effect: '...*an improvement in the condition of a patient that occurs in response to treatment but cannot be considered due to the specific treatment used.*'

PubMed (US National Library of Health 2014) introduced 'placebo effect' as a MeSH in 1990 and defines it as:

> *An effect usually, but not necessarily, beneficial that is attributable to an expectation that the regimen will have an effect, i.e., the effect is due to the power of suggestion.*

Dr Howard Brody MD (2000a, p. 14) has written on this topic and defines the placebo both broadly and succinctly as follows:

> *In medical research, a placebo is an intervention designed to mimic the modality or process being studied, but without any of its non-symbolic healing properties (i.e. serving only as a symbol), so as to serve as a control in double-blind trials. In therapeutic healing, a placebo is a treatment modality or a process administered with the belief that it possesses the ability to affect the body only by virtue of its symbolic value.*

A placebo isn't always a sugar pill, though that is typically what we associate with the word. For example, there have been sham surgeries where the patient is anesthetized and an incision is made, but no surgery actually takes place. The patient (participant/volunteer) wakes up not knowing if surgery was actually performed. Ultrasound is a very easy procedure with which to conduct double-blind placebo tests. The machine can be rigged so that the practitioner and patient both think that it is on and working when it is actually not. Placebos are not always completely inert either. For example, placebo trials testing psychotherapeutic techniques have seen college professors with no psychotherapeutic training sitting in on sessions with students who believed that they were with a psychotherapist. As you can imagine, double-blinding (where neither the practitioner nor the participant know which is the placebo) is much harder to achieve with many procedures than is single blinding.

The second half of Brody's definition, which applies to therapeutic healing, is what health practitioners are most concerned with, since it involves application of the placebo effect. Our goal, as health care practitioners, is not to deceive the patient, but to recognize the *special nature* of the relationship between healer and patient. The placebo effect is one aspect of that relationship that allows us to engage and augment the patient's own healing system, just as doctors and other practitioners have done for thousands of years. We are not just a person to our patients...we are also very much a symbol. Techniques described in Part 2 will help you to refine your patients' symbolic perception of you, thus increasing your effect on their healing systems. The last definition is the placebo effect itself, or placebo response (both terms will be used interchangeably in this book). Once again, we will refer to Dr Brody's succinct definition (Brody 2000a, p.9):

A change in the body that occurs as a result of the symbolic significance which one attributes to an event or object in the healing environment.

In an interview of Ted Kaptchuk, Director of The Program in Placebo Studies and the Therapeutic Encounter at Harvard Medical School (Voices of BIDMC Research at Harvard Medical School, 2012), the interviewer asked, 'What is the placebo effect?'. Kaptchuk's answer was probably one of the most insightful answers that you could get on the subject:

The placebo effect is the positive benefits people receive when they're on placebo treatment. The problem with that definition is that it doesn't make sense. How could something that has no effect have an effect if it's an inert substance? An inert substance can't have an effect.

I would say a placebo not only hides real treatment but hides the art of medicine; the caring for a patient. So a placebo is about:

- *the attention*
- *the eye gaze*
- *the warmth*
- *the compassion*
- *the confidence of the physician in a doctor-patient relationship.*

I would say that the placebo is about the symbols of medicine, like:

- *the diploma on the wall*
- *the prescription pad*
- *and the stethoscope.*

I would say that a placebo is about the routine rituals; the procedures of medicine;

- *waiting in the doctor's office*
- *talking*
- *disrobing*
- *being examined*
- *putting your clothes back on*
- *getting a diagnosis*
- *and then being prescribed pills, injections or procedures.*

Ultimately I think the placebo effect is about imagination, hope and trust in the clinical encounter

Looking at these definitions, we can see that one of our tasks, as medical professionals, is to manage the healing environment, such that the correct symbols are present to maximize the placebo effect for our patients at large and for each specific patient as well. As we will soon see, this could be anything from the professional appearance of your office setting, to their perception of your professional competence, to your ability to tune into each patient's needs, fears and circumstances, and your aptitude for managing their expectations.

ENTER THE PLACEBO

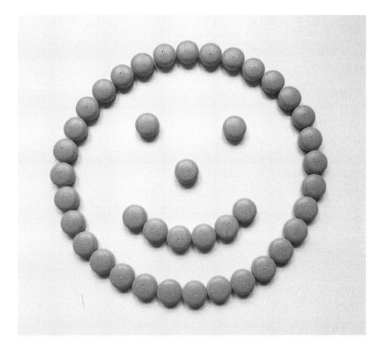

Fig. 1.1

Notable placebo studies

Here are some studies that highlight the amazing power of placebos. We will look at many more studies to illustrate other concepts in future sections, but what follows should help to 'wet your whistle' and prepare you to embrace the amazing power of what is, in your patient's eyes, basically a symbol.

- A systematic review of various wart treatment modalities saw placebo results typically averaging 27% cure rate, with one study exhibiting a 73% cure rate from inert dye paint. The modality considered 'best' by these authors were topical treatments containing salicylic acid, but even in these studies the placebo group experienced a 48% remission rate (Gibbs & Harvey 2006). The author's words, 'Cure rates with placebo preparations are variable, but nevertheless considerable.'
- In a study testing whether the relationship between exercise and health is moderated by one's mindset, 84 female room attendants were measured on objective physiological health variables affected by exercise. Those in the 'informed' condition were told that the work they do (cleaning hotel rooms) is good exercise and satisfies the Surgeon General's recommendations for an active lifestyle. Subjects in the control group

were not given this information. Although actual behavior did not change, 4 weeks after the intervention, the informed group perceived themselves to be getting significantly more exercise than before. As a result, compared with the control group, they showed a decrease in weight, blood pressure, body fat, waist-to-hip ratio, and body mass index. Researchers said, 'These results support the hypothesis that exercise affects health in part or in whole via the placebo effect' (Crum & Langer 2007).

- In a study of patients hospitalized with peptic ulcers, 70% showed excellent results lasting over a period of one year when given an injection of distilled water and told that it was a new medication that would definitely cure them. The second group was given an injection of distilled water and told that it was an experimental medication yet to be proven. This group saw only 25% improvement (Volgyesi 1954).
- In one study, women who believed it was very likely that they would have severe nausea from chemotherapy were *five times* more likely to experience severe nausea than fellow patients who thought its occurrence would be very unlikely (Roscoe et al. 2004).
- One-third of all post-surgical patients and people suffering traumatic pain experience at least 50% reduction in pain from placebos. Morphine produces similar results (50% reduction in pain) in about three-quarters of patients. Still an impressive showing for the placebo (Evans 1985).
- Patients suffering pain after wisdom-tooth extraction got just as much symptomatic and inflammatory relief from a placebo application of ultrasound as from an actual ultrasound treatment in this double-blinded study. The control group doing self-massage with the coupling cream did not experience these effects (Hashish et al. 1986).
- A 1998 study of depression saw a 200% improvement in persons receiving a placebo, when compared with a no-treatment group. The third group, which received the active medication, saw only 33% improvement over the placebo group (Kirsh & Sapirstein, 1998).
- Fifty-two percent of the colitis patients treated with placebo in 11 different trials reported feeling better, and 50% of the inflamed intestines were measured as improved when assessed with a sigmoidoscope (Meyers & Janowitz 1989).
- A study of rheumatoid arthritis patients using placebos saw a 50% reduction in the number of inflamed joints as well as a 50% reduction in swelling and tenderness in 40% of the participants (Tilley et al. 1995).
- The placebo has been consistently found in study after study over the last 50 years to be equivalent to psychotherapy in its response rate (Brown 2013).
- Conditions that respond well to psychotherapy also respond well to placebos. Mental illnesses that do not see improvement with

psychoanalysis, such as serious depression or schizophrenia, do not see improvement with a placebo either.

- Pharmaceutical companies that have studied the placebo to minimize its effect on their studies have been confounded by the fact that the placebo effect has actually been getting stronger in the last few decades (Silberman 2009)!
- A placebo treatment is unquestionably not the same as no-treatment. This has also been show in multiple studies (Brown 2013, Kaptchuk et al. 2010).
- One study randomly divided pacemaker recipients into two groups; in only one group were the pacemakers turned on. All patients were much better than baseline, by very nearly the same amount, after 8 weeks (Linde et al. 1999).
- A 2002 study of 180 patients with osteoarthritis of the knee were randomly assigned to receive arthroscopic débridement, arthroscopic lavage, or placebo surgery. Patients in the placebo group received only skin incisions then underwent a simulated debridement without insertion of the arthroscope. Outcomes were assessed over a 24-month period for pain, function, an objective test of walking and stair climbing. At no point did either of the intervention groups report less pain or better function than the placebo group (Moseley et al. 2002).
- Study participants using placebo pills and who were informed that the pills they were taking were inert, saw substantial improvement of symptoms over the no-treatment group (Kaptchuk et al. 2010).
- Withdrawal symptoms can also occur after placebo treatment. In a Women's Health Initiative study of hormone replacement therapy for menopause, women had been on placebo for an average of 5.7 years. After discontinuation 40.5% of the women using placebos reported moderate or severe withdrawal symptoms versus 63.3% of those on hormone replacement (Ockene et al. 2005).
- In a number of studies, patients who took all their prescribed placebos did significantly better than those who took only 80% of them (these results mimicked those in the active treatment groups; this has been shown for studies of heart attack survivors, post-chemotherapy infections, treatment of schizophrenia, and others) (Moerman 2006).
- Sixty percent of ulcer patients given placebo treatment in Germany showed healed ulcers (on repeat endoscopy) after a month, while only 20% of Dutch and Danes were better (Moerman 2006).
- A study that intended to look at the use of antipsychotic drugs to treat aggressive challenging behavior in intellectually disabled patients found that placebos actually worked better than drugs. The largest decrease in the measured behavior was in the placebo group with a decrease of 79% from baseline versus 58% for risperidone and 65% for haloperidol

(Tyrer 2008). What this means is that the antipsychotic medications drugs actually decreased the placebo effect of taking a drug for this purpose.

Interesting phenomenon surrounding the placebo response

There are many interesting phenomena surrounding the placebo effect in respect to what enhances and suppresses the actual response to the placebo pill or treatment. The following effects have been documented in research studies. They are not all laid in stone, as there has been some variability in the findings, but the trends indicate the following:

- The effects of a placebo increase if the pill is physically larger, and yet smaller than normal sized pills also appear to have a more powerful effect (Buckalew & Ross 1981, Thompson 2005).
- Warmer-colored pills work better as stimulants, while cool-colored pills work better as depressants (de Craen et al. 1996).
- The effects will increase if the placebo is taken with increased frequency (conditioning theory) (de Craen et al. 1999).
- Increased frequency of visits to the attending health professional increase the effectiveness of the placebo (conditioning theory) (Thompson 2005).
- Being told that a placebo will decrease pain will decrease most people's experience of pain, and yet being told that that same placebo makes pain worse will increase most people's experience of pain (the nocebo effect) (Thompson 2005).
- A placebo can be viewed as a symbol. The more significant the symbol, the more powerful the effect is likely to be. Surgery is at the high end of that scale. The scale looks something like this:
  - Capsules surpass tablets (Hussain & Ahad 1970).
  - Injections are seen to be more effective than drugs administered orally (Grenfell et al. 1961).
  - Injections that sting work better than injections that do not sting (Ernst 2001).
  - Medical treatment machines are better than injections (Kaptchuk et al. 2000).
  - Sham surgery is considered the most powerful placebo (Kirsh 2010).
- New or novel treatments (or drugs) often surpass older ones (Shapiro & Shapiro 2000).
- The severity of intervention influences the placebo response. With increased pain, there is increased placebo response (Levine et al. 1979). A 2001 review found that invasive, uncomfortable, sophisticated or painful interventions tended to enhance the placebo effect (Ernst 2001).
- A placebo administered by a doctor is more potent than a placebo administered by a clerk. Even less effective is a placebo sent via postal delivery (Thompson 2005).

- Brand name placebos work better than generic placebos (Branthwaite & Cooper 1981).
- More expensive placebos tend to be more powerful than discounted ones (Waber et al. 2008).
- It is well established that people who adhere to their drug schedules experience better outcomes. It is the same with placebos. The better that people adhere to their drug schedule, the better their outcome. This was even shown inpatient mortality figures (Simpson et al. 2006).
- People have actually experienced withdrawal symptoms after long-term use of placebos (Ockene et al. 2005).
- Placebos have been shown to be geographically and culturally sensitive (variable) (Moerman 1983).

This information is just a sampling of what is to come. Many studies will be presented later in the book to elucidate specific concepts. I hope that you find yourself curious to learn more about this amazing phenomenon.*

---

*If you find the above information interesting, I recommend the documentary, *Placebo: Cracking the Code.* This 1-hour video looks at many interesting aspects of the effects and interviews patients, doctors and lead research-ers in the field. A simple Google search will yield several sites which allow you to view this documentary for free.

A HISTORICAL PERSPECTIVE

The history of medical treatment until relatively recently was the history of the placebo.

Arthur K. Shapiro MD
(Shapiro 1959, p. 303)

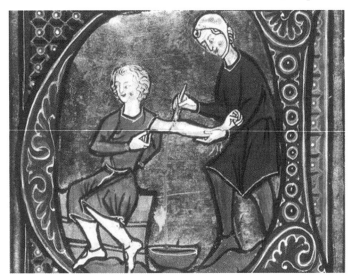

Fig. 1.2

Western medicine is now rooted in the scientific approach, but not so very long ago medicine was based more on intuition, fashion, social mores or religious beliefs and restrictions. Mind you, even with all of our advances there is still a strong desire to return to natural alternatives, whether tested or not. A humorous illustration of this is shown in Box 1.1.

A short history of medicine

I have an earache…

2000 BC – Here, eat this root.

1000 AD – That root is heathen. Here, say this prayer.

1850 AD – That prayer is superstition. Drink this potion.

1940 AD – That potion is snake oil. Here, swallow this pill.

1985 AD – That pill is ineffective. Here, take this antibiotic.

2000 AD – That antibiotic is artificial. Here, eat this root.

Box 1.1

Pre-20th century

Until the 20th century, most medications prescribed by physicians were what we now consider to be pharmacologically inert, and if not, often harmful. Physicians over the centuries were therefore inadvertently prescribing placebos or worse, and were **still** held in high regard as healers (Frank & Frank 1991). That physicians were held in high regard before the 20th century, armed largely with placebos, tells you just how powerful the placebo effect can be.

How long has the placebo been around? It has probably been available to those battling pain, injury and illness as long as man has had language, since it uses belief (in part) to turn on inner healing. The word placebo ('I will please' in Latin) entered the English language by way of a peculiar mistranslation of the 116th Psalm that read, 'I will please the Lord', rather than the more correct 'I will walk before the Lord'. In the medieval Catholic liturgy, this verse opened the Vespers for the Dead. Because professional mourners were sometimes hired to sing vespers, 'to sing placebos' came to be a derogatory phrase describing a servile flatterer. By the early 19th century, 'placebo' had come to mean a medicine given 'more to please than to benefit the patient'.

Henry Beecher

The placebo developed legitimacy in Western medicine due to a push from Dr Henry K. Beecher in the mid-1950s. Beecher served as an anesthetist in World War II. As is the case in times of war, supplies sometimes fell short. On one occasion Beecher had to perform surgery on a soldier but morphine supplies were exhausted. Not only would this be very painful to the patient, but also more importantly, cardiac shock is a very serious risk when operating without anesthetic. Fortunately for all parties involved, an ingenious nurse gave the patient a saline injection and told him that it was morphine. The patient settled down immediately, allowing Beecher to perform surgery. What was amazing was that not only did the patient feel little pain, but also more importantly, he did not go into full-blown shock. These same circumstances were repeated on several other occasions during Beecher's tour as a physician and on multiple occasions a saline injection seemed to do the job of an anesthetic. Beecher was so impressed with the power of a placebo that when he returned to America he convinced a group of colleagues at Harvard to study the phenomenon.

As is often the case in history, similar ideas and movements appear synchronously. At Cornell, Harry Gold had been studying the use of placebos in treating angina and was also convinced of the power of the placebo and began his own work in the area. Louis Lasagna was another contemporary of Beecher's and a pioneer in this area who worked with Beecher. This is not to say that use of placebos began then, but this was the beginning of scientific interest in them. Dylan Evan states in his book *Placebo – Mind over Matter in Modern Medicine* (Evans 2004, p. 2) that:

> *Although doctors had been quietly using sugar pills and water injections as standard operating practice to placate desperate patients for many years*

before Beecher started running his studies, few regarded the practice worthy of research.

Placebo use in clinical trials

In 1955, Beecher published an article in the *Journal of the American Medical Association* entitled 'The powerful placebo' (Beecher 1955).In this, Beecher put forth a persuasive argument for use of the placebo in clinical trials, claiming that the placebo could 'produce gross physical change'. The medical establishment stood up and listened to Beecher. Within a few years the randomized, placebo-controlled clinical trial was born. Beecher's argument was basically this; any drug being used or brought onto the market needs to be tested to determine its efficacy. The clinical trial could do this. However, what do you compare a drug against...no treatment? If 35% of people get better just taking a sugar pill then why not use a placebo as a baseline to compare against? This appeared to raise the bar for any drug being tested, and seemed more humane for the control group than having a 'no treatment' control group.

Now just to backtrack a bit and to be completely transparent on this matter, Beecher came to these conclusions by examining 15 studies. We know now that some of his statistical methods were sloppy and the range of conditions in these studies was limited to the common cold, coughs, anxiety, seasickness, headaches, angina and postoperative pain. He also misquoted findings from 10 of the trials. Furthermore, only one of these studies had a 'no treatment' group, without which you cannot categorically say that improvement was entirely due to the placebo. Improvement could have been due to the natural course of the illness, spontaneous remission of the illness, fluctuation in symptoms etc. Now if you are feeling anxious about spending money on this book on the placebo effect after seeing the flaws in Beecher's studies do not worry. The placebo effect is very real, and many other studies that would follow showed some dramatic and fascinating results. At any rate, doctors, researchers and regulators of that era jumped on the Beecher bandwagon due to a strong need to regulate and manage the emerging pharmaceutical industry. The medical establishment was ripe and ready to embrace the placebo in clinical trials.

Interestingly enough, the concept of a clinical trial goes back much further than this. In the 14th century, King Frederic II of Sicily decided to study the effects of digestion on his knights. Frederick had two knights eat identical meals, and then he ordered one of them to bed and the other out hunting. After a few hours he had them both killed and then autopsied their alimentary canals. Low and behold, digestion had proceeded further in the knight who relaxed (Greenhalgh 2001) (I'm guessing that he didn't know that he was about to be slaughtered). I somehow doubt that Frederick's knights were overly delighted to see the birth of the comparative method, or that they thought 'birth' was the best word to use in this particular case.

Anyway, history trundled along until the birth of statistics in the 18th century, without which the results of trials could not be effectively analyzed. The acceptance of statistics was very slow and painful, and it wasn't really until the first half of the 20th century that there was even acceptance of comparative methods. The term clinical trial does not appear in medical literature until the early 1930s. It wasn't until Linford Rees presented his results comparing electro-convulsive therapy with insulin-induced coma to the American Medico-Psychological Association in 1949 that the concept of the randomized clinical trial was brought to the forefront of the medical community (Healy 1997).

Enter Henry Beecher and the placebo. Now we have something to compare a drug or a therapy against. For testing drugs, it is a simple matter of dispensing an identical pill containing an inert substance. Other therapies require more creativity in designing the placebo, but for many therapies, a placebo can be constructed once researchers agree on what the active component of the therapy is and then design a procedure that somehow removes it without the participants' knowledge. The point here is that we now have the birth of the modern clinical trial, with all of the elements necessary to test new drugs in a scientific manner. These elements include double-blinding (neither the participant nor the clinician know which is the active drug), randomization (study members are randomly assigned to either the active therapy or the placebo), and placebo control (meaning that there must always be a control group, which receives no active therapy, just a placebo). Well guess what? Even in these meticulously designed studies, you typically see some very interesting results from the placebo group.

Evidence-based medicine arrives

The latter part of the 20th century brought us evidence-based medicine (EBM), which is the great litmus test for all medical modalities these days because it attempts to separate the chaff from the grain in medical treatments. One major goal of EBM is to weed out ineffective and harmful treatments, and help to protect the public from 'snake oil' salespersons who rely exclusively on the placebo effect. It is a tremendous advance in the critical analysis of treatments available today, whether pharmaceutical or not.

The scientific approach, which has now been adopted without abandon, has many benefits over previous approaches in medicine; however, it is not necessarily the 'be all and end all'. It clearly loses out to intuition as the shortest distance between two points, and even people in the research field agree that intuition is invaluable in the area of developing a hypothesis, and in understanding what phenomenon presents itself in any given study. However, if you want to prove your hypothesis, you need to use the scientific method. Before science, all that we had to base our treatment choice and protocols on was anecdotal evidence. This type of evidence makes for wonderful parlor stories, but can be very misleading, since the sample size is '1', very few standards are typically followed, and stories are usually highly colored. For example, use of bloodletting was ubiquitous in western medical practice for almost 3000 years! Virtually every doctor practicing could testify to its efficacy from his own experience, and tell hundreds of anecdotal stories of how a given patient improved after being bled. As it turns out these patients got better despite the therapy, rather than because of it. That's not to say that the placebo effect wasn't at play here. It most certainly was if the patient and doctor both believed that this procedure could cure the person.

At the other end of the scale from anecdotal evidence are systematic reviews and meta-analyses, due to their rigorous standards, the number of participants and the in-depth analysis. The only problem with this type of evidence is that this researcher has potentially never left their office to produce the study, nor talked to one patient or the researchers involved in the study. This is not to suggest that meta-analyses are not extremely important, but there is a clear risk of something getting lost in the translation when the researcher does not speak to the parties involved in a study. As with everything else in life, a healthy balance is the best approach. As a practitioner, for example, a sensible approach might involve reading current studies on the pathology in question, as well as a meta-analysis on the topic, and then balance that information with anecdotal evidence from your own practice.

David and Goliath

One final thing to be aware of is the almost prohibitive cost of conducting a clinical trial. A 2012 report on this subject entitled 'Price indexes for clinical trial research: a feasibility study' (Berndt & Cockburn 2013) puts the total grant cost per patient at $16567, with an average annual growth rate of 7.5%. Total grant cost per patient is the total amount paid by the sponsor of a study under its contract with the site, divided by the number of patients planned to be enrolled at that site. Authors of this report focused on the total grant cost per patient as the economically meaningful unit of analysis for understanding price trends in clinical trials. One can immediately see that if you are trying to evaluate the efficacy of a vitamin, or an herbal remedy, or a manual intervention, for which there is typically no patent available, then without a very substantial grant from somewhere, no research is likely to take place because of the prohibitive cost of the venture. So when you hear someone say that there is no evidence to support the efficacy of a non-patentable approach (e.g. research in whole food nutrition, or vitamins or a manual therapy intervention) versus the evidence supporting a pharmaceutical intervention, or a patentable product, then keep in mind the David and Goliath factor. Big pharma has a massive amount of money, and it has methods of recovering its R & D dollars. The more natural approaches to health management have no means by which to recover research dollars, so are therefore put at a rather distinct disadvantage.

Informed consent and patients' rights

The other significant event happening in clinical trials in the second half of the 20th century was the appearance of patients' rights. Originally trial participants were not necessarily informed that a placebo was being used. There was a paternalistic sensibility that had a long and illustrious history in the medical profession. The sense was 'we know best' when it came to informing patients and research candidates about the possible dangers or informing patients of possible side-effects of treatments. This pretty much was how things were done since Hippocrates' time with the Hippocratic Oath being the guiding principle being used to justify this paternalistic attitude. However comparative trials were beginning to show all of the cracks in the body of knowledge known as *materia medica*. This caused the founder of modern pharmacology Sir John Gaddum to once remark that the materia medica was the only body of knowledge that had become smaller as it had advanced. Doctors, researchers and the public at large became increasingly aware in the latter part of the 20th century that the power paradigm was shifting. Currently any procedure that involves potentially administering a placebo requires informed consent from the participant. Informed consent became enshrined in the US as a result of the *Consumer Bill of Rights*, introduced in 1962 by President John F. Kennedy. It established peoples' rights to safety, to be informed, to choose, and to be heard.

Surgery as a placebo

Needless to say, some rather interesting but (now) unethical experiments were performed before this time, not the least of which was sham surgeries performed in two different studies in the mid-1950s (Diamond et al. 1958, Cobb et al. 1959). In the early 1950s, thousands of mammary ligation surgeries were performed on patients with angina pectoris. This was a routine medical procedure that involved tying specific arteries with the belief that this would encourage more flow to the heart, or cause sprouting of new blood vessels. When pathologists found no evidence of new blood vessels appearing, the proposed mechanism was brought into question. Two doctors, independently decided to carry out placebo-controlled trials with one group receiving the mammary ligation surgery, and the control group receiving sham surgery where the chest was cut partly open, but no arterial occlusion was performed. The results of both studies were similar. In both the control group and the mammary ligation group, approximately 75% of *all patients* reported substantially lower pain levels, had greatly increased exercise tolerance, and had less need for vasodilation drugs. There was, in fact, no statistical difference in the results of the surgery group or the control group! No matter how you view these studies, the results were incredibly impressive and surprising. What was the response of the medical community? Mammary ligation as a treatment for angina was quickly abandoned, yet surprisingly there was no large-scale interest in this dramatic illustration of the placebo effect. I think that this study is fascinating on many levels because:

1. Although this study would be considered unethical by today's standards in that patients were not informed that they might receive a placebo, in retrospect, no harm was actually done and the patient was spared major surgery. The end result was that the inefficacy of a surgical procedure was brought to light by a placebo procedure.

2. The critical need for EBM that fortunately is now the standard in medical practice is well illustrated here as well. Thankfully, due to modern evidenced-based practice, surgeons are not as quick to perform procedures these days unless they are reasonably sure that they can improve the patient's health or symptoms.

3. Finally, as we will see later, the more powerful the symbol, the greater the placebo effect tends to be, with surgery being at the top end of the scale. This study illustrates that fact well, and shows us the incredible power of the placebo.

Now to look at how placebos work, let's first examine the concept of belief.

THE NATURE OF BELIEF

I wouldn't have seen it if I hadn't believed it.

Marshall McLuhan

Reality is merely an illusion, albeit a very persistent one.

Albert Einstein

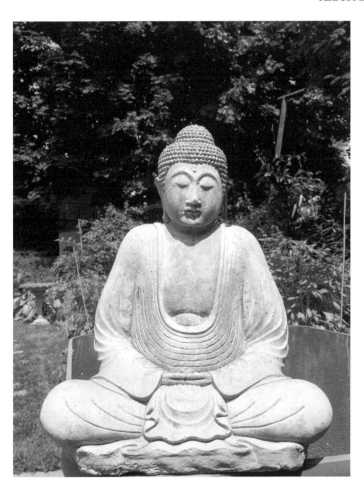

Fig. 1.3

One of the opening phrases of the Dhammapada, one of the most revered Buddhist scriptures is: *'Our life is the creation of our mind'*. This is not just a statement made to open you up to new possibilities, it is also what science tells us is actually happening in our brain. Belief is an abstract notion developed within our own mind by conscious and unconscious thoughts. How do we develop or create our personal view of the world and our own reality? Well, our brain can't really reach out and touch the outside world directly. It communicates, as you know, with receptors that respond to light, pressure, temperature, chemicals, and so on. These messages are then transmitted to the brain. The brain receives a massive amount of information every second, and from all of this information it has to decide what is important, and what is not. From the information that is deemed important, our reality or our personal view of the world is constructed. At the same time, the brain is also managing homeostasis by sending and receiving both neural and chemical messages throughout the body as it monitors every single bodily function. Most of this happens at an unconscious level, however there is conclusive evidence that the conscious mind can step in and augment or override many of these autonomic processes (Paul-Labrador et al. 2006)

We all tend to take for granted that when our senses perceive something, we are actually seeing, smelling, tasting, touching or hearing something. However, as educated health professionals we know enough neurology to realize that this is not really the case. In sight, for example, photons of light stimulate photoreceptors in our eyes, which then communicate with neurons by way of neuropeptides at synaptic junctions, which then in turn carry information to the brain. The brain processes the information, then based on conscious processes and past information decides just what it is seeing. It is really nothing short of a miracle how each one of our senses cooperates with the brain in this wonderful orchestration called 'perception'. All metaphors aside, the point being stressed here is that when we look at something, we are not actually 'seeing' the object; we are actually seeing a picture in our mind, created by our brain. Worth noting is that there are many steps along the way, and room for interpretation at one or more of these steps. All of our other senses operate in a similar manner.

This might seem like splitting hairs to you, but it is important to recognize that interpretation, previous experience, and conscious decision all go into creating our personal realities, whether this is simply perceiving something directly with our senses, or constructing reality through conscious thought. We do not want to get too far out on a limb with this topic, but it is important that you fully comprehend that both you and your patient have actually constructed your own personal realities, that there is a *plasticity* to perception, and that the 'black and white' world isn't quite so black and white as we often assume it is.

Research into the brain has progressed dramatically in the last few decades. This amazing organ comprises about 100 billion neurons. Each neuron is able to communicate with between 1000 and 6000 other neurons. (That`s about 100 trillion connections!) One observed feature of the brain is its ability to essentially rewire itself, or at least to give new priority to pathways that were previously unused (Karni 1995). Every time you create a new habit, or begin a new task, you actually build new neural circuits. The more you repeat the habit, the more this pathway is reinforced or prioritized. A study of rats that were raised in cages with toys and mazes saw them develop more neural connections than their neighbors in empty cages (Benson 1997). This has broad implications in the area of illness and negative thought patterns. None of us need be trapped in an endless loop, doomed to repeat our old ways. We can make changes and develop new healthier patterns of thought.

As we can change our beliefs, we change our reality. One great quote from 1960s' media guru Marshall McLuhan was, *'I wouldn't have seen it if I hadn't believed it'*, turning the old phrase 'I wouldn't have believed it if I hadn't seen it with my own two eyes' on its head. This, in a nutshell, is the nature of belief, and we see this illustrated every day in others and ourselves. For example, on more than one occasion, I have walked right past my car in a parking lot because I was positive that I had parked it in another place. I wasn't even open to the possibility of my two-ton car being right in front of my own eyes, so it wasn't. Examples such as this speak volumes about the nature of belief. The reason we discuss belief is that in most cases of placebo response the patient has developed a belief in the treatment that he or she is being given will be effective. See Boxes 1.2 and 1.3 for a few studies that elucidate this point.

Lose weight by changing your mind

A Harvard University study of hotel workers (mentioned earlier) conducted by Alia Crum elucidates the incredible power of the mind in creating a placebo effect (Crum & Langer 2007). This study involved workers in seven hotels and looked at whether the relationship between exercise and health is moderated by one's mindset. Hotel room attendants clean on average 15 rooms a day, and engage in exerting activities that clearly meet and exceed the US Surgeon General's exercise requirements. Room attendants may not perceive their work as exercise. Each of seven hotels was randomly assigned to one of two conditions: informed or control. Subjects in the informed condition received a write-up discussing the benefits of exercise and were informed that their daily housekeeping work satisfied the CDC's recommendations for an active lifestyle. The informed group were also given an information sheet which gave specific details of the average calorie expenditure for various activities and informed them that it was clear that they were easily meeting and even exceeding the Surgeon General's recommendations. This sheet, written in both English and Spanish, was read and explained to the subjects and then posted on the bulletin board in their lounge. These subjects were told that the research-ers were interested in getting information on their health so that they could study ways to improve it. Subjects in the control group were given all the same informa-tion as those in the informed group except they did not receive information about how their work is good exercise until after the second set of measures was taken. The participants who 'believed' their jobs gave them adequate exercise showed a decrease in weight, blood pressure, body fat, waist-to-hip ratio, and body mass index. The group who did not adopt this belief system saw none of these changes.

Box 1.2

What is pertinent about the above study is that the activity level in neither group in this study had changed. The only thing that had changed was the belief system of the test group.

A more recent Harvard study by Alia Crum and colleagues looked at the mind's ability to affect the production of ghrelin, a hormone that is secreted in the gut (Crum et al. 2011). Ghrelin is called the hunger hormone, because when it is secreted it signals the brain to seek out food. Ghrelin also slows down our metabolism, so this hormone plays an important role on weight maintenance weight loss. Interestingly enough, the brain appears to have the ability to augment or suppress the production of ghrelin. The following experiment was devised to test the mind's ability to mediate the production of ghrelin. On two separate occasions, 46 participants consumed a 380-calorie milkshake under the pretense that it was either a 620-calorie 'indulgent' shake or a 140-calorie 'sensible' shake. Ghrelin levels were measured via intravenous blood samples at three time points: baseline, anticipatory, and post-consumption. During the first interval, participants were asked to view and rate the (misleading) label of the shake. During the second interval, participants were asked to drink and rate the milkshake. The ghrelin levels dropped about three times more when people were consuming the indulgent shake (or thought they were consuming the indulgent shake), compared with the people who drank the sensible shake (or thought that's what they were drinking). The mindset of indulgence produced a dramatically steeper decline in ghrelin after consuming the shake, whereas the mindset of sensibility produced a relatively flat ghrelin response. Participants' satiety was consistent with what they believed they were consuming rather than the actual nutritional value of what they consumed. This experiment demonstrates one of the mechanisms by which our belief system plays a role in weight management.

Box 1.3

One other example of belief systems in weight loss is the system spearheaded by Jon Gabriel. His method focuses on visualization to lose weight. He claims to have lost over 220 lbs primarily by using visualization techniques. After failing at every diet that he tried, he vowed to never go on a diet again (a bold move for someone who weighed over 400 lbs). After searching for alternative methods of weight loss, he stumbled upon visualization and finally achieved the success that he had never achieved by dieting. He has attracted thousands of followers who also claim that the essential reason that they have been able to lose weight and keep it off is by altering their belief system.

Belief and depression

In 2002, a study compared the performance of *Hypericum perforatum* (St. John's Wort), sertraline (Zoloft) and placebo in a group of 340 adults with major depressive disorder. The initial study saw no major differences in response in either group. In 2011, another group of researchers published a paper, which reanalyzed the original data to determine whether patients who believed they were receiving active therapy rather than placebo obtained greater improvement, independent of treatment. In the original study, participants were asked to guess their assigned treatment after 8 weeks. This information was factored into the second paper. What the researchers found was that while the assigned treatment had no significant effect on clinical improvement, the patient's belief system around what pill they were taking was significantly associated with improvement. Among subjects who guessed placebo, clinical improvement was small despite that fact the there was a fairly even distribution of subjects who were actually on sertraline, *Hypercium* or placebo. Among subjects who guessed *Hypericum*, improvement was large no matter what pill they were actually on (again, there was a fairly even distribution. Among subjects who guessed sertraline, those who received placebo or sertraline had large improvements, but those who received *Hypericum* had significantly less improvement. It seems very evident that these patients' belief system was the major factor at play in this study; but let's allow the researchers in this study have the final word:

> *Patient beliefs regarding treatment may have a stronger association with clinical outcome than the actual medication received, and the strength of this association may depend upon the particular combination of treatment guessed and treatment received.*

(Chen et al. 2011)

Dylan Evans

Dylan Evans is a British academic and author who has written books on emotion and the placebo effect as well as the theories of Jacques Lacan. Evans studied linguistics and later he received his doctorate in philosophy from the London School of Economics. His book *The Placebo Effect* sets the highest bar over any book that I have read for attributing any recorded phenomenon to the placebo effect. Among persons studying and supporting this phenomenon, he is probably one of the most skeptical. For Dylan Evans, the placebo effect could best be described as the belief effect. He argues that there are basically three ways by which we acquire beliefs:

1. *Voice of authority*; for example, your doctor tells you something, or any expert in any field imparts information that you take on faith.
2. *Direct experience* (with previous exposure or conditioning being one form of experience where we learn that if we do 'A' then typically 'B' happens).

But if experience begins to tell us that the voice of authority is wrong, we will eventually reject the opinion.

3. *Logic*, which can lead us to develop new beliefs (based upon experience) or to reject existing beliefs by noticing inconsistencies in our existing beliefs.

He raises this argument in part to support his theory of the belief effect, but also to reject claims by certain persons in the self-help field who suggest that all you have to do is believe. He points out that if that were true then we would eventually have to ignore (#2) our direct experience, and (#3) logic, if our experience told us differently. This would seem to make sense to me and would also explain the tendency for placebo effects to taper off over time in most long-term studies.

Bruce Lipton

Bruce Lipton has spent a good portion of his life exploring the connection between belief systems and biology. In his book, *The Biology of Belief*, he cites many examples and likely mechanisms by which our thoughts affect gene expression. Lipton's background is in cell biology, teaching the subject to medical students. Lipton sees the cell membrane as the actual place where perception and many decisions about all cellular (and therefore organism) processes take place. The rising field of epigenetics seems to support Lipton's theory that control for most processes within organism do not take place in the DNA, but rather somewhere else. DNA sets limitations, but is more of a library than a blueprint or a contractor. Epigenetics is 'functionally relevant modifications to the genome that do not involve a change in the nucleotide sequence'. Examples of such modifications are DNA methylation and histone modification, both of which serve to regulate gene expression without altering the underlying DNA sequence. These changes may remain through cell divisions for the remainder of the cell's life and may also last for multiple generations. However, there is no change in the underlying DNA sequence of the organism; instead, non-genetic factors cause the organism's genes to behave (or 'express themselves') differently. A clear example of epigenetics is a study of prostate cancer patients who underwent a change in diet and lifestyle for 90 days. This study found that this change triggered the activity of over 500 genes, many of which inhibited biological processes critical to formation of their tumors (Ornish et al. 2008).

Another emerging field that also supports Lipton's theories is the field of signal transduction. Signal transduction refers to the ability of a cell membrane to act like a switch for molecules that attach to the surface of the cell. This process occurs when an extracellular molecule activates a cell surface receptor. This receptor in turn alters intracellular molecules creating a response. Both the field of signal transduction and epigenetics supports Lipton's hypothesis that the DNA was not the control center. What this means, among other things, is that gene expression can be altered by environment and by experience. Lipton believes that it is then a very small step to believe that our thoughts can change DNA expression.

See Box 1.4 for an example of a study on this. This is a powerful notion for you and your patient to absorb. It means that by thoughts alone, you can actually change your body's response to illness. Multiple studies have shown once again that meditation (Box 1.5) can affect the body's immune response.

A 2009 study of 44 meditation subjects supported Lipton's idea. Participants were actually able to produce physiological changes in their brain structure by creating new neural pathways just by conscious thinking to support this notion (Luder et al. 2009). Changes in brain physiology from meditation alone have also been observed and measured in other studies (Lazar et al. 2005, Hölzel et al. 2008).

Box 1.4

In one 2003 study, 25 subjects meditated for 8 weeks. A 16-person wait-list control group was tested at the same points in time as the meditators. At the end of the 8-week period, subjects in both groups were vaccinated with influenza vaccine. They found time significant increases in left-sided anterior activation, a pattern previously associated with positive affect, in the meditators compared with the non-meditators. They also found significant increases in antibody titers to influenza vaccine among subjects in the meditation compared with those in the wait-list control group. Finally, the magnitude of increase in left-sided activation predicted the magnitude of antibody titer rise to the vaccine (Davidson 2003).

Box 1.5

So it would seem that the conscious mind definitely has the ability to step in and make changes to internal physiologic processes, but how does one go about applying this theory? While changing one's belief system is important, unfortunately we conduct most of our day under subconscious control. It has been said that only 5% of what we do is under conscious control (Bargh 2009), the rest is subconscious or unconscious programming, most of which was acquired by the age of six. If your patient is stuck in their healing or behavior patterns and doesn't seem to be able to break out of them, it is likely due to subconscious or unconscious programming that is playing out. Lipton refers to this area as a big room with a giant tape recorder/player with no- one at the controls. It is possible to get in and change this programming, but often thinking positive thoughts or changing conscious beliefs is not enough. We will discuss this topic more in the next section and toward the end of the book in the section entitled, 'Where do we go from here?'.

Practitioner's belief system

One interesting take on the placebo effect is that our bodies are probably pro-grammed to not engage in a full immune response, because our immune sys-tem requires vast amounts of energy. As a result, we allocate the body's limited resources as needed and the body will limit resources sent to our immune system depending upon the severity of the threat. From this viewpoint, as practitioners, we are helping the patient to turn on resources and healing capabilities that every one of our patients already have. If you believe that your patient already has strong healing power, you will project that belief on to them, whether consciously or unconsciously.

This section could go on and on, but let's not get too far out on a limb. However, before we move ahead, one important point needs to be emphasized at this time. You should always be cognizant of your own beliefs as a therapist/practitioner. You transmit all sorts of signals to your patients, whether you realize it or not, both consciously and unconsciously. Studies show that the practitioner's beliefs affect the therapeutic outcome, even in the case of a research assistant knowingly handing out a placebo versus and active medication. This is why studies are now double-blinded, so that the clinician's belief system does not affect the outcome of the study. We will examine this extremely interesting topic in Part 2.

BODY/MIND MEDICINE

On the basis of these recent insights, it is clear that the placebo response represents an excellent model to understand mind-body interactions, whereby a complex mental activity can change body physiology.

Fabrizio Benedetti (2012),
Professor of Physiology and Neuroscience,
University of Turin Medical School

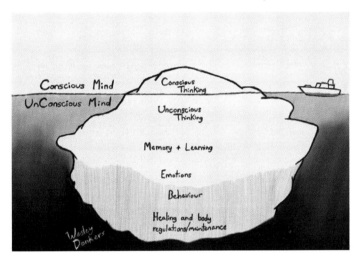

Fig. 1.4

The body and the mind: are they separate?

Many years ago, I read Ken Dychtwald's book, *Bodymind*. Admittedly, the title drew me to the work. This book introduced me to bioenergetics and other esoteric approaches to the body–mind complex. However, more than anything, it helped me to let go of the idea of separating mind from body. It seems natural in conversation to separate mind from body to some degree. René Descartes is the 'whipping boy' commonly cited as the reason for this system of thought, due to his theory of dualism. Descartes was no slouch though, and is still considered one of the most important Western philosophers of the past few centuries. Much more than a philosopher, his work on physics, physiology and math was also incredibly profound. His mathematical theories have had powerful lasting effects, and are a part of everyday usage in modern geometry, calculus, as well as optics. What he has come under fire for mostly is his dualistic theory of the human body, which saw the body was a physical entity that adheres to the laws of physics; whereas the mind (or soul) on the other hand was considered a nonmaterial entity that does not follow the laws of physics. Descartes argued that only humans have minds, and that the mind interacts with pineal gland to affect the body. Like many great thinkers, he was right about many things, but was not infallible. It turns out that all animals have pineal glands, and all sentient beings are now clearly considered to have minds. Separating the mind from the body may serve a purpose in some specific circumstance, but just from a philosophical viewpoint, any separation or disconnection from the whole can be viewed as a root of disease. It is only my personal opinion, but I believe that true health involves a healthy connection to all things around one's self. It is perhaps a scary concept when carried to the extreme, since 'all things' include those things (and those people) that our own value system may view as good or evil. But really, I don't see how it can actually be any other way. However, rather than going down this road of philosophy and personal opinion, I will return to slightly more tangible ideas.

I will make the assumption here that most of us working in the manual therapy field are not so much Cartesian-minded, seeing the body parts and systems as being separate from one another, as we are holistically oriented, seeing the body and mind as basically inseparable and all systems within it as integrated. This is our intuitive sense as bodyworkers, and modern science reaffirms that belief. I will, however, readily accept though that there will always be people on both sides of the fence on this matter and these two following quotes spaced almost 2000 years apart illustrate this ongoing debate.

> *This is the great error of our day in the treatment of the human body, that physicians separate the soul from the body.*

> Plato, in reference to Hippocrates' approach.

> *Unfortunately, the proponents of these two opposed views [holistic and allopathic] have tended to generate more heat than light. Too often each side has assumed the truth of its own position without providing evidence, as if it were obvious.*

> (Evans 2004, p. 17)

The fact is, our brain does *not* operate in a vacuum. Neural tissue reaches into and communicates with virtually every other tissue of the body. The discovery in the 1980s that our brain communicates directly and indirectly with the immune system led to the very interesting and developing field of psycho-neuroimmunology. Since neural tissue reaches every nook and cranny of the body, a simple thought can change your physiology, and numerous studies support this fact.

Candace Pert

Another interesting fact about the mind–body link came out of Dr Candace Pert's work on the biology of emotion. Her earlier work led to the discovery of endorphins. Pert originally hypothesized that neurotransmitters associated with strong emotion would only be found in the limbic system of the brain. Instead what she found was that these chemicals are ubiquitous throughout the body. So in fact, the whole body experiences emotion, not just the brain. It is difficult to shed the Cartesian way of viewing the body, but with each new discovery we can see that the concept of separating mind from body is a completely arbitrary and, largely, a mistaken idea. As you let go of this separation, the concept of mind affecting body, or placebo effect (or whatever you choose to call it) falls very comfortably into place. This point is being emphasized because as a practitioner if you do not genuinely believe in the placebo effect in your practice and in your patients (and in yourself for that matter), you will not see therapeutic outcomes that are as positive as if you sincerely believe in this healing phenomenon.

The unconscious and the subconscious mind

A further interesting topic in the area of body–mind medicine is the *unconscious* mind. While ill-equipped to speak on this topic because none of my training as a massage therapist included education in this area, it is important to address it at this time. I recall Stuart Taws* at his seminar saying that there are both conscious and unconscious elements to any injury and the unconscious mind makes decisions about how *safe* our environment is or about how *safe* a movement is, or is not. As he spoke those words, I felt a penny drop while considering the many other factors that are at play in the therapeutic process. I was also aware though that I know almost nothing about the 'unconscious'. Despite tremendous intellectual curiosity in this area, it is difficult to have personal insight into areas that the conscious mind cannot (by definition) reach. In my post-secondary school years, I was fascinated by Carl Jung's insights into the unconscious, but still as a practitioner, theory is of little use if one cannot apply it in some way. Before going further, let us clarify the terms 'unconscious' and 'subconscious'. There appears to be varied definitions even within the psychiatric community on this matter (Miller 2010) but we need to come to some agreement on this if we are to have a fruitful discussion, so these terms will be described and clarified in this paragraph. *Unconscious* is the term usually used in psychology to refer to the thoughts we have that are 'out of reach' of our consciousness.

A traumatic childhood event, a repressed memory, or a very distant memory that we can't 'access' at our choosing are examples of unconscious memories. Memory of these events can be triggered by psychoanalytical methods or by events such as a scent or a familiar place. The unconscious contains not just memories but also thoughts. These unconscious thoughts are part of our programming that we have adopted and can contain anything, such as underlying assumptions about failure or success in life or when performing tasks. The major

*Stuart Taws developed Soft Tissue Release©, a holistic approach to addressing both neural and soft tissue restrictions.

difference with the subconscious mind is that we can choose to remember events or thoughts that it contains. The subconscious part of your mind can be viewed as the part of your conscious mind that which is not part of your momentary conscious processes, for example: your address, your phone number or your first pet's name. Before reading this, you were not conscious (thinking right now) of these facts, but should someone ask you for them, you are able to bring them to the conscious level by pulling them from your subconscious. For the purposes of our discussion, this is the basic difference between subconscious and unconscious thoughts.

The other very important aspect of the unconscious and subconscious from a strictly neurological perspective is just how many processes within the body are controlled at a sub-or non-conscious level. Most of what goes on in our bodies does not require consciousness. This involves everything from heart rate, blood pressure, digestion, healing, immune system activity, thermoregulation, even most motor control and breathing to name some of the more obvious functions. We are all able to sleep at night, so obviously are able to hand the entire ship over to unconscious processes. However, many processes are a blend of conscious and unconscious control. Let's look at something such as motor control. When you are learning a task, such as walking for example, there is a tremendous amount of conscious involvement; however, once the task is mastered most of the activity is relegated to subconscious processes. Breathing is another obvious example where subconscious processes manage it very well, but the conscious mind can step in at a moment's notice and alter breathing patterns. As it turns out, most bodily processes allow for some degree of conscious intervention; some obviously more than others.

So let's see how this applies to what we do. There is a tremendous amount of guarding that can take place after any injury, and one might assume that guarding is the conscious mind at play, and to some degree it is. However, if you tell your patient that the tissue in a given area of their body has healed completely and they believe in your expertise, then their conscious mind has accepted it. If they are still guarding the area then clearly there are subconscious and possibly unconscious elements at play. Their 'instinct' is telling them to protect the area. Many therapies that you can employ will address this component of injury, directly reprogramming the nervous system or essentially reprogramming the conscious, subconscious and unconscious mind simultaneously. Some examples of these modalities are neuro-linguistic programming, passive stretch therapy, Feldenkrais, the Alexander Technique, Trigenics, Neuromuscular Integration and Structural Alignment (NISA), and Neuromuscular Therapy, just to name a few. The goal in almost all of these therapies is to either reprogram movement, or to tell the mind that 'it is okay to move again', essentially removing the *block* between mind and body. This too is clearly a portion of what is going on with the placebo effect. The block is somehow lifted, allowing the body–mind system to do what it already knows how to do ... that is, heal itself.

Ingrid Bacci

Ingrid Bacci PhD has written several books on chronic pain management and is deeply rooted in mind/body approaches. Her body-centered approaches to managing stress and chronic pain include a plethora of practical examples for any practitioner looking for new techniques or for patients looking for self-help. In her book *Effortless Pain Relief* (Bacci 2005), the following quote applies to our discussion here:

> *The mind is not a function of the brain, but a flow of information passing through the body that takes place mostly out of our conscious awareness. The subconscious mind is actually the body itself.*

This is an interesting way to picture the psychological concept of subconscious (or unconscious). The subconscious and unconscious minds are, in fact, much more than just the brain. They exist in and truly are the whole body. Just as consciousness includes body awareness, subconsciousness includes body information flowing below the consciousness radar, and unconsciousness includes all body memories and experiences. Once you embrace the body and the mind as inextricably intertwined, it is natural to assume that the mind affects our health, and therefore healing.

Conclusion

The point of this section (much like the rest of this book) is to assist you as a health professional in breaking down barriers that you might have between the mind and the body. If you begin to see the mind as the body and vice versa, you will see improved therapeutic outcomes with your patients. Rather than delve too deeply into body-mind concepts here for which I am ill-equipped, I suggest some of the following books for anyone wishing to explore this topic. Keep in mind that body-mind books can be quite conceptual in nature or they can be more scientifically-based, depending upon the author. By the same token you may an analytical thinker, or you may think rather conceptually. To pursue reading in this area, I suggest that you find a book that suits your style of thinking.

FURTHER READING

Bacci I (2005) Effortless pain relief. New York, Free Press, Simon & Schuster
   Very practical book with lots of examples of how to immediately apply her approach

Chopra D (1990) Quantum healing: exploring the frontiers of mind/body medicine. New York, Bantam Books
   A classic book on the topic of body-mind medicine

Gallagher S (2006) How the body shapes the mind. New York, Oxford University Press

Pert C (1999) Molecules of emotion: why you feel the way you feel. New York, Simon and Schuster

Sarno JE (1998) The mindbody prescription. New York, Warner Books
   An old classic. Dr Sarno tends to be a voice crying in the wilderness with his (over)diagnosis of tension myositis syndrome, but he definitely strikes a chord

Sternberg E (2001) The balance within: the science connecting health and emotions.

PERFORMANCE OF THE PLACEBO

Variability

The medical establishment has used placebos for the last half-century in clinical trials as a baseline for testing drugs to determine the efficacy of treatments (particularly drugs), since any given treatment must, at the very least, outperform a placebo to be considered a valid therapy. So, just how well do placebos perform? The answer is 'pretty much all over the map'. When McQuay and Carroll examined pain relief scores from five placebo-controlled trials, they found individual variances from 0–100% (McQuay et al. 1995).

Medical anthropologist Daniel Moerman was interested in the placebo effect variance from a cultural standpoint. He examined 31 studies of identical design of the same drug (cimetidine) against a placebo (Moerman 1983; this drug was tested in the 1970s to treat stomach ulcers before the discovery of *Helicobacter pylori*). An endoscope was used to view participants' stomachs after 1 month. The trials took place in many different countries. The responses to the active drug (cimetidine) were fairly uniform across all the studies. The placebo arm, on the other hand, varied from 10% in Denmark to 90% in Germany and anywhere in between in other countries. Interestingly enough, the overall average ended up at 30% (the magic number that you hear most often quoted concerning the placebo effect; Evans 2004).

One can only speculate as to why such variation was seen in these studies of identical design, but presumably attitudinal, situational and personality differences might account for this rather large variance. Either way, the variability of results seen in these 31 studies is quite remarkable.

Typically in drug studies, responses from the placebo arm are much more variable than the drug being tested. The extreme example of this would be the aforementioned Moerman study where the active drug success rates were 70–75% compared with 10–90% for the placebo arm. It would appear that placebo performance in drug studies depends upon several factors such as study design, attitudes of researchers, attitudes of participants, the pathology being studied and even the country or culture where the study is taking place. The variation is so broad that it is a statistician's nightmare to come up with one number that people can all agree on. The response rate quoted most often is 35%. Dr Henry K. Beecher, a pioneer in this field, put forth this number in 1955, but even in his studies the numbers varied from 15% to 58% (Evans 2004). Add to that, a few of his methods and a bit of his math has since fallen into question, but the number has stuck, and is still often quoted to this day.

On the upside

In a study of five different surgical procedures, where expectations of participants were heightened, 70% of patients showed good to excellent responses

(Roberts et al. 1993). Conditions involved in this review included bronchial asthma, herpes simplex cold sores and duodenal ulcers. These same surgical procedures were later found to have little efficacy and were abandoned. However, in the early years patient outcomes were very good, presumably due to patient expectation. We will examine the matter of patient expectations in Part 2.

One study, which looked at placebos for pain management, reviewed 75 articles and found a response rate of almost 60%! The study team found the response rate to placebos 'strikingly high on average' (Turner et al. 1994). Clearly, as manual practitioners, this is an area that we should examine. It is in our patients` interest that we attempt to maximize their healing potential and help them out of pain. Dylan Evans, who sets an extremely rigorous standard for evaluating placebo trials in his book, *Placebo: Mind Over Matter in Modern Medicine*, discounting all placebo trials without a no-treatment arm, states categorically after reviewing many placebo pain trials that, '*Placebo anaesthesia is real*'(Evans 2004a, p. 28). He also states (Evans 2004a, p. 30):

> *…nobody yet has found a kind of pain that is completely unresponsive to placebos, which does suggest that they work across the board.*

Is the placebo effect getting stronger?

It has been suggested that placebo effects appear to be getting stronger in recent decades (Silberman 2009). On the surface this seems a fascinating notion to consider. How could a placebo effect be getting stronger? Well, no one knows for sure but there are several reasons put forth.

1. Earlier clinical trials were not constructed as well. Although studies were theoretically double-blinded, in many studies a large number of both clinicians and the participants were able to correctly guess which medication was the active medication and which was the placebo. If participants in a study guessed that they were on a placebo they would theoretically be less likely to believe that it would help with their symptoms. Modern studies are constructed better so that it is harder for study participants to guess if they are on a placebo, so are more apt to believe that their placebo is in fact active.
2. Another likely reason is that current drugs being tested nowadays tend to have slightly reduced side-effects. This, coupled with better trial methodology, will make it harder for trial participants to guess if they are on an active drug. There has even been experimentation with placebos with side-effects. These so-called placebos are actually pharmacologically active, but not for the condition being tested. This makes it even harder for participants to guess if their pill is actually the active medication or a placebo.
3. One other potential reason for the improved performance of the placebo actually lies (oddly enough) in the tremendous market success of the

pharmaceutical industry. When you run a drug trial you are looking for 'therapeutic virgins' – potential volunteers who were not already medicated with one or another drug. As more and more of the North American population uses statins, antidepressants, or blood pressure drugs, for example, drug trials are increasingly moving offshore to find un-medicated participants. These trials have increasingly moved into Africa, India, China, and the former Soviet Union. However, what we do know about the placebo effect is that it varies (sometimes dramatically) across cultural lines. So, in other countries, cultural dynamics can boost the placebo response. A patient's hope of getting better, and their expectation of expert care, is quite high in underprivileged societies that have poor health care. This is a ripe environment for placebo effects.

4. The cost of running drug trials has also driven many of them offshore, and for the reasons stated above, the placebo effect can be dramatically different in another country or culture.

5. Add to that, doctors in many foreign countries are actually paid to fill up trial rosters quickly, which may motivate them to recruit patients with milder forms of illness that are known to respond better to placebos.

Many pre-1990 studies do not accurately display the true power of placebos unless the trial was constructed in such a manner that the participants were unable to guess whether or not they were actually on a placebo. One way that dedicated researchers are trying to overcome this phenomenon (as mentioned earlier) is to construct trials where the placebo contains active ingredients which create body sensations but that do not knowingly cause any effects that would alter the phenomenon being tested (i.e. blood pressure, blood sugar etc.). All in all, this would suggest that placebos are likely more powerful than we have typically been able to measure until recently. Herbert Benson reports in his book, *Timeless Healing: the Power of Biology and Belief*, that his reviews indicate that placebos have '*substantial impact*' in the area of chest pain, fatigue, dizziness, headache, back pain, abdominal pain, numbness, impotence, weight loss, cough and constipation (Benson 1997). Could the placebo effect be even larger than we think? Interestingly enough, one review of 26 studies found that in 23 studies, where researchers happened to ask, both patients and physicians did better than chance at guessing who was on the placebo (Fisher & Greenberg 1993). In one study, 78% of patients and 87% of psychiatrists correctly guessed who was receiving the active drug (Rabkin et al. 1986). As suggested, these findings are one of the arguments for 'active placebos', placebos with some side-effects, which would be more likely to 'fool' the research participant, yielding more accurate test results.

Built-in biases within the system

What the placebo is not is a panacea. There are areas where placebos do not perform well at all. When these conditions are included in large meta-analyses and lumped in with other conditions where placebos do perform well (such as in the Hrobjartsson & Gotzsche study (2001)) placebos can be misinterpreted as having a minor effect, as poor placebo performance in certain conditions lowers the statistical mean. Certainly, this is a very poor way to evaluate the placebo. There is no drug on the market, including wonder drugs of the past that could pass the test of curing all diseases. As great as penicillin is, it is useless at treating lower back pain. It is likewise unreasonable to expect that a placebo should cure any and all human ills, as well. This standard would never be applied to any drug or any modality so why would one expect this of a placebo? As a practitioner, you would typically not employ a technique for dealing with carpal tunnel syndrome to treat temporomandibular joint dysfunction, unless you were convinced of a connection between the two conditions. By the same token, you would be disappointed to read a peer-reviewed article debunking your carpal tunnel treatment because it did not help with TMJ dysfunction.

Another fact to consider is that *many studies are never even published* because either the placebo outperforms the drug, or the drug's performance is not statistically significant against the placebo. Take this 2003 headline from the National Cancer Institute as an example, 'Researchers push for publication, registration of all clinical trials' (Reynolds 2003). Some advocates of EBM are pushing to have all drug trials published. They feel that the underreporting of clinical trials in journals and registries is undermining the progress of medical science and breaching an ethical obligation to patients. This issue appears to gaining more traction and has many valid issues. What we see of placebo performance, for example, are only the trials where the placebo was out-performed by the drug in question.

Pain and inflammation

As manual practitioners, we see a lot of acute and chronic inflammation. The acute inflammatory response typically manifests as tumor (swelling), rubor (redness), calor (heat) and dolor (pain). This is not an area that one might intuitively expect to see a marked placebo effect, and yet a number of studies have shown placebos to be quite effective in this area. One oft-quoted study is a trial where postoperative dental patients experiencing inflammation and pain after wisdom-tooth extraction got just as much symptomatic and inflammatory relief from a placebo application of ultrasound as from an actual ultrasound treatment in this double-blinded study. Researchers had made adjustments to the ultrasound machine so that neither the technicians nor the patients knew who was receiving the placebo (Hashish et al. 1986). The control group self-massaging with the exact same coupling (ultrasound) gel did not experience these effects.

As mentioned in my introductory section, studies have found that roughly one-third of all post-surgical patients and people suffering traumatic pain experience at least 50% reduction in pain from placebos. Morphine is effective in about three-quarters of patients but typically also reduces pain by 50% (Evans 1985).

Still, this is not bad for a sugar pill. A study of rheumatoid arthritis patients using placebos saw a 50% reduction in the number of inflamed joints as well as a 50% reduction in swelling and tenderness in 40% of the participants (Tilley et al. 1995). No matter how you interpret these results, this is a very real and impressive showing for placebos. Even the placebo effect's harshest critics note impressive results from placebos in the area of headaches, postoperative pain and sore knees (Hrobjartsson & Gotzsche 2001). Likewise, Dylan Evans (2004) states:

> *Of all the claims made for the placebo response, those that emphasize its power to relieve pain are the most well established.*

One interesting study with a third arm (no-treatment) group compared placebos with buprenorphine, a powerful pain drug, on cancer patients who had undergone a thoracotomy and lobectomy. On the first day patients were all given buprenorphine for their pain at 30-minute intervals until the pain was reduced. The next day when their pain returned, patients were randomly given either salt injections or no medication at all. Those patients receiving no treatment saw their pain levels increase, while those receiving the placebo injection saw 'significant' decrease in pain over the next hour. One theme that seems to occur in placebo responses, particularly in the area of pain, is that placebos are more effective if the body has 'learned' from an initial encounter. This is what is termed 'conditioning'. The placebo attempts to mimic that condition.

Function

Function is another area of special interest for manual practitioners. People come to see us as much for functional improvement as for pain relief. The two are usually linked, but not always, of course. Some approaches, such as osteopathy, focus on function, assuming that pain will follow suit. Massage, on the other hand, has traditionally focused on reducing pain, assuming that increased function will follow. The fact that there are so many approaches to bodywork is highly suggestive of involvement of the placebo effect. In all likelihood, the placebo effect is much more involved than any of our egos as practitioners would like to think. We would like to think that it is that special technique that gives us such good results; however, it is just as likely that our confidence in that technique is part of the reason that it is so often successful. To me it seems rather interesting when talking to other health professionals to find that they can get excellent results, sometimes doing the exact opposite to what others would do for a particular condition.

A 2008 meta-analysis of osteoarthritis studies looked at 198 trials with 193 placebo groups (16364 patients) and 14 untreated control groups (1167 patients). This study (Zhang et al. 2008) concluded:

> *Placebo is effective in the treatment of OA, especially for pain, stiffness and self-reported function.*

So yes, placebos do work, and they seem to work well in the area of musculo-skeletal dysfunction.

Conditions reporting the greatest placebo effects

One question that is often asked of me is, 'What conditions respond best to place-bos?' Interestingly enough the placebo has been consistently found over the last 50 years to be equivalent to psychotherapy in its response rate in study after study (Brown 2013). Conditions that respond well to psychotherapy also respond well to placebos (anxiety and panic disorders, mild to moderate depression). Mental ill-nesses that do not see improvement with psychoanalysis like serious depression or schizophrenia do not see improvement with a placebo.

The most concentrated research on the placebo effect has looked at the neuro-biological mechanisms of the placebo response around pain and analgesia; there are also new models emerging around the respiratory and cardiovascular system, the immune and endocrine system, Parkinson's disease, and depression (Col-loca et al. 2005). Placebos have also been studied and appear to be fairly powerful with asthma, Crohn's disease, ulcers, irritable bowel syndrome (IBS) and arthritis. However, the readership of this book is more interested in musculoskeletal issues. Here I have the pleasure of telling you that the placebo response is very high in the areas of acute and chronic pain (including headaches), in inflammation and related function. That is likely because of the psychobiological pathways involved as we will see later. This is very good news for manual practitioners wanting to improve outcomes for their patients.

The placebo effect in manual therapy

As you well know, manual therapy takes in a broad number of modalities, from a number of professions, treating many conditions, so there is no clear answer in this matter. There are conflicting individual studies that point in different direc-tions, and study design is poor in many of the trials. As a result, we will look at a few systematic reviews (these examine and synthesize the essential findings from multiple studies) on manual therapy that been published from 2010 onward. The good news from one perspective is that we see a clear indication that the placebo effect is a notable component of treatment success. The bad news is that it is very common to see comments in the conclusions of most systematic reviews concern-ing poor conduct methodology and reporting quality in the individual studies. All in all research in the area of manual therapy is still in its infancy. It is impossible to perform double-blind trials, and even single-blinding can be challenging with most modalities. Comments in several systematic reviews suggest future compar-ative trials as the best manner to conduct studies.

A 2010 review of evidence, entitled *'Effectiveness of manual therapies: the UK evidence report'* considered 49 recent relevant systematic reviews, 16 evidence-based clinical guidelines, plus an additional 46 RCT that had not yet been included in systematic reviews and guidelines. The authors looked at 26 categories of conditions containing RCT evidence for the use of manual therapy: 13 musculo-skeletal conditions, four types of chronic headache and nine non-musculoskeletal conditions. Once again, the authors spoke of involvement of contextual effects, another research term describing the effect that the practitioner-patient relationship plays in therapeutic outcomes. In their conclusions, the authors state (Bronfort et al. 2010):

> *Additionally, there is substantial evidence to show that the ritual of the patient practitioner interaction has a therapeutic effect in itself separate from any specific effects of the treatment applied. This phenomenon is termed contextual effects. The contextual or, as it is often called, non-specific effect of the therapeutic encounter can be quite different depending on the type of provider, the explanation or diagnosis given, the provider's enthusiasm, and the patient's expectations.*

The 2011 systematic review in the preface entitled, 'Placebo response to manual therapy: something out of nothing?' reviewed 94 research papers on manual therapy (Bialosky et al. 2011). Authors of this study clearly felt that the placebo accounted for a component of success in these studies. A quote from the conclusions of this study stated:

> *We suggest that manual therapists conceptualize placebo not only as a comparative intervention, but also as a potential active mechanism to partially account for treatment effects associated with manual therapy. We are not suggesting manual therapists include known sham or ineffective interventions in their clinical practice, but take steps to maximize placebo responses to reduce pain.*

A 2010 systematic review entitled *'Complementary and alternative therapies for back pain II'* (Furlan et al. 2010) looked at 265 RCTs and five non-RCTs. The size of this review inevitably led to a large number of conclusions, but no particular therapy performed strongly in this report. Placebo treatments were consistently better than no-treatment, but only in some cases did the active treatment perform better than the placebo or sham treatment. The authors state that stronger efforts are warranted in the future to improve the conduct methodology and reporting quality of primary studies of complementary and alternative medicine.

A 2012 paper entitled *'A systematic review and meta-analysis of efficacy, cost-effectiveness, and safety of selected complementary and alternative medicine for neck and low-back pain'* (Furlan et al. 2012) looked at 147 RCTs and five non-RCTs. This report found that complementary and alternative medicine (CAM) treatments were significantly more efficacious than no treatment, placebo pills, or usual care in reducing pain immediately or at short-term after treatment. What researchers did note was that these therapies did not significantly reduce disability compared to sham treatments. Their analysis also indicated that none of the CAM treatments was shown to be superior to one another.

The poorest results of manual therapy against placebos appear in a 2013 review of 20 RCTs that examined spinal manipulation therapy (SMT) in adults with acute low back pain (Rubinstein et al. 2013). The primary outcomes of this study were pain, functional status and perceived recovery. Secondary outcomes were return-to-work and quality of life. The researchers concluded that SMT was no more effective for acute low back pain than inert interventions, sham SMT or as adjunct therapy. They also stated that SMT also seems to be no better than other recommended therapies, but also stated that the relatively few numbers of studies that met their research criteria limited their evaluation of other therapies. Overall, this 2013 update of the Cochrane Review paints placebos as being as powerful as spinal manipulation in treating low back pain.

Overall, I would say that the systematic review of studies to date is very humbling for those of us working in manual therapy and complementary alternative medicine. No specific manual therapy shines in any of these reports. It would appear additionally that many studies lack proper design and reporting. These therapies often seem to be able to out-perform placebo pills in the short haul, but do not appear to be able to out-perform sham treatments, at least not on disability scales. Finally, there doesn't seem to be evidence of long-term benefits from CAM treatments indicated in these reviews. This is not to say that there are not long-term benefits and that these treatments are not efficacious, but clearly additional, well designed, comparative studies need to be performed. Phrased in another manner, CAM treatments and manual therapy treatments do not appear to perform better than sham treatments where the active ingredient of knowledgeable touch is removed. The evidence to date therefore points to a notable placebo effect in CAM treatments, and in manual therapy.

Conclusion

Certainly it would seem that the placebo effect is real and measurable. It would also appear that in the field of manual therapy, the placebo effect appears to be a strong component of the treatment, and appears to affect therapeutic outcomes to a substantial degree. The placebo effect is substantial in the areas of pain, musculoskeletal pain, impaired function, acute injury and chronic inflammation with all of its manifestations. Considering the power of the placebo effect and its role in therapeutic outcomes, it would almost be foolish not to become knowledgeable about this phenomenon. In fact, it would be prudent to add its application in some form or another to your arsenal of modalities that you presently use as a health professional, as you try to maximize your patients' health and healing capabilities.

DO PLACEBO EFFECTS LAST?

It is easy enough for most of us to imagine temporary, subjective improvements from placebos but are real changes seen, and do they last? Once again, placebo results vary across the board, but on the whole, both subjective and objective changes are often seen, and some results last well beyond the life of the study. For example, the peptic ulcer trial (Volgyesi 1954) mentioned earlier saw tissue changes that lasted for the course of the study (one full year). In his book *The Placebo Effect and Health*, Grant Thompson MD states that in separate trials for treatment of panic, angina and rheumatoid arthritis, the placebo effect was shown to last for 30 months (Thompson 2005).

Pavlovian extinction

Conditioning studies seem to indicate that if the expected outcome is achieved, whether through placebo, active drug, or ritual, for that matter, positive imprinting will reinforce the behavior. The term Pavlovian extinction refers to the falloff in the effect or learned behavior that occurs once an animal no longer gets the reinforcement (positive or negative) said effect or behavior. After Pavlovian extinction, a placebo loses its symbolic value and, therefore, its power. In most conditioning studies, once the stimulus is removed, extinction begins to set in. It is worth noting that many people in the medical community are now advocating use of placebos in conjunction with active medicines in certain cases where either the drug is very expensive or the side-effects of the drug affect the patient's quality of life. Multiple conditioning studies have shown that placebos are effective in treating many disorders when used in conjunction with active placebos. This can cut people's drug costs in half in areas where it has been shown to be effective. Some cancer drugs affect the patient's quality of life. Once again in this area, placebos have been shown to still be effective while also minimizing the side-effects of the medication in question. It is worth noting that in some studies participants were fully aware that their drug regime included both active and placebo medication. Multiple studies show that placebos still work even when the participants know that they may be taking a placebo. This is the case in any clinical trial, because participants are told from the outset that they may be taking a placebo.

Maintaining effects though ritual, habit or belief

Theoretically the placebo effect, through conditioning and expectation, could continue for a lifetime in humans. Consider someone you have known who lived to a ripe old age and had to eat at a specific time, or have everything 'just so' or else they just wouldn't 'feel right'. Incorporation of ritual through conditioning is probably older than written history itself, and the conditioning theory of placebos involves that same concept. If the placebo effect is linked to a given behaviour and the person exhibits that behaviour then the correct stimulus is in place.

Consider the Crum el al 2007 study mentioned earlier on page 13, linking lifestyle with weight loss. In this study, subjects simply adopting a belief system allowed them to lose weight with no behavioural changes. Researchers said, 'These results support the hypothesis that exercise affects health in part or in whole via the placebo effect' (Crum & Langer 2007). What this study lacked for our purposes was longer term follow-up to see whether the effects lasted, but the logic and the implication was that if the mindset was in place, the response would continue.

Effects that last for the duration of the study

A 1986 study of 35 patients with angina pectoris with placebo (apart from short-acting nitroglycerin) as the only anti-angina treatment involved a 6-month follow-up (Boissel et al. 1986). In 27 patients, the placebo treatment was said to be a success. No severe cardiac event occurred. The number of angina attacks per week decreased by 77% during the entire 6 months.

Exercise test improvement was also seen. These effects lasted for the entire duration of the study. Once again, the only limitation was the length of the study.

In 2002 the knee debridement sham surgery study (mentioned earlier) took place. All 180 patients had osteoarthritis of the knee and were then randomly assigned to receive one of three procedures; either arthroscopic debridement, arthroscopic lavage, or placebo surgery. Outcomes were assessed at multiple points over a 24-month period with the use of five self-reported scores – three on scales for pain and two on scales for function – and one objective test of walking and stair climbing. A total of 165 patients completed the trial. During the full 24 months of this study neither of the intervention groups reported less pain or better function than the placebo group (Moseley et al. 2002).

Another more recent study looked at the long-term benefits of rosiglitazone, a drug used to treat psoriasis, over a 96-week period (Ellis et al. 2007). The drug did not perform well, but fortunately the study was published in the *American Journal of Clinical Dermatology* under the title 'Placebo response in two long-term randomized psoriasis studies that were negative for rosiglitazone'. What this study did find was that the placebo responders' improvement lasted for the full duration of the study.

Here once again we need to determine just what the placebo effect is. I have had several cases personally, as I am sure you have, where a patient begins a course of treatments and then after one treatment reports to be symptom-free and remains symptom-free. I know this to be the case, because many of these people continued to see me for monthly massage and report full remission from the specific pathology or malady in question. Although this is anecdotal, not evidence-based information, it suggests to me that a degree of placebo effect was in play because the pathology ran an extremely short course, based on normal healing times. There are many reported cases in the media where people with serious illness suddenly go into remission and claim that it was the power of belief, these people are for all intents 'cured'. Once again, this is all anecdotal, but there are thousands of these cases out there and at some point a thousand anecdotes become evidence.

In 2008, Khan and colleagues conducted a meta-analysis on eight placebo-controlled antidepressant trials that included a total of 3063 patients. They found research where patients were continued on placebo for more than 12 weeks and examined whether they relapsed back into depression or not. The researchers found that four out of five people of those receiving placebo continued to be depression-free 4 months after their initial treatment. A full 75% of them remained depression-free on their follow-up visit, which occurred anywhere from 6 months to a year later (Khan et al. 2008).

A 2-year study of benign prostate hyperplasia (Nickel et al. 1996) was conducted at 28 centers across Canada, involving 613 patients. Participants were given finasteride or a placebo. Doctors found that the 303 men on the placebo pills were doing better, even though their prostates had grown, on average, by 8.4%. Although an enlarged prostate can impede urine flow, the latter was actually improved for the men taking the placebo. Some participants were so impressed that they didn't want to stop taking the pills.

To be fair on the matter of lasting results, let us recognize that there are few treatments or medications that have long-term lasting results. For example, millions of people take blood pressure, diabetes, or anti-clotting medication twice daily and unless a miracle arrives, will continue to take those pills for the rest of their lives. If they cease taking the treatment or medication, the underlying pathology will once again have an effect upon their health. Another example is the soft tissue treatments that I perform as a massage therapist. These treatments will increase a patient's range of motion and decrease their symptoms of work-related cumulative trauma, but if the patient returns to work and makes no changes in work style or ergonomics, these improvements are not likely to last. Likewise a treatment designed to calm the sympathetic nervous system will quickly be reversed if the patient immediately returns to a high-stress setting. So, criticisms levelled at the lasting effects of any given treatment, whether placebo or not need to be considered in a relative manner.

Trial length limitations

Another matter evident from clinical trials is that there is virtually no long-term follow-up. Any clinical trial has a finite life; very few exceed 1 year. At the end of the study, the cards are put on the table (so to speak) and the participant finds out whether or not they were on a given drug. Once it has been revealed to the patient that he or she has received a placebo, the 'jig is up'. Any effect, positive or negative is likely to cease at that point. If the patients believe that they were not actually receiving an active treatment, their symptoms will typically return. There is the matter of study design, but also of cost and practicality. The longer a study runs, typically the more it will cost. Admittedly some of the most revealing studies that have been done (placebo or not) are cohort studies of large groups over long periods of time such as the 1976 Nurses' Health Study that tracked multiple health indicators in a population of 121700 female registered nurses. This exceptional study is still ongoing. Any study of this magnitude will necessarily be government-sponsored. Studies of this sort do not typically have multiple treatment arms, so they need to be constructed in such a manner that statisticians can make inferences of placebo effects from the information gathered.

At this point you might be wondering how on earth you could incorporate this into your treatment? We will deal with this shortly in another section on ethics, and in subsequent sections. Don't worry! There are completely ethical ways of including placebo effects in your treatments that do not involve any degree of deception on your part that can still leave a lasting placebo effect.

OBJECTIVE RESULTS FROM PLACEBOS

Results from placebos are not just in the mind of the patient. Very real and measurable changes occur, and these changes have been documented in thousands of studies. Here are some examples of those studies:

- In the case of sham mammary ligation surgery (Diamond et al. 1958, Cobb et al. 1959) mentioned earlier, exercise tolerance was increased and use of vasodilation drugs was decreased by up to 75%.
- The aforementioned peptic ulcer trial (Volgyesi 1954) saw tissue changes that were endoscopically verified.
- The wisdom-tooth extraction ultrasound trial (Hashish et al. 1986) mentioned earlier produced reductions in swelling and healing time.
- Herbert Benson and his team performed a placebo study on angina pectoris patients and saw improvements in 60–80% of participants in exercise endurance, nitro-glycerine use and ECG results (Benson & McCallie 1979).
- Other studies have found an increase in natural killer cell function with saline injections when subjects were first conditioned with adrenaline injections (Kirschbaum et al. 1992).
- A Canadian study found placebos could temporarily increase dopamine levels in Parkinson patients (de la Fuente-Fernandez et al. 2001).
- Dylan Evans' list of conditions most influenced by placebos includes: inflammation, stomach ulcers, anxiety, depression and virtually all types of pain (Evans 2004).
- Conditioning studies performed on animals have seen results such as immune cell depression (Ader & Cohen 1975) and blood pressure alteration when a placebo was linked to active medications, and then administered separately at a later point in time. This is particularly interesting in that (presumably) the belief system need not be involved where animal conditioning is concerned.
- Placebo-induced immune system suppression has also been proven in humans in various conditioning studies (Albring et al. 2012, Schedlowski & Pacheco-López 2010).
- The bona fide investigation into the mechanism of the placebo effect currently taking place at several medical universities has revealed many very real, measurable physiological changes which are taking place (Benedetti & Amanzio 2013, Pollo et al. 2011, Meissner 2011). There will be more of this information in the section on Biological Pathways and Theories.
- A 2011 review of current literature found that 'recent research has revealed that these placebo-induced biochemical and cellular changes in a patient's brain are very similar to those induced by drugs' (Benedetti & Amanzio 2011).

These studies all indicate that real physiological changes happen when placebos or placebo treatments are administered. In particular, the inflammatory response appears to respond to the placebo effect. This is particularly useful in manual therapy where we see a tremendous amount of acute and chronic phase inflammation presenting in our patients.

Pain, on the other hand, is a subjective symptom. It is experienced personally and attempts at measuring it objectively have not achieved great success. However, once again, this is good news for those of us working in manual therapy. The subjectivity of pain makes it especially responsive to suggestion and the placebo effect. In fact, multiple studies show cultural differences in interpretation of the quality and severity of pain (Moerman 2000, Sternbach & Tursky 1965, Bates et al. 1993, Wolff & Langley 1968), further supporting the view that pain is a subjective experience that is alterable.

Another study showing the subjectivity and relative nature of pain compared soldiers injured in battle (Anzio beachhead) versus civilian populations with similar tissue damage (Beecher 1956). This study found that 90% of the civilian population reported pain strong enough to request a narcotic, as compared with only 25% of the soldiers. One interpretation here is that a hospital stay for soldiers was a welcome escape from the very real possibility of death in combat, so most felt very content to be recuperating in a hospital bed. In essence, their pain meant something very different for them.

Effects of placebos are real and here to stay. In 2011, Harvard created an institute dedicated wholly to the study of placebos, the Program in Placebo Studies and the Therapeutic Encounter (PiPS). It is based at the Beth Israel Deaconess Medical Center, and Ted Kaptchuk, a prominent figure in placebo studies, was named its director. Its purpose is to bring together researchers who are examining the placebo response and the impact of medical ritual, the patient–physician relationship and the power of imagination, hope, trust, persuasion, compassion and empathic witnessing in the healing process. PiPS research is multi-disciplinary and extremely inclusive spanning molecular biology, neuroscience and clinical care, as well as interdisciplinary, ranging from the basic sciences to psychology to the history of medicine. If Harvard is devoting an institute dedicating to studying this phenomenon, it would be safe to assume that the placebo effect is real. This should also lead to future studies that can tease out what is happening when a placebo is administered.

A 2011 review of current evidence entitled 'The placebo response: how words and rituals change the patient's brain' was undertaken at Department of Neuroscience, University of Turin Medical School by Fabrizio Benedetti, a leader in the field neurobiology of placebos. The following quote speaks directly to anyone working in a clinical environment (Benedetti & Amanzio 2011):

The placebo effect, or response, has evolved from being thought of as a nuisance in clinical and pharmacological research to a biological phenomenon worthy of scientific investigation in its own right. The study of the placebo effect and of its negative counterpart, the nocebo effect, is basically the study of the psychosocial context around the treatment and the patient, and it plays a crucial role in the therapeutic outcome.

The study's conclusion states:

This recent research has revealed that these placebo-induced biochemical and cellular changes in a patient's brain are very similar to those induced by drugs. This new way of thinking may have profound implications both for clinical trials and for medical practice.

So we see here that one of the leaders in this field views placebo effects on par with drug effects physiologically, and that they play a crucial role in the therapeutic outcome. This alone should indicate the importance of this topic in your practice.

Reiterating an earlier quote by Dylan Evans, noting after reviewing hundreds of studies (Evans 2004, p. 30):

Nobody yet has found a kind of pain that is completely unresponsive to placebos, which does suggest that they work across the board.

So, in conclusion we can see that placebos not only work in a subjective manner, affecting the patient's belief system, but clearly the placebo effect produces real, objective, measurable changes in the body.

THE NOCEBO

Be careful about reading health books. You may die of a misprint.

Mark Twain

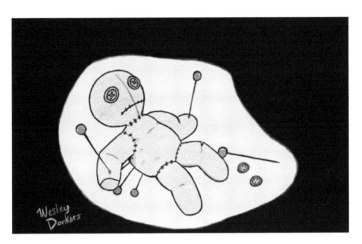

Fig. 1.5

I am sure that everyone reading this book can think of examples of both positive and negative thoughts affecting their lives. The fact that placebos can have ill effects (termed the nocebo effect) as well as beneficial should, upon reflection, come as no surprise. If the mind does in fact have power to affect our health, clearly different thoughts could either boost our state of health or impair it. There are few things in this world that have only positive effect, and the placebo effect is no exception. To consider the power of the placebo effect, look at the following examples where people experienced negative instead of positive outcomes:

- When given sugar water but told that it was an emetic, 80% of patients in one study responded by vomiting (Hahn 1997).
- A review of 77 publications (Pogge 1963) revealed side-effects such as drowsiness, headaches, nervousness, insomnia, nausea, and constipation are among the commonly reported side-effects from taking placebos.
- Another systematic review found negative side-effects such as nausea, diarrhoea and skin eruptions from taking placebos (Wolf & Pinsky 1954).
- Another example of the nocebo effect is the famous Japanese lacquer tree experiment (Ikema & Nakagawa 1962). In Japan, the lacquer tree causes skin reactions similar to poison ivy. Persons walking under these trees or past lacquer processing factories were occasionally developing skin reactions. Researchers were surprised at this in that the quantities of allergen that these people were being exposed to would have been

extremely small. A study was designed where 57 high school students were blindfolded, and then exposed to the lacquer tree leaves on one arm and the benign chestnut tree leaves on the other. The twist was that they actually applied the opposite leaf that they indicated. Interestingly enough, in over 50% of cases, the arm with the chestnut leaves reacted within minutes by developing itching, redness, swelling and eventually papules. Interestingly enough, very few persons exposed to the lacquer tree leaves developed an allergic reaction, despite the fact that many of these boys had previously been sensitized to lacquer tree leaves.

- Another case of the nocebo effect involves asthma patients receiving a bronchodilator, isoproterenol, then given different messages at different intervals. Researchers measured both the rate of flow and the total volume of air for each participant. When subjects were told that they were receiving a bronchoconstrictor, 20% of participants saw decreased volume and airflow (Luparello et al. 1970).

- The most dramatic nocebo effect is the lethal consequences on some individuals who have been given a voodoo curse. Voodoo death is a phrase coined by eminent British physiologist Walter Cannon in 1942 (Cannon 2002). In many cultures, from Africa to South America, Asia and Australia, competent authorities have reported cases in which a person has died within a few days of a voodoo curse being put upon them. As you might suspect, these curses do not seem to work unless the person is aware that the curse has been placed upon them, so presumably it is the belief system that is involved in voodoo death. Proof once again that this phenomenon involves the victim's belief system is that voodoo doctors appear to have lost their power as individuals within those cultures adopt Western values and beliefs.

- A 2003 cross-sectional survey (Ockene et al. 2005) of 8405 women at 40 clinical centers who had been taking estrogen plus progesterone or placebo as a part of the Women's Health Initiative was conducted in 1996. This famous study was stopped in July 2002, after investigators found that the associated health risks of the combination hormone therapy outweighed the benefits. The aforementioned cross-sectional survey was an exit survey that was performed in roughly eight months after the stop date. Moderate or severe withdrawal symptoms were reported by 40.5% of those on placebo compared to 63.3% of those on hormone replacement.

- A 2012 review entitled 'Nocebo phenomena in medicine: their relevance in everyday clinical practice' (Häuser et al. 2012) looked at published studies to that date including nocebo effects. Their conclusion was that these effects are very real and that clinicians face an ethical dilemma in that they are required not only to inform patients of the potential complications of treatment, but also to minimize the likelihood of these complications. They suggest that the clinician emphasize the fact that the proposed treatment is usually well tolerated, or else obtain the patient's permission to inform less than fully about its possible side-effects. They recommend communication training in medical school, residency training, and continuing medical education would be desirable so that physicians can better exploit the power of words to patients' benefit, rather than their detriment. This of course is why you are reading this book!

The most likely trigger for many side-effects from participants taking placebos in drug trials is the long list of side-effects that participants of clinical trials have to read while signing the informed consent forms. There are undoubtedly other reasons as well, from normal fluctuations in participant's health or other social factors that could be present. In the case of the Women's Health Initiative estrogen plus progestin trial (mentioned above) this was stopped in July 2002, after investigators found that the associated health risks of the combination hormone therapy outweighed the benefits. It is reasonable to speculate that the media hype surrounding this study played into some participants' minds and played a role in the nocebo effect. What is also of note here is that the placebo (nocebo) effect was barely mentioned in the report, or its conclusions. It was teased out by other researchers who looked more closely at the data. This is often the case with the placebo arm in many studies. It is typically downplayed because the focus is always on the active medication.

Informed consent and the nocebo effect

The seeds of nocebo symptoms are indeed planted in their heads at some point in time. For example, if you ever listened to a commercial for a pharmaceutical drug on television and you hear all of the side-effects and cautions that these companies are legally required to state, you would actually wonder who would take such a drug. The necessary transparency that is required in today's medical environment has the definite tendency to produce the nocebo effect, so it is critical that you properly word potential side-effects of your treatments in such a way that you minimize their effect on your patient. Your informed consent statement that you are required to clearly state before obtaining consent for any treatment indicating any potential side-effects can plant the seeds for those side-effects, so it must be done judiciously. They will not teach you this in school because they are more concerned with you passing the board examinations and as such they would prefer that you err on the side of overstatement. Every word that you say potentially plants a seed, so be careful to choose your words wisely so that you can maximize the placebo effect and minimize the nocebo effect.

CRITICISM OF THE PLACEBO EFFECT

The reader should be made aware that there is a small community of persons who don't believe in the placebo effect at all. This group is clearly a minority, but it is important to consider their concerns. Arguments put forth against the placebo effect suggest that the healing rates seen are due to spontaneous remission of the illness, fluctuation in symptoms, the natural course of the illness, statistical regression to the mean, and poor study design. Let us look at these issues one at a time.

Spontaneous remission

Spontaneous remission sounds suspiciously like the ability of the body to heal itself. This criticism sounds somewhat like a desperate attempt at semantics to try to discredit the placebo effect. I will challenge this point vigorously because the best thing that any one of us would hope for is that each patient who visited us suddenly had spontaneous remission of their illness. This does happen, and although it is the exception to the rule, it must be recognized that healing has taken place whether the allopathic model can explain it or not. Just like the placebo effect has long been discounted, spontaneous healing has been discounted because it doesn't fit into the model. But if it does happen, the problem is with the model, not with spontaneous healing. What has definitely happened in these instances is that the patient's health outcome has been dramatically improved and their own body has healed itself. Spontaneous remission (SR), like the placebo effect, appears to be highly variable.

Some of the highest recorded rates of SR are seen in variant angina with 45 out of 100 patients suddenly improving (Walters et al. 1983). In cancers the rate is highly variable with some cancers spontaneously improving more frequently than others. One controversial study suggested that invasive breast cancers showed an SR rate of over 20% (Zahl et al. 2008). (This conclusion was drawn comparing two different groups of women in four Norwegian counties. The first group had early screening and the second group did not. Early screening detected 22% more incidences, yet the overall rates of incidence at the end of 6 years were similar in both groups.) Generally numbers such as 1 in 100 000 are loosely thrown around concerning SR in cancer, but as indicated, you really have to look at a specific disease or specific cancer if you want to attempt to find out what the SR rate is. I was surprised to see that in PubMed's database, as of June 2014, that 20 082 papers contained the phrase 'spontaneous remission' in the paper. 'Spontaneous remission' was actually found in the title of 595 research papers, so the mainstream research community has not ignored this topic. If you insert the term 'spontaneous regression' (which refers to a temporary remission) then even more papers appear. The research community is aware that this phenomenon exists, but it is even harder to understand than the placebo effect. In many cases SR occurs after the body has experienced an acute infection and fever. Some people will label SR as a miracle (which it undoubtedly is from a mystical frame of reference) but this doesn't help us to understand the mechanism. The point to be made here is that yes, SR does occur; it has been well documented, but it is not well understood. This may not be the placebo effect, but if it is not then I would suggest that it is either a first cousin, or maybe the father or the godfather of the placebo effect. If the body is suddenly healing itself, then perhaps it would be best that we do not let skeptics steer the agenda towards ignoring the phenomenon as a statistical anomaly, but rather let science study the phenomenon and attempt to determine why this is happening.

Fluctuation in symptoms

One valid concern of the critics is fluctuation in symptoms. Our bodies are not static machines. They are a complex organization of over 3.72×1013 cells (Bianconi et al. 2013), all trying to achieve homeostasis individually and collectively. We are always in a state of flux, so our state of health is always waxing and waning. This could account for part of the statistical variation seen when data is collected during and at the end of a study. However, what studies consistently show is that the placebo effect is more at play with some pathologies than with others. For some conditions it is almost non-existent. If there was variation in symptoms and this accounted for the placebo effect, would we not expect to see this across the board with all conditions, rather than only in specific pathologies?

Natural course of the illness

The thrust of this argument is that some people are just getting better due to the natural course of their illness. This makes sense, and there is no way to dispute this without including a third study arm; a no-treatment group. While natural course of the illness may account for some of the study noise seen in research studies, placebo effects are actually quite high in some instances (even outperforming drugs in some cases), and almost non-existent in others. If the natural course of the illness is the reason for this statistical phenomenon, one would expect to see placebo responses to be reasonably similar across many conditions. Instead, the placebo responses vary wildly across many conditions and even across multiple studies of the same condition. As well, we typically see improvement in the placebo arm of a study when compared against a 'no-treatment' arm. If we are talking about natural progression of the disease, then we would not expect to see a statistical difference between these two groups.

Statistical regression to the mean

Statistical regression to the mean is a complex phenomenon that probably only statisticians really understand; however, it is possible to get a handle on the basic concept. The theory goes that if a statistical variable is extreme on its first measurement, it will tend to be closer to the average on its second measurement and, paradoxically, if it is extreme on its second measurement, it will tend to have been closer to the average on its first. Here's an example. If a researcher were to give a large group of people a test of some sort and selected the top-performing 5%, these people would be likely to score less well on average if re-tested. Similarly, the bottom 5% would be likely to score better on a retest. In either case, the extremes of the distribution are likely to 'regress to the mean' due to simple luck and natural random variation in the results. What this means in the medical world is that study participants with the worst symptoms will tend to regress toward a more normal measurement if the initial measurement taken at the outset of the study was extreme. This phenomenon is always at play in statistics but this still does not explain why you see very strong placebo responses to certain conditions and very poor responses to other conditions. Certainly some of their statistical concerns are valid in that the complementary health community is often quick to embrace anything out of the norm and is often guilty of accepting information that supports their viewpoint, without giving it the proper critical analysis. Critical thinking is important, but sometimes it can be carried to an extreme to simply reject anything that doesn't fit into the current medical model.

Poor study design

One criticism levelled against drawing 'placebo effect' conclusions from drug studies is that most of these trials lack a no-treatment 'arm'. Without inclusion of this arm in a study, it is impossible to say definitively that the improvements seen were the placebo effect. The third 'no-treatment arm' is not done in drug studies partly because of cost, but mostly for ethical reasons. If you have a person with an illness and you withhold treatment, this is basically inhumane. It has long been established that a placebo performs better than no treatment, so the placebo arm of a study is still receiving treatment. Now that the placebo is being studied in earnest, there have been a number of very interesting and creative studies done that include a no-treatment arm. Poor study design can happen at any time and these do not contribute to good science. One of the most common design problems is having a sample size which is too small. There are so many other areas where a study can go off the rails, but these days a clinical trial is so expensive to conduct and there are so many hoops to jump that the issue of bad study design is far less an issue. No one is interested in giving a group of researchers tens of thousands of dollars for a study unless it can pass the many stages of initial approval and will eventually withstand the rigors of peer review.

Hrobjartsson and Gotzsche

In the late 1990s two researchers, Hrobjartsson and Gotzsche, set out to prove that the placebo effect was not real. They isolated 130 studies with three treatment arms (out of which 114 provided relevant data) enabling a proper comparison between the placebo group and the no-treatment group (Hrobjartsson & Gotzsche 2001). These studies looked at over 40 different conditions from asthma, to smoking addiction, to menopause symptoms, and even marital discord. Their samples measured the placebo effects in two manners; either in a binary fashion (yes or no, + or -), or on a continuum. The results from the binary studies were not statistically significant so this was played up in the meta-analysis conclusions. Also, the researchers averaged the placebo effect over all these conditions and concluded that the placebo effect was not apparent. This was the 'sound bite' that the press grabbed on to. However, the studies that measured patients' responses on a continuum revealed a very different story. These studies showed a '*significant*' placebo effect in several medical conditions. Clearly, this is the fairer way to evaluate the placebo. The placebo is not a panacea. It does not cure all illnesses and medical complaints. No researcher has ever put this notion forth, so seems a rather ridiculous standard to set for the placebo.

As mentioned previously, if you had a modality that you believed in, such as ultrasound, or massage, or chiropractic manipulation for example, you would not suggest that with it you could cure everything from a lumbar strain, to a herniated disk, to a brain tumor. It might work well on one pathology, a limited degree on another and then not at all on yet another. It would be absurd to attack or discount any modality because it could not be used to treat all pathologies. This is where Hrobjartsson and Gotzsche's criticism of the placebo effect is not even remotely fair. There is no drug on the market that would show significant results over 40 different conditions. Dylan Evans, whose book, *Placebo: Mind over Matter in Modern Medicine*, has an extremely critical eye where the placebo is concerned. He takes absolutely no leap of faith in his book as he examines the literature on the placebos. His conclusion from looking at the studies in Hrobjartsson and Gotzsche's meta-analysis is: '*These studies then do provide good evidence that placebos can produce clinical benefits*' (Evans 2004a, p. 26). Some of the results of studies without the third treatment arm are so impressive (e.g. where sometimes as many as 70% of participants experience effects with sham artery ligation; Diamond et al. 1958, Cobb et al. 1959), the viewpoint that there is no placebo effect sounds far more like a 'flat earth' opinion than a logical conclusion.

Conclusion

The placebo effect is a very difficult concept to quantify, since we don't really know what is causing this phenomenon. The term admittedly tends to be a catch-all phrase for improvement in symptoms over the course of any given study, so there is undoubtedly some over-enthusiasm on the part of some individuals to attribute health improvement to this phenomenon. There is a degree of truth in all of the points levelled against the placebo effect, but still the placebo effect emerges as a potent factor in the improvement of the symptoms in the conditions that we as manual practitioners see in our day-to-day practice. Some of the criticism is simply semantics, and my position is that most of us in our respective professions just want to see health and symptom improvement in our patients and are happy to leave the business of labelling this healing phenomenon to others.

BIOLOGICAL PATHWAYS AND THEORIES

On the basis of these recent insights, it is clear that the placebo response represents an excellent model to understand mind-body interactions, whereby a complex mental activity can change body physiology. Psychiatry and psychology, as disciplines investigating mental events, are at the very heart of the problem, for they use words and verbal suggestions to influence the course of a disease. Psychiatry, for example, has in its hands at least two therapeutic tools: words and drugs. Interestingly, what has emerged from recent placebo research is that words and drugs may use the very same mechanisms and the very same biochemical pathways.

(Benedetti 2012)

Current theories

To begin, just what is the placebo effect, and why does it even exist? This seems like a simple enough question, but if the answer was simple, then it is unlikely that we would see so many books and papers exploring the phenomenon, nor would we see tens of millions of research dollars spent trying to understand the mechanism. There are some interesting theories that have been developed. The biochemical pathways may give us some clues as to what is going on. For example, the placebo effect can increase cortisol production. This was first discovered accidentally in trials meant to test the efficacy of ultrasound after wisdom tooth extraction. It was shown using sham ultrasound that people could actually reduce the inflammatory response by belief alone (Hashish et al. 1986).Since then, various experiments and trials have linked the placebo effect with cortisol production in other contexts, such as in reducing postoperative swelling. However, cortisol can cause problems as well as solve them. Under stress, the body increases cortisol production, which suppresses all aspects of the immune system, not just inflammation. This, of course, can lower resistance to disease, so as you can see it is not in our systemic long-term benefit to have an exaggerated immune response if not required. Conversely, many other studies show that the placebo effect can reduce or dampen cortisol production, which will reduce sympathetic nervous system activity, effectively taking the brakes off the immune system, allowing it to do its job. Based on this observation one theory is that the placebo effect is a mechanism allowing for conscious intervention allowing an individual to augment or dampen, or in other words to mediate aspects of the immune system.

Another theory held by psychologist Nicholas Humphrey at Cambridge University, UK, speaks to energy allocation within the body. He argues that humans have evolved a highly sophisticated 'health management system' designed to control the expenditure of critical resources in order to maximize survival chances. Therefore, the thinking is that the placebo effect is an emergent property of that internal system, intended to avoid investing too many resources in an immune response to a relatively minor infection. However, when required, one can consciously intervene to ramp up the immune and healing response so that the body can redirect resources to healing when no immediate threats are perceived.

We can imagine another theory if we look at pain for a moment. Pain evolved to restrict unnecessary activity and to encourage rest because the tissue involved is either injured or rebuilding itself. The placebo effect appears to be quite effective at dampening pain, but the pain exists for a reason, and that is to restrict activity. However, an individual can consciously assess the potential risks (e.g. knowing that an injury needs to heal, but needing to escape imminent danger) and more or less choose to ignore the pain, for survival reasons. In this case, the placebo effect might delay healing in favor of movement. This speaks to the idea of the placebo effect being a mechanism, which may have evolved to allow conscious intervention into the internal health management system, which can yield survival benefits based upon perceived immediate threats.

However, why does the placebo effect seem more noticeable in the interplay between an authority figure and a patient/participant? Fabrizio Benedetti speculates that health management began to evolve in a social context among the leading non-human primates. Benedetti has spent the bulk of his lifetime studying the placebo effect. His take is that this 'endogenous health care system' can be activated by interaction with other members of the group yielding the evolutionary advantage of recovering from a disease and/or improve your quality of life. He sees trust as being an implicit aspect of this contract, where the individual can put his or her care in the hands of another member of the group so that their personal energy can be spent on healing, rather than on survival. It is worth noting at this time that in non-human primates, some members of the social group show altruistic behaviours, by taking care of sick group-mates. In primitive cultures, this role would have been performed by the shaman. In modern society, this role would be filled by a health care professional.

It would also follow from Benedetti's theory that if a member of the group becomes elevated in status and increased trust develops in this person, then one might expect to see an increased placebo effect. The same would hold true for a group such as the medical profession. As the profession or person becomes elevated in status, we would see increased placebo effect. From what has been observed, this does indeed seem to be the case. This is all speculation of course, but this is exactly how theories begin to be formulated. Philip Hunter, a freelance science and technology writer, whose thoughts on this subject extends this line of thinking (supporting the evolutionary advantage of the placebo effect or endogenous health care system) by saying (Hunter 2007):

Thus, the role of endogenous health care management seems to be to identify when to override natural caution through a combination of risk assessment and reassurance by a trusted group member. The question in medical practice is how to exploit this and reinforce clinical or surgical therapies by reassuring the patient.

Theories such as these are all speculative. Nothing is remotely definitive on this topic, but it is fun to speculate as to why the placebo effect exists at all. What is becoming a bit clearer is that something is definitely going on both neurologically and chemically when the placebo effect is manifesting. What follows is a very basic look at what happens inside the body when the placebo effect is observed.

Biological pathways

Involvement of the prefrontal cortex

What is known for sure is that if an individual lacks prefrontal control, there is limited to no placebo response. The prefrontal cortex brain region is intimately involved in planning complex cognitive behavior, personality expression, decision-making, and moderating social behavior. This brain region is considered to be the center of orchestration of thoughts and actions in accordance with internal goals. One of the features of Alzheimer's disease is the impairment of prefrontal executive control. Benedetti and co-workers (2006b) found that a clear disruption of the placebo response occurred when reduced connectivity of the prefrontal lobes with the rest of the brain was present.

Definitions

Well it's time for some more definitions, because the water is about to get a bit muddier. Up until now, you may have read words like model, mechanism, pathways and felt as if you had a handle on things. If so then I commend you; however, the words become increasingly confusing as you delve deeper into the research. In this section, we are going to look at the biological pathways that appear to be at play when a placebo response is elicited. There are several 'models' proposed. These include neuro-endocrine pathways, inflammatory pathways, endorphin pathways, and psychoneuroimmunological pathways. Now you will notice that we use the word 'pathway' here, but the research literature also uses the word 'mechanism' in these instances. This is fine, but this same literature will then use the word 'mechanism' to describe the psychological phenomenon at play, which then actually needs a mechanism of action. This can be quite confusing when one considers that we are examining a topic that requires a certain degree of mental gymnastics to begin with. 'Mechanism' for the purposes of definition, then, is a broader term that includes the psychosocial trigger or phenomenon creating/surrounding the placebo effect, but it also includes the biological pathway.

In the literature, it seems that the word 'pathways' appears (for the most part) to exclude psychological phenomenon – the actual triggers of the placebo effect – so this is the word that we will use to describe what is going on after some trigger has set the placebo effect in motion. This section is about the theories and the models concerning what is happening in the body to bring about the placebo effect, i.e. healing response.

Just to reiterate and clarify, here are some working definitions:

Model – a proposed, yet to be proven, mechanism for the placebo effect

Mechanism – everything involved from start to finish including psychosocial factors, psycho-emotional factors which initiate the biological processes (e.g. expectancy, conditioning, meaning), and all biological processes involved in production and manifestation of the effect

Pathway – the neurobiological pathway (e.g. neural, endocrine, immunological, inflammatory) that the body uses to create the effect.

With these definitions in mind, hopefully you find the following quote from Fabrizio Benedetti illuminating to the discussion that we are about to embark upon, and you will get a chance to use your new definitions!

> *The placebo effect is a psychobiological phenomenon that can be attributable to different mechanisms, including expectation of clinical improvement and Pavlovian conditioning. Thus, we have to look for different mechanisms in different conditions, because there is not a single placebo effect but many. So far, most of the neurobiological mechanisms underlying this complex phenomenon have been studied in the field of pain and analgesia, although recent investigations have successfully been performed in the immune system, motor disorders, and depression. Overall, the placebo effect appears to be a very good model to understand how a complex mental activity, such as expectancy, interacts with different neuronal systems.*

(Benedetti et al. 2005)

So just how does the placebo effect work? This field of inquiry has exploded in recent decades. Of all of my sections that are likely to become out of date with the passing of time, this one will be the first! There are several reasons for the surge of research into this area. One reason (as mentioned earlier) is that pharmaceutical companies have a tremendous investment in understanding placebo mechanisms, and that is because the placebo is their direct 'competition' in every drug trial, and recently they have been losing edge to the placebo in the area of psychotherapeutic drugs. The major reason for this progress is that it is only recently that we have gained access to the diagnostic and imaging tools to look at the mechanisms. A parallel field of psychoneuroimmunology has also been moving ahead in leaps and bounds because of the advances in technology and it has added much to what we now know about the placebo effect. You will read about this later in this section.

Few placebo trials until recently were linked to pathway and mechanism theories, so advancement in placebo triggers versus placebo mechanisms has progressed and continues to advance somewhat independently. Studies indicate that placebo-mediated pain could involve any one or more of the following endogenous substances; opioids, cannabinoids, dopamine or cholecystokinin depending upon the circumstances. These substances can modulate pain perception in different directions. Positive verbal suggestions can lead to positive expectations that, in turn, activate either opioid or cannabinoid systems to create an analgesic placebo response. Conversely, negative verbal suggestions can lead to negative expectations, which would activate cholecystokinin and deactivate dopamine to create a hyperalgesic nocebo response. Current research suggests that these biochemical events would take place within a pain-modulating network that involves both cortical and subcortical regions (Tracey 2010).

Brain scanning techniques have allowed conclusive proof of the placebo effect and studies in the early part of the 21st century have revealed various brain structures and regions to be involved in placebo responses. Scott et al. (2007) have shown activation of the nucleus accumbens causing dopamine release. Petrovic and colleagues (2005) showed that the rostral anterior cingulate cortex and the lateral orbitofrontal cortex are involved in both emotional placebo and placebo analgesia. Kong and co-workers (2006) found involvement of bilateral rostral anterior cingulate cortex, lateral prefrontal cortex, right anterior insula, supramarginal gyrus, and left inferior parietal lobule in placebo analgesia. Zubieta et al. (2005) found involvement of the pregenual and subgenual rostral anterior cingulate, the dorsolateral prefrontal cortex, the insular cortex, and the nucleus accumbens in placebo analgesia. While these studies have added to the mountain of proof concerning the validity of the placebo response, they have also shown how incredibly complicated this response is. Because of the nature of experimentation, these studies can only connect small dots of what is likely a maze of processes involving every system of the body (not just neural) when one's body moves from injury or disease back to homeostasis. These studies largely look at one piece of the puzzle such as pain mediation. One thing that has emerged from studies of patients suffering from dementia of the Alzheimer type is that the prefrontal cortex of the brain is definitely involved in placebo responses where expectation was involved. It was found that if prefrontal functioning was impaired, expectation-mediated placebo responses are reduced or totally lacking (Benedetti et al. 2006b).

We will not delve too deeply into the area of pathways and mechanisms in this section, firstly because little is conclusively known about the mechanisms. What is known is that there are multiple pathways. Secondly, what is known tends to be highly technical (you know...scientist-type stuff, big words and all that!!). And thirdly, it is doubtful that at this time you will be able to apply knowledge about the details of these pathways into your practice. What you can glean from the research is what basic pathways are involved. Once you grasp the concept of the pathway, there are definite inferences that we can make that have practical implications for you as a practitioner. Since this book is intended to be practical, not theoretical, we will try not to get lost in the trees, but rather I will paint a picture of the forest by touching on the proposed theories. Then, if you are sufficiently intrigued, you can pursue research available on this topic. One recent paper well worth a read is Benedetti's 2011 review of the evidence to date entitled, 'How placebos change the patient's brain' (Benedetti et al. 2011; the full text is currently available to the public).

The more inquisitive reader can search articles on this topic through PubMed (http://www.ncbi.nlm.nih.gov/pubmed), a free database maintained by the National Institutes of Health and the United States National Library of Medicine. It accesses the MEDLINE database of references and abstracts on life sciences and biomedical topics. This is your primary resource for most medical research. Abstracts are provided for every study. The full text of a number of studies is available. If you can't access the full text of an article you can try your local library or university. They may have full access. Being a non-academic myself, I was in this same situation; however, living in a university town I was able to access these journals through the university library.

There are several competing, or perhaps complementary theories concerning placebo response pathways. These include:

- Endorphin pathways
- The parasympathetic nervous system
- A psychoneuroimmunological pathway
- The acute phase inflammatory response.

The endorphin pathway

Endorphins are naturally occurring pain modulators in the body that are similar in shape and property to the opiates (e.g. morphine). They are manufactured primarily in the periaqueductal grey matter and the rostroventral medulla regions of the brain. Moderate endorphin release has been shown to reduce pain, and higher concentrations are associated with euphoria. A few studies have been designed that have shown involvement of this pathway with placebos. Researchers designed a study where participants were receiving pain relief from taking a placebo. Then participants were administered naloxone that bonded to endorphin receptors sites on cell surfaces, preventing endorphins from attaching. After the naloxone injection, the pain-relieving quality of the placebo immediately diminished (Levine et al. 1978). Brain research, as was mentioned earlier, has advanced a lot in recent decades. Modern diagnostic equipment now allows us to look inside the living brain. Brain scans of subjects experiencing pain relief from taking a placebo show μ-opioid receptors in the brain being activated (Zubieta et al. 2005).

Clearly, the endorphin pathway is involved in the placebo effect, especially where pain modulation is happening. This pathway may or may not be involved in healing, but is definitely involved in blocking pain. The fact that the placebo effect seems to be so powerful in the area of pain modulation, coupled with the fact that opiates are the strongest pain medication known, also supports this theory.

Sympathetic/parasympathetic pathway

Another popular theory is activation of the parasympathetic nervous system, or rather, deactivation of the sympathetic nervous system. Our sympathetic nervous system prepares us for action, but chronic stimulation of this system is associated with (Brody 2000a):

- Hypertension
- Arteriosclerosis
- Cardiac distress cardiac arrest
- Osteoporosis
- Memory loss
- Accelerated ageing
- Stomach ulcers
- Fibromyalgia and chronic pain syndromes
- Eczema
- Vulnerability to infections.

The primary brain centers at the origin of sympathetic pathway are the amygdala, hippocampus and the hypothalamus. Interestingly enough, these structures are also a primary part of the limbic system. If you remember your schooling then you probably remember needing to know about the limbic system (then quickly forgot about it). Emotion involves the entire nervous system of course, but the limbic system is primarily responsible for our emotional life (and has a lot to do with the formation of memories). The limbic system is actually a complex set of structures that lies on both sides of the thalamus, just under the cerebrum. It includes the hypothalamus, the hippocampus, the amygdala, and several other nearby areas. Interestingly enough this is also the area that revs up our sympathetic responses to stimuli whether real or simply perceived.

The amygdala and hippocampus are both very sensitive to any emotions that we are experiencing, and are intimately connected with the cortex, or thinking area of the brain. Any thought can produce changes in the amygdala and hippocampus, which along with the hypothalamus can begin a cascade of events that leads to the increase or decrease of the fight or flight response, depending upon the emotional charge of the thought. The hypothalamus, which lies immediately below the amygdala and hippocampus, sits outside of the blood–brain barrier, and as such is very sensitive to any external influences in the bloodstream. Initiation of the sympathetic nervous system begins a cascade of events that result in stimulation of our adrenal glands. Collectively this system is known as the hypothalamo–pituitary–adrenal axis or HPA. From the hypothalamus, there are two pathways, neural and endocrine. The endocrine pathway (which travels via the pituitary gland) signals the adrenal cortex to release cortisol, which, among many other things, suppresses the immune system and the inflammatory response. The neural pathway signals the adrenal medulla to release catecholamines (not the least of which is adrenaline), which are known to increase heart rate, blood pressure, breathing and metabolic rate. In addition to these symptoms, our sympathetic nervous system increases muscle tone, which as you know can manifest as musculoskeletal pain. This may appear in classic areas such as the lumbar or cervical spine or the shoulder girdle, or in specific areas where the patient has predisposition to dysfunction. Continued stressful circumstances can potentiate amygdala(e) functioning, allowing it to become more powerful – some might even say wilful – over time, sometimes exerting subcortical control over our human cortical reasoning. This is well worth remembering as a practitioner. Because of the neuroplasticity of the brain, any area that gets overstimulated will potentiate and undergo physical changes. The overstimulated HPA axis tends to feedback into itself. The important take-home message here is that unhealthy patterns can be eventually replaced with healthy patterns. An exaggerated sympathetic response can eventually be tamed, but the habit needs to be broken.

So reducing the stimulation of the sympathetic pathway, allowing the parasympathetic pathway to emerge via the HPA axis, could account for placebo success with generalized musculoskeletal pain, specific pain such as headaches, cervical or lumbar pain. This pathway could also account for placebo success with hypertension, chronic pain and stomach ulcers, as well as bolstering of the immune system and normalization of blood sugar levels.

While the sympathetic/parasympathetic pathway is very well understood, placebo involvement at this point is still being studied, but more and more studies link it to the placebo effect. Fabrizio Benedetti states in his 2006a study entitled, 'The biochemical and neuro-endocrine bases of the hyperalgesic nocebo effect':

> *By studying experimental ischemic arm pain in healthy volunteers and by using a neuropharmacological approach, we found that verbally induced nocebo hyperalgesia was associated to hyperactivity of the hypothalamic–pituitary–adrenal (HPA) axis, as assessed by means of adrenocorticotropic hormone and cortisol plasma concentrations. Both nocebo hyperalgesia and HPA hyperactivity were antagonized by the benzodiazepine diazepam, suggesting that anxiety played a major role in these effects.*

This finding supports the HPA axis theory and also indicates that there are direct clinical implications for us as practitioners.

What has been extremely well studied is meditation. Clearly the parasympathetic pathway is the mechanism stimulated by the meditative state, as indicated by Benson (1997, p.131):

- Decreased metabolic rate
- Decreased blood pressure
- Decreased heart rate
- Decreased rate of breathing
- Decreased muscle tension
- Increased slow brain waves.

We will learn more about the benefits of mediation in the final section of Part 2 where we discuss methods that your patients can employ to maximize their own healing response.

Psychoneuroimmunological pathway

Okay, this is the biggest word that you will see in this book! The immune system is deeply complex in every manner, whether one examines the manufacturing of its basic components, its ability to sense a perceived threat, the myriad sentinels that it uses to watch and react to invaders, the complex internal signalling taking place, or the armies that it can produce and employ to battle specific threats. (Hence the really big word!) The immune system has been described as being an intelligence of its own, comparable to the brain (Ewald 2000). Certainly, it is amazingly intelligent, and the discovery in the 1980s of a rich supply of nerves linking the brain with the immune system led to the fascinating new field of study known as psychoneuroimmunology (PNI).

PNI has uncovered not only much of the internal signalling within the immune system itself, but the feedback systems back and forth between it and the brain. Like the sympathetic nervous system response, the HPA loop is involved with its neural and endocrinal branches. The branch appears, once again in the deep emotional centers of the brain with the endocrine branch traveling via the pituitary gland. The neural branch, once again, uses the autonomic pathways. Although, this communication takes place at an unconscious level, there is potential for conscious influence in either pathway in that higher brain centres in the cerebral cortex also communicate with these emotional centres. The hypothalamus, sitting outside the blood–brain barrier, immediately senses presence of immune system release of Interleukin-1, Interleukin-6 and tumor necrosis factor, informing the brain of threats and of immune system activity.

Immune system cells, as it turns, out are studded with receptor sites for neuropeptides associated with emotional states. In other words, your immune system reacts to, among other things, how you are feeling. So as you can see, there is a lot of information passing back and forth from the brain to the immune system allowing for fine-tuning, checks and balances. Involvement of the hypothalamus and pituitary gland in this loop has caused some researchers to speculate that there is an ideal 'set point' for the immune system, to keep it at a certain level of readiness (Schwartz 1994, Barak 2006). Too high or too low a set point, according to this theory, could cause an individual to be more prone to certain conditions. However, at this point, it is only speculation.

Howard Brody suggests that PNI theory is the most likely explanation of what is happening with the placebo effect (Brody 2000a) in that endorphins, catecholamines, and cortisol (used in the previous two systems) are all monitored by the hypothalamus and as such are part of the psychoneuroimmunological feedback loop.

While much has been uncovered in PNI research, much still has yet to be proven before it can be definitively linked to the placebo effect. At this point is still a matter of conjecture and debate.

The acute phase inflammatory response

Dylan Evans has proposed yet another mechanism, the acute phase response. Evans is a lone voice, but in his book, *Placebo: Mind Over Matter in Modern Medicine*, he presents a detailed argument for his theory. Evans states that the conditions where the placebo effect is most pronounced (pain, swelling, ulcers, depression, anxiety) all involve the acute phase inflammatory response. He reminds us that this response goes beyond the classic signs of inflammation (tumor, rubor, calor and dolor), but is now recognized to include a suite of symptoms known as 'sickness behaviour' (Kent et al. 1992). Sickness behaviour includes lethargy, apathy, loss of appetite and increased sensitivity to pain. He also reminds us the chemicals such as Interleukin-1β are involved in the acute phase feedback loop, as is the hypothalamus-pituitary gland-adrenal gland loop. Signs of depression are remarkably similar to sickness behaviour and there are strong links established between depression and anxiety. Evans details the biochemical arguments for seeing these as inflammatory conditions as well. Rather than try to detail his theory here in this book, any readers interested in Dylan Evans' take on placebos and their possible mechanism would be encouraged to pick up a copy of his book.

Conclusion

When considering the topic of placebo pathways and mechanisms, I am reminded of two mantras that my college pathology professor (an MD himself) would oft repeat. Firstly, *'Almost every disease process begins with inflammation'*, and secondly, *'When there is more than one theory about what is going on, there is probably some truth in each theory.'* I have found both of these statements to be very helpful in understanding what is going on in the body, and in keeping an open mind as to what else might be going on. It certainly appears that the HPA axis is involved in the placebo effect, and undoubtedly, the immune response is being summoned. The immune system is incredibly complex and involves everything from the initial acute phase response and detection of non-self to attack and defense of the body. The brain appears to be able monitor what the immune system is doing and affect its actions as well. This might be the broadest way of describing our understanding of the placebo effect at this time in scientific terms.

If one definitive placebo pathway was ever uncovered, it might be beneficial in terms of maximizing the placebo effect and predicting other ways that it might work to our benefit. However, in the end it may just be a lot of shadow boxing, since we are talking about people's belief systems. Belief is not a static thing, and mental processes are without a doubt, incredibly complex. Any clear answer in the area of pathways and mechanisms is not likely to be forthcoming any time soon.

THE PLACEBO RESPONDER

An individual who trusts a member of his own social group, whether a shaman or a modern doctor, has surely an advantage over those who lack this mental disposition. This pure social interaction can, in some circumstances, be as powerful as the action of a pharmacological agent.

Fabrizio Benedetti MD,
Professor of Physiology and Neuroscience,
University of Turin Medical School

Is there such a thing as a placebo responder... a type of person that consistently responds well to placebos? When placebos were first used for research in the 1950s, researchers looked for the factors that caused people to respond to placebos. Their goal, in part, was to find these traits or factors and then weed out these research subjects from trials to the end of removing the unpredictable 'placebo wildcard' which seemed to be skewing research results (Brody 2000a). They looked at age, gender, personality traits, and education. Some of these studies were actually quite interesting to look at both in their design and their findings, but they are now 50 years old or more and subsequent studies produced contradictory results, so let's look at more recent research.

From what you will learn about the placebo effect in this book, it is only in the augmented group in the study (Box 1.6) that you would expect to see a strong placebo response.

A 2009 study (Kelley 2009) looked at patient and practitioner influences on the placebo effect in irritable bowel syndrome. In it, 289 patients were randomized for 3 weeks to:

1. Waitlist (n=96): patient symptoms were monitored periodically but no treatment was delivered
2. Limited (n=97): placebo acupuncture was delivered twice a week by a neutral practitioner, and
3. Augmented (n=96): placebo acupuncture was delivered twice a week by a warm, empathic practitioner.

They randomly assigned participants to one of three groups. It was found that **patient extraversion, agreeableness, openness to experience, and female gender** were associated with a stronger placebo response, but only in the augmented group.

Box 1.6

In the present age of marked political correctness, people may look askance at studies which try to determine which individuals or groups are more 'suggestible' such as the above study or Daniel Moerman's study (mentioned above in the section, 'Performance of the placebo'), which looked at different cultural responses to and interpretation of pain. However, as long as the intent is to understand mechanisms at play, not to create an argument for discrimination, there is no reason to discourage or fear this type of research. It would appear that the placebo response is typically higher in some cultures where people are more apt to be open and trusting, and is typically lower where the culture is more insular or one of suspicion (Evans 2004). In the earlier part of the 20th century, the thinking was that a person who was more apt to respond to placebos was more impressionable or somehow a 'weaker' individual. In reality, virtually all people show placebo response in the right circumstances. As well, it has been shown that an individual that responds well in one situation may fail to respond in another. Factors affecting placebo response are more apt to be specific to the situation or environment (Frank & Frank 1991, Brody 2000a). One experiment that illustrated this was a study of obstetrical patients given placebos to reduce pain from each of three different causes (Liberman 1964; labor pain, after-labor pain and self-induced pain). In all three situations, placebos provided more relief than the no-treatment group; however, there was no statistical correlation between particular individuals across the three situations.

Acquiescence

Clinical psychologists Seymour Fisher and Roger Greenburg found one personality trait that was more placebo-responsive, which they termed '*acquiescence*'(Fisher & Greenberg 1997, Fisher & Fisher 1963). People scoring high acquiescence scores were typically described as being open, trusting, uninhibited and 'other-focused'. Faced with a problematic situation, persons with this trait prefer to cope in ways that involve linkages with those around them, rather than in solitary ways. Interestingly, people scoring high acquiescence scores also respond better to active medications as well (Fisher & Greenberg 1997). Conversely, individuals who are mistrustful and isolated tend to be poor placebo reactors (Lasagna et al. 1954). If true, this might suggest that some of your 'difficult' patients will continue to be a challenge where the placebo effect is concerned. However, if you look at the gambit of techniques in Part 2 that you can apply, hopefully you will find ways to get even your challenging patients to turn on their inner healer.

A similar psychological concept to acquiescence is a psychological term known as 'Locus of control' (Rotter 1990). Patients with an external locus of control would be considered more acquiescent. To quote Jerome Frank (Frank & Frank 1991):

> *A personality trait that is termed locus of control seems to influence relative responsiveness to different forms of therapy. Persons with a predominantly*

internal locus of control attribute favourable or unfavourable life events to their own efforts or enduring personal characteristics. In contrast persons with external locus of control attribute life events primarily to chance, fate, or powerful others.

A 1978 study by Liberman, which demonstrated the association between '*mastery orientation*' (a concept very similar to locus of control) and response to placebos, showed that subjects with an external focus improved dramatically more when given a placebo, than the internally focused group.

The concepts of acquiescence, locus of control, and mastery orientation all speak loud and clear to me about the concept of *trust* in placebo responsiveness. If you want to access the inner healer in your patient, they must trust you and your abilities. This is clearly easier inpatients with an external locus of control, but it is essential that you develop trust with your inwardly focused, shy, cautious patients, by whatever manner possible.

Children, on the whole, appear to be more responsive to placebos than are adults. They have been shown to have higher than average response rates for conditions such as attention deficit hyperactivity disorder (ADHD), migraine headaches, depression, anxiety, and asthma (Brown 2013). One can speculate as to why this is, but it does appear on surface to fit into the acquiescence theory. When one thinks of a child, words like open, trusting, uninhibited often come to mind. These same words describe acquiescence.

Anxiety

Anxiety level of the patient also consistently affects placebo response. The more anxious the subject, the stronger the placebo response tends to be (Evans 1974). This strongly suggests the parasympathetic nervous system as a pathway involved in the placebo response. It is also suggestive of how to treat your patients, especially those with increased levels of anxiety. Consider this quote from a 1997 study (Schweizer & Rickels 1997) on anxiolytics (drugs that combat anxiety):

The development of new treatments for generalized anxiety disorder increasingly has been sabotaged by a high placebo-response rate. As a consequence, and in contrast to the surge of approvals for new antidepressants, only one new anxiolytic has been approved by the U.S. Food and Drug Administration in the past 15 years.

Pharmaceutical companies have had trouble bringing new drugs to the market because of high placebo response rates. Sadly, the public has not been made aware that anxiety is largely controllable without drugs. Put another way, very few of the drugs tested have been able to beat placebos in treating anxiety, and those that do, necessarily contain side-effects.

In relaying the factors around placebo responsiveness to a friend in an entirely different profession, he told me of his experience with this same concept. As a professional engineering consultant, he has been called into a few situations where anxiety levels were running very high due to the complex nature of the problems, the time pressures involved and the ever-present economic constraints. His response in these situations is to say, '*Okay everybody, I'm here. This may not be an easy problem to solve, but it is doable. This is my area of expertise, and I will not leave until we have solved this problem.*' He said that you can see the anxiety level drop immediately, and suddenly big impossible problems become bite-sized manageable problems. This really is the placebo effect in action. A professional walked in the room. Trust was quickly established (trust in his ability to solve the problem and trust that he will not leave them in the lurch until the situation has been resolved). Immediately fears were allayed and the HPA axis begins sending healing signals to the body as it moved out of sympathetic mode.

Ted Kaptchuk, director of Program in Placebo Studies and the Therapeutic Encounter at Harvard, wrote a paper in 2008 entitled, "Do 'placebo responders' exist?" (Kaptchuk 2008a). This publication looks at papers and research into this topic since the 1950s and suggests that the research on this topic is now old enough to be considered 'medical history' and points to some flaws in the methodology employed. He draws no clear conclusions about the 'placebo responder,' but he does suggest that new studies need to be performed and suggests a methodology to employ. There is clearly a difference between a cold research setting and a warm clinical setting with a caring practitioner. In the cold setting, it would seem that anyone could be a responder, but there is little predictability about who the responder might be. In the warm, empathic clinical setting, it would seem that we might see that some of the aforementioned traits such as anxiety, acquiescence, patient extraversion, agreeableness, and openness to experience might be qualities inpatients that might respond better to the techniques suggested in Part 2 of this book.

Where there's a need, there's a market, and one product that has appeared to capitalize on this desire to weed out the placebo responders to lower the cost of drug trials. It uses a web-based software program that uses a neurocognitive approach to determine which subjects are 'placebo responders.' It claims to improve the success rate and reduce the cost of clinical trials by weeding out such individuals. Even if this software or any other method for reducing/eliminating the placebo effect does work, many might find the idea somewhat distasteful. The whole concept brought by Beecher in the 1950s was that drugs should at the very least be able to beat a placebo. If the placebo effect is eliminated from drug trials, but a placebo pill is still used to determine drug's efficacy, are the results valid? The world is full of placebo responders. You and I, for example, are two responders, and if or when we take these drugs, we are likely to experience any number of placebo effects as well as the drug effect, so it does not appear to be in the public interest to remove this phenomenon from drug trials.

Recent research

Just to muddy things up a little bit more, a 2014 study (Darragh et al. 2014) looked at personality traits associated with higher placebo responses and found some confounding results when compared with other research over the previous decade. Their study involved 63 healthy volunteers and exposed them to two psychosocial stress tests. Prior to the second test, the placebo group received an intranasal spray of 'serotonin' (placebo) with the suggestion that it would enhance recovery. Subjective stress, heart rate and heart rate variability were measured. Surprisingly in this study, lower optimism score and less empathic concern predicted greater perceived benefits from the placebo treatment. Lower overall drive, fun-seeking, and sensation-seeking were related to a greater physiological response to the manipulation. Multivariate analyses revealed lower optimism and behavioural drive to be predictive of responding to the placebo manipulation. The research team agrees that a cluster of traits characterized by behavioural drive, extraversion, optimism and novelty or fun-seeking appears to be germane to placebo responsiveness, but they suggest that contextual stimuli may generate different patterns of responding. Researchers in this study suggest that rather than a 'placebo personality' it may be that responsiveness is better typified by a two faceted transactional model, in which different personality facets respond to different contextual contingencies.

In other words, this researcher suggests that perhaps traits like optimism, drive, and extraversion might be important to consider when looking for a placebo responder, but apparently in some situations higher drive is associated with higher responsiveness, and in some cases lower drive triggers a stronger response. Likewise with the other traits discussed.

Conclusion

As with many aspects of human behaviour, research often shows conflicting information, and it is not always easy to sort out what is really going on. Looking for a placebo responder is not likely to help us as practitioners. Looking for a placebo responder or a personality trait that lends itself to response is of more use to the research community. It makes sense to minimize the placebo effect in these situations. The practitioner is treating anyone and everyone that passes through their door, so we are not trying to selectively weed out, or to look for these specific traits in individuals.

If there is one lesson to be learned from the topic of placebo responder, it is in the area of trust. Jerome Frank sums up the qualities of the placebo responder as such (Frank & Frank 1991, pp 137-138):

> *In general, the placebo reactors tend to be more anxious, can let themselves depend on others for help, can readily accept others in their socially defined roles.*

Your acute awareness of the importance of **trust** in the practitioner/patient relationship is critical for all patients, but especially for those with a strong internal locus of control. Trust is at the heart of the practitioner/patient relationship and it is also essential in helping to trigger the inner healing system of your patient. As well, effectively dealing with a patient's anxiety is also extremely helpful in triggering the patient's healing systems. You can help your patients alleviate their anxiety in many ways through explanation of their pathology, lending them your ear, teaching coping mechanisms etc. We will discuss a variety of techniques and methods that you can employ in Part 2, which will help you access the patient's inner healer.

ETHICS AND INFORMED CONSENT

In this section, we will explore the ethics surrounding your decision as a health care practitioner to maximize the placebo effect in your practice. At first glance, it may seem to you that if you use the placebo effect on your patient without their knowledge, it is deeply unethical, and you may be right, but like all ethical issues, things are rarely black and white. On the other hand, you might be looking at this and thinking:

A. *This placebo stuff is quite benign,* or

B. *I am only acting in the patient's best interest,* or

C. *I was already employing some of the techniques described in this book without even realizing that they might be the placebo effect.*

Of these scenarios, 'B' is the least defensible. The idea that any treatment is in the patient's best interest and therefore the practitioner doesn't need to tell the patient is indefensible in the 21st century. The age of medical paternalism has passed. On the other hand, you might be saying to yourself, *'I thought that it was just my basic personality to be confident, honest, trustworthy etc. I never thought of this as the placebo effect.'* There is no quick answer here, but we do need to dissect things somewhat to examine the ethical considerations around this phenomenon and try to arrive at some conclusions.

To begin with, if you knowingly employ the techniques described in this book to augment your patients' healing system, and you genuinely believe in the placebo effect, you should fully expect that it will improve patient outcomes. You will personally have to decide what you will do with this realization. You will also see in Part 2 that *everyone* uses aspects of the placebo effect to some degree in their everyday life, and every practitioner is already getting a placebo response from his or her patients. The placebo effect flows out of a healthy trusting relationship with anyone, but really comes in to play in a trust relationship where one individual has expertise and/or power that the other does not have. As always, it is good to take a historical perspective on an issue to see how we arrived at where we are today. At the heart of this matter lies informed consent, so let's look at how it has changed throughout history.

Physician knows best?

The medical profession has enjoyed a long and illustrious history of treating patients in a paternalistic manner. Since the time of Hippocrates, the clear sense of physicians was 'the physician knows best', whether it involved informing patients about potions that they were taking or the possible side-effects of any treatments received; even if this included the risk of death (bloodletting being the classic example). This is not to say that physicians in general did not have the best interests of the patient in mind. Clearly, they did, and the Hippocratic Oath outlined that guiding principle. For millennia, this oath justified the paternalistic attitude of physicians.

Research, even as recent as the early part of the 20th century, was known to involve such things as using cigarettes to entice prisoners into taking part in experiments on altered dietary regimes (Evans 2004). The growth of personal liberties and individual rights that had developed over the last few centuries in the West was as an important factor in bringing about the concept of informed consent, but the atrocities of Nazi experiments on prisoners brought forth in the 1947 Nuremberg trials caused the world to stand up and take notice of this matter. The trial of 23 German physicians and scientists saw testimony of witnesses of Nazi hospitals and camps detailing experiments where Jews and other prisoners were subjected to freezing temperatures and high altitudes, infected with malaria and typhus, injected with drugs and poison; all against their will (Evans 2004). These atrocities highlighted just how far the slippery slope could go, and before long, the concept of informed consent became a cornerstone of modern medicine. As mentioned earlier, informed consent became enshrined into American law in 1962 with the *Consumer Bill of Rights*. It established people's rights to safety, to be informed, to choose, and to be heard. The 1964 World Medical Association Declaration of Helsinki enshrined the individual's rights into its code of ethics. It stated that when participating in research, an individual's consent should be in writing, and that the well-being of the human subject should take precedence over the interests of science and society. The new paradigm has the individual rights trumping all other concerns.

Backing up 100 years, doctors at the end of the 19th century and the beginning of the 20th century were becoming increasingly aware that much of their arsenal of remedies was slowly being proved useless at best, and if not, then downright harmful. This caused the founder of modern pharmacology Sir John Gaddum to once quip that the *materia medica* was the only body of knowledge that had become smaller as it had advanced. The ethical dilemma for doctors was: do they go on using these 'placebos' (remedies that had been proven useless) and if so do they inform their patients about the results of the research?

Ethics in the 21st century

Dylan Evans points out that health care providers working in alternative medicine face similar dilemmas today due to the growing body of evidence of the placebo effect, and the ready access to information on the internet. To quote Evans, *'There is a rapidly accumulating body of scientific evidence which strongly suggests that many forms of psychotherapy and alternative medicine may be pure placebos'* (Evans 2004, p. 184). This is not to suggest for one minute that these treatments are not beneficial. The question in point is: does the patient have a right to be informed that they are in fact receiving a placebo? The ethical dilemma exists due to your duty to care for your patients and see that they receive the best medical treatment possible on the one hand and your patient's right to be informed on the other. If we were talking about doling out a placebo pill, few of us would be ethically challenged. Clearly the patient needs to be informed. If it is a treatment that research and conventional wisdom see as pure placebo (e.g. ear candling or ionic foot baths) then once again, no real challenge exists. You must inform the patient before using the treatment that studies show that the treatment compares comparably to placebo. The next few scenarios present the ethical dilemmas that you might face as a health care practitioner.

1. What if the treatment is viewed both by the profession and the public at large as being entirely valid, but there is no evidence-based research to back it up as having efficacy? Walter Brown points out in the introduction to his book, *The placebo effect in clinical practice*, that 'some experts estimate that less than 50% of the treatments routinely used by physicians have actually been proven effective in careful studies' (Brown 2013, p. 2). Much of the evidence for manual therapy is quite shaky even though we all see reasonably consistent patient improvement, and our patients tell others of our wonderful healing abilities. However, even though you operate from logic, and explain the logic of the treatment to the patient, the research may not be there to back up the efficacy of your chosen modality or treatment. It is important to recognize that in the field of manual therapy very few of the modalities that we employ have been tested in double-blind trials. This is because there have not yet been methods devised to create a placebo chiropractic adjustment, or placebo muscle energy technique, or myofascial technique for example. Of the very few modalities employed by manual practitioners where a blinded placebo treatment has been developed (e.g. ultrasound, acupuncture), few results have shown them to perform well against the placebo treatment. At best, the modalities typically employed in manual therapy have been examined in comparative trials against other treatments. While we all believe that our treatments are efficacious, this is based largely on our own intuitive sense, rather than on science. It is important to remember that this is exactly how doctors felt hundreds of years ago when they were treating illness by bleeding patients and using all manner of concoctions that have now been proven useless or even harmful. Like us, these doctors had many patients that improved with these treatments, bolstering the doctor's confidence that the treatment was efficacious. What is being suggested here is while you may be convinced that your treatment is not a placebo, that with the exception of a very few modalities, you have no proof that this is the case.

2. What if the treatment is viewed both by the profession and the public at large as being entirely valid, even though research to date indicates that the treatment does not outperform a placebo? This appears to be

the case with anti-anxiety medication and with antidepressant drugs as well except in the most severely depressed or severely anxious patients. Acupuncture rarely outperforms placebos, but thousands of clinics across North America perform acupuncture every day. This is not to knock acupuncture, but the consistent evidence of its ability to outperform placebos is not present. Psychotherapy, likewise, is on par with placebo for many conditions in multiple studies (Brown 2013). Areas where placebos perform well, psychotherapy performs well. Conditions unresponsive to placebos like OCD or schizophrenia do not respond well to placebos or psychotherapy. Do you burst the patient's bubble in these situations?

3. What if a portion of your treatment is due to the proven effects of the therapy, and a portion is due to the placebo effect. This is a category probably most of us fit into. As you have probably already figured out by reading this book, unless you are rude, condescending and cold and are perceived by your patients as an incompetent nincompoop, a part of your success with your patients is due to the placebo effect. This should already be clear to you, and if it is not, then it will become clear in the sections ahead. Do you need to inform your patients that part of the reason that they are getting better is because they like and trust you both personally and professionally?

4. After reading this book you choose to enhance your treatments with techniques described in this book, knowing that you are employing the placebo effect. Do you then carry on in the patient's best interest, never informing them that perhaps they hold the keys to their own kingdom of health, or do you inform them that some of their improvement may in fact be due to their faith in you?

Like all matters of ethics, I cannot provide quick and easy answers for you on these scenarios. I have my own thoughts on each scenario, but it is best that you work through and arrive at your own conclusion as to what you should do. I will provide you with enough information in this section and throughout the book for you to make an informed ethical decision on your own. If you are reading this section with a group, then now would be a good time for a discussion.

If we were to take the lead from the first few thousand years of medicine, we could say, 'Let's just keep this among ourselves. The patient only stands to benefit from this, and after all, what harm is being done?' Well, this just simply is not the paradigm under which modern medicine operates. In the present age, the patients have rights to know the details of, and consent to, any treatment that they are undergoing. Furthermore, we are operating from an evidence-based model, which should preclude us engaging in a treatment that is pure placebo.

So, let us begin with the easiest ethical dilemma. If you are actually distributing or recommending a placebo, you must disclose this fact. Personally, I can think of no instance in my practice where I would employ a pure placebo, but there may be some instances where a practitioner might recommend them. The strongest argument might be to use them in conjunction with active treatments/medications that are either very expensive, or that have serious side-effects. Examples of these circumstances are illustrated in paragraphs that follow. As it turns out, there are tactful ways of getting proper informed consent for placebos without losing the placebo effect in most instances.

Informing the patient that he or she actually holds the keys to their health is not an entirely new concept. Two thousand years ago when Christ was doing faith healing he was quoted as saying, 'Your faith alone has healed you'. As is described in several other sections of this book, open administration of placebos still produces a placebo response; it is mostly a matter of phrasing the topic in the correct manner. Just because you are honest about what you believe is going on, the placebo effect will not necessarily evaporate. However, some tact is in order so that the patient gets the correct message concerning this phenomenon. For example, I recall visiting my family doctor many years ago, and as he prescribed a certain medication for me he said, 'This medication will help with this issue; however your body will have to do the rest. Ultimately all healing comes from within.' That statement says quite a bit, and in fact there is also a pretty strong hint that the placebo effect aka inner healing was what would ultimately cure me. In that statement my doctor also subtly handled informed consent around the placebo effect, while also reinforcing the effect at the same time. This is one way to handle informed consent around the placebo effect as a health care provider. It is unlikely that we will ever be able to separate the placebo effect from any of our treatments, so if we are to act ethically and with transparency, it would be wise for each and every one of us to develop some phrase, such as the one that my doctor gave me, to inform our patients that their own belief system/inner healer/placebo response is a key player in their health and recovery. In fact it would be wise to inform your patient that even as a health practitioner with years of experience, you still take a back seat to the patient's own inner healing system. This is not only a great way to promote the patient's own inner healing abilities, it is also good for you to let your ego take a back seat to what is really going on.

The American Medical Association's opinion statement (Box 1.7) appears to address the concerns that many ethicists would have around this subject. There is recognition of the importance of the trust relationship that exists and it gives the practitioner latitude to use techniques to improve therapeutic outcomes. The question of how to broach the subject of informed consent is not covered, and this is important in that it must be tactful but honest.

AMA Opinion Statement

In 2007 The American Medical Association tackled this subject directly with a position statement. Opinion 8.083 – Placebo Use in Clinical Practice states:

...Physicians may use placebos for diagnosis or treatment only if the patient is informed of and agrees to its use.... The physician need neither identify the placebo nor seek specific consent before its administration. In this way, the physician respects the patient's autonomy and fosters a trusting relationship, while the patient still may benefit from the placebo effect. A placebo must not be given merely to mollify a difficult patient, because doing so serves the convenience of the physician more than it promotes the patient's welfare. Physicians can avoid using a placebo, yet produce a placebo-like effect through the skillful use of reassurance and encouragement. In this way, the physician builds respect and trust, promotes the patient-physician relationship, and improves health outcomes.

Box 1.7

Placebos without deception

A 2007 study by Karen Chung and colleagues at University of Florida examined an interesting question. For her doctoral thesis, Chung looked at the after-effect of individuals' placebo responses on their future ability to experience a placebo response. This was the first study to ask this sort of question. They examined two different groups, one with IBS and another with experimental pain. Chung and colleagues discovered that there were **no differences in future pain responses between participants who were told that they experienced a placebo response versus those who were not told.** The conclusions of the researchers were:

These studies suggest the placebo response persists even after revelation of a personal placebo response and placebo use does not appear to cause adverse effects on mood and other attitude variables assessed.

This study supports the idea that patient awareness of the placebo response does not necessarily negate its effects. You need not dance around the fact that as a clinician, there is likely to be a placebo component to any useful therapy.

Note that the researchers in the study in Box 1.8 did not just say, 'We are going to give you a sugar pill'. They presented the context of the placebo so that:

1. *There was no deception about the fact that it was a placebo* and
2. *They were informed that clinical studies showed that there had been significant improvement in others with the same condition who had taken the same pills* (or followed that same course of treatment) *through mind–body self-healing processes.*

A 2010 Harvard study, 'Placebos without deception: a randomized controlled trial in irritable bowel syndrome', conducted by Kaptchuk and colleagues (2010), provides useful insight into using placebos with informed consent. This study involved 80 participants diagnosed with IBS, a condition known to respond to placebos. The study was designed to test whether open-label placebo (non-deceptive and non-concealed administration) is superior to a no-treatment control. Patients were randomized to either open-label placebo pills presented as:

placebo pills made of an inert substance, like sugar pills, that have been shown in clinical studies to produce significant improvement in IBS symptoms through mind-body self-healing processes

…or no-treatment controls with the same quality of interaction with providers. What they found was that the open-label placebo produced significantly higher improvement scores both in subjective and objective measurement scores than the no-treatment group.

Box 1.8

It is worth noting that in some studies, participants were fully aware that their drug regime includes both active and placebo medication. In a three-armed study on ADHD in children (Sandler et al. 2008), one arm received an optimal dose of medication for 2 months, the second arm received an optimal dose for 1 month then a 50% optimum for the next month, and the third arm received an optimal dose for 1 month plus a visually distinctive placebo (and were told that it was a placebo); then for the second month they received 50% of the optimum does plus once again a placebo. Parents were asked post-study if they would be interested in having their children take dose extenders (combination of placebo and active medication) in the future. Surprisingly 71% said yes to the idea. Parents felt that the dose extender would result in fewer side-effects and allow the medication to last longer.

A 2011 survey asked an interesting question: 344 university students were asked if they would agree to use a placebo as a first line of defense if they became depressed. The survey found that 70% would agree to the use of a placebo and 73% said that they would agree to placebo use for other conditions (Nitzan et al. 2011).

Another study looked at 81 patients and 107 healthy subjects (Feffer et al. 2011). Patients were recruited from an out-patient clinic and were diagnosed as either in the past or present as suffering from a depressive episode. All subjects were briefed thoroughly about the efficacy, potential benefits and limitations of placebo in treating depression and then completed a self-report questionnaire. In all 64% of the patients expressed consent to use placebo in case they suffer again from depressive symptoms, compared to 79% of healthy subjects. In both groups over 70% of the subjects did not perceive prescribing placebo as a deceit or as an act that diminishes the patients' autonomy. The authors of the study concluded that among other things the findings question some of the ethical justification of excluding placebo from the clinical practice and call for further discussion on the subject.

Proper phrasing around the placebo

When these studies were performed, the phrasing of a placebo was important. Notice that the participants were 'briefed thoroughly about the efficacy, potential benefits and limitations of placebo in treating depression'. This is full disclosure that allows the participant to make an informed decision. Calling it a sugar pill is also honest, but does not allow the patient to really make an informed choice and will in no way call upon the patient's body's own ability to heal itself. So as you can see, you really don't need to dance around the subject of any of your treatments that have a partial or strong placebo component. If your patient is to ask you about the efficacy of any given treatment, I would recommend that you approach the subject head-on with the known efficacy of the treatment, the limitations, and the properly worded statement indicating that many people with this condition have shown improvement using this treatment modality by engaging their own internal healing systems that each and every one of us has been blessed with.

Written consent

All health care providers ask patients to fill out detailed health histories that typically have the patient sign some form of release or consent. While it is important for all health care providers to know that they need to obtain express consent for each and every treatment that they provide at the time that they are providing the treatment, the topic of placebo effect can actually be tactfully addressed on the patient intake form. In fact, it would probably be great if every intake form of every health provider across the country addressed the topic. This would remove negative stigma attached to the placebo effect and serve all patients better, in that it would empower them in the area of their own health. An example of the phrasing might be:

Any medical intervention has limits. Beyond that, the body must bring itself back into balance. As a patient, I am aware that my health is largely my own responsibility. Furthermore I have been made aware that my relationship with my health care provider, my beliefs, attitudes, lifestyle and diet can either augment or impair this healing process. Signed _____.

If you feel that getting things in writing is too much, then you can and should regularly provide the basic content of the above message verbally with your patient.

The phrasing could be done any number of different ways, the key element being that the patient must be made aware that their own belief system, and the therapeutic relationship with you (or any health care provider), is a part of their healing response. This statement speaks volumes and handles informed consent around this matter without 'bursting the bubble'. This, coupled with your commitment to professionalism, which involves always placing the patient's interest before your own, should always act as your guiding light toward ethical decision-making and behaviour as a health professional.

Part 2

Concepts and Application

There is no reason that we cannot have both the real medicine and the very best placebo. And there is no reason why real medicine itself cannot be the very best placebo, if it sends the right symbolic messages to our inner pharmacy.

Howard Brody MD
(Brody 2000a, p. 48)

INTRODUCTION TO PART 2

One important reminder of why we are looking so closely at the placebo effect in this book is that every clinical trial that tests the effectiveness of a drug or a treatment is designed to minimize the placebo effect. The reason for this is that the placebo effect is coming to play in all therapeutic treatments. The aim of Part 2 is to attempt to understand and then maximize this effect. To quote Daniel Moerman:

> *It is not too hard to see that placebos can be meaningful, and people can respond to such meaning in important ways – producing dopamine in Parkinson's disease; producing endorphins inpatients in pain – but the key thing here is that if the inert pill is meaningful, so is the active one. That is, meaning (placebo-based) responses are always there.*

This portion of the book will be more treatment-focused. If you are more practically minded rather than theory-based, and you stuck it out through Part 1, then thank you. If you have just joined us for Part 2, then I welcome you. You should find something to sink your teeth into in this section of the book. Every section in Part 2 introduces you to a different concept, each of which has been shown to improve your patient's response to your treatment. The general format for these sections is to first discuss the research behind the concept so that you are confident that you are working from an evidence-based model. We will then look at ways for you to implement the theory into your practice so that you can maximize the healing/placebo response in your patients.

According to experts, the placebo effect is initiated and mediated by one or more of the following psychoneural constructs

- Conditioning
- Expectancy and hope
- Meaning.

Conditioning refers to what the mind or body has learned from prior exposure to a given stimulus (either positive or negative). Conditioning appears to work on animals as well as humans in some very interesting ways, and is probably the only concept that is measurable on animals in that expectancy and meaning would require anthropomorphising, which would all but invalidate the research. Conditioning is also unique in that it is also referential to the past only.

Expectancy refers to just what the patient expects out of the experience; sort of a self-fulfilled prophesy concept. Expectancy is future-referenced, while conditioning is based on past experience, and yet as you will see it is quite difficult to tease these two concepts apart in clinical trials. There have been some experiments that have actually separated it from expectancy and conditioning, so we will look at those later. Hope is not really the same as expectancy, but is lumped in to this category because it is future-referenced.

Meaning is perhaps the mother of all placebo theories. Many stimuli and concepts flow into meaning and of course for the patient almost all thoughts and actions flow from meaning. Meaning could be described as something which for the patient is referenced partly from past experience (or lack thereof), which takes in all aspects of the present healing environment, all of the patients future expectations, then assembles meaning from all of the information assembled. Brody (2008) describes meaning as whether or not an individual feels:

1. Listened to and has received adequate explanation for the illness that makes sense
2. Care and concern being expressed by the healer and others in the environment
3. An enhanced sense of mastery over the illness or its symptoms.

While this description makes sense, it could also be argued very easily that expectations and hope have meaning to the individual and that conditioning is a method of learning, and that all learning eventually has to have meaning. Meaning might be the big umbrella that encompasses all theories about why the placebo effect manifests itself.

While meaning is a tremendously interesting and abstract notion, it is not a section title in Part 2. Instead, the abstract notion of 'meaning' has been broken down into a number of specific concepts. As well, any concept to which the patient gives meaning and that has been shown to enhance healing is included in this section. The point could be raised whether or not some of these concepts raised are in fact the placebo effect, to which I would have to respond, 'Does it really matter?' . It is at those points in particular in this book that I am least concerned with the label 'placebo effect'. Ultimately, I believe that as health practitioners we are not concerned with semantics about whether or not we are actually turning on the *placebo effect per se*, as long as we are accessing and activating our patients' internal healing systems. My understanding of science and medicine is that it is not necessarily required that mechanism always be understood, as much as the fact that the results should be repeatable. For example, what is the mechanism of acupuncture or of trigger point therapy? We have some idea of what is going on, but at the moment, all that we have are theories. This does not stop us from employing a modality if we can get repeatable results. The same holds for the concepts presented in Part 2.

While nothing about this is an exact science, there is some evidence that different placebo response effectors appear to be cumulative, meaning that if proper conditioning has been established, and the patient's expectations are high, and the other aspects of the treatment are interpreted as being helpful, then each effect will add to the other. Two of the strongest and widely accepted theories around the placebo effect involve expectation and conditioning. As a practitioner, you can expect to see improved response from your patient if you employ lessons from several of the following sections rather than choosing one concept and working only with that one.

The final section of Part 2 presents a smorgasbord of ideas for your patient to use toward the goal of augmenting their own healing systems. It is not intended to be a complete and definitive list, as much as it is a selection of techniques and ideas from which you could pick when suggesting homecare for your patient.

As you read the following sections and put them into practice you will undoubtedly discover other methods and ways to implement these concepts. When you do, I welcome you to contact me with any suggestions and feedback that you might have that would enhance future editions of this book. I would very much appreciate any comments or suggestions that you, as a reader and health care provider would have concerning any aspect of this book. I can be contacted via the contact link on my website at www.fultonmassagetherapy.com

CONDITIONING

The reflection of the current social paradigm tells us we are largely determined by conditioning and conditions.

Stephen R. Covey (Covey 2004)

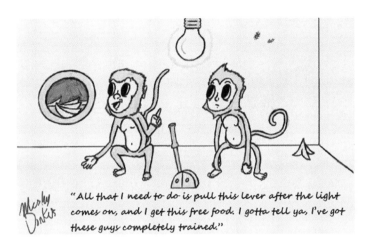

"All that I need to do is pull this lever after the light comes on, and I get this free food. I gotta tell ya, I've got these guys completely trained."

Fig. 2.1

The conditioning theory is the most well-established and quantifiable of the placebo theories and has been proven by a multitude of both human and non-human animal studies (Wickramasekera 1980, Boileau et al. 2007). The fact that placebo conditioning works on animals is very interesting indeed. While we should not be surprised to find that other animals have their own *natural health care management system* (to borrow a phrase from the preface) as well, it is rather interesting to look at the concept of belief at this time. It is highly unlikely that an animal's belief system is coming into play with immune system conditioning studies, when it is unlikely that animals even know what an immune system is. This is also the case for a percentage of humans as well whose immune systems have responded to conditioning, so something other than belief is likely causing the effect in these instances. As of yet, we do not understand the biological underpinnings of conditioning; what is important here is that placebo conditioning works.

Soon after Pavlov developed his conditioning theory by getting dogs to salivate at the sound of a bell, or any other stimulus associated with food, other Russian researchers were able to conduct immune system conditioning on guinea pigs. Guinea pigs, when injected with an inflammatory chemical, developed swelling and redness. The animals were then given a neutral stimulus before the injection on a conditioning schedule. Eventually the neutral stimulus (which at this point would be called a conditioned stimulus) produced redness and swelling (Martin 1997). This took place in the second decade of the 20th century; however, the rest of the world largely ignored these findings (world wars have a way of distracting people!). Placebo conditioning theory would sit still for another 50 years until momentum was gathered around this topic.

In the 1970s the proverbial ball was then picked up by psychologist Dr Robert Ader and immunologist Nicholas Cohen. Ader and Cohen were studying learned taste aversion when they stumbled upon the placebo effect accidentally (Ader & Cohen 1975). To quote Dylan Evans:

> *By repeatedly injecting rats with cyclophosphamide (a drug that induces nausea) whenever they drank sweetened water. Ader and Cohen succeeded in training the rats to avoid sweet-water. Unfortunately for the poor rats, however, it seems that their immune systems had been affected too, and they began to die in unexpectedly large numbers. Besides inducing nausea, cyclophosphamide also suppresses the immune system. So Ader and Cohen had inadvertently conditioned the rats to suppress their own immune responses whenever they drank the sweetened water. In fact, the more sweet-water the rats consumed, the more likely they were to die.**

(Evans 2004, p. 100)

This experiment illustrated three rather interesting facts about placebo conditioning that are now well recognized:

1. The immune system could be conditioned by use of a placebo
2. Increase in placebo use (frequency) increases the effectiveness of a placebo
3. The effects of placebo conditioning can be so dramatic that it can lead to death of experimental animals.

Another interesting point about this study was that the rats had been broken up into several different groups, with each group being given a different reinforcement schedule. Ader and Cohen found that the group with the reinforcement schedule most closely linked to cyclophosphamide saw the most marked responses, adding further credence to the conditioning theory.

---

*The father of conditioning theory is Russian psychologist, Ivan Pavlov, who noticed that dogs salivated at the sight of food. He therefore began introducing other stimuli that did not cause dogs to salivate and began timing their appearance or sound just before or around the time of the appearance of food. Lo and behold, this previously neutral stimulus began to make dogs salivate. This is classic Pavlovian conditioning. Using Pavlov's dogs as an example, I will explain some conditioning jargon. In classical conditioning training, a naturally occurring unconditioned response (i.e. salivation), which happens in the presence of an unconditioned stimulus (the food), is linked to a neutral stimulus (the bell) through a reinforcement schedule. Over time the neutral stimulus becomes a conditioned stimulus, eliciting a response similar to the unconditioned stimulus. If the conditioned stimulus is then continued without reinforcement, the conditioned response eventually fades. This is termed (Pavlovian) extinction.

Two more interesting facts that came out of subsequent placebo research by Ader's were that:

1. Placebos are more effective when they follow active and effective therapies (Ader 2000)
2. Proven active drug therapies have been found less effective when they follow ineffective treatments (Ader 2000).

One documented application of Ader's research was a young girl, 'Ruth', who at 11 years of age developed systemic lupus erythematosus (SLE) (lupus) (Brody 2000a). Two years later she was suffering from a severe exacerbation of the illness that was causing kidney damage, hypertension and bleeding. Her doctors prescribed cyclophosphamide to suppress her overactive immune system, but unfortunately, the medication has many toxic side-effects. Her mother knew of Dr Ader's cyclophosphamide studies and wondered about trying something similar on her daughter. Her physicians agreed to the trial using a full dose of cyclophosphamide for the first 3 months with cod liver along with rose perfume. In subsequent months, she was administered cod liver oil and rose perfume, but only received the cyclophosphamide during every third session. Over the course of a year, Ruth's SLE went into remission. While this incident is simply an anecdote, subsequent research has demonstrated the efficacy of placebos when used in conditioning schedules to reduce the side-effects of drugs.

One example of a conditioned placebo response used by some physicians to this day is the prescription of antibiotics for a common cold, which is viral, not bacterial in nature (Brody 2000a). Patients who have previously improved by taking antibiotics have in fact been exposed to a conditioning reinforcement schedule. This is not the only factor at play here; there is also the expectation of the patient and the symbol of the doctor as a medical authority as well.

A 1990 study looked at a group of women receiving chemotherapy for cancer (Bovbjerg et al. 1990). Chemotherapy is known to suppress the immune system, so researchers decided to measure immune system activity several days before their scheduled chemotherapy and again just before their chemotherapy session. A number of participants showed significant drops in immune activity, simply by being in the environment where they were about to receive their injection. Their immune system had 'learned' to suppress itself, presumably by the sights, sounds and smells of the hospital environment.

In 1999, a study paired gamma interferon injections in humans with an oral placebo (Longo et al. 1999). Gamma interferon is known to increase macrophage activity. Participants in the study group were then slowly weaned off their injections but still given an oral placebo. At the end of the study, the group receiving only placebos still exhibited increased macrophage activity.

---

*On a personal note, I cringe at the thought that much of the advancement of medical knowledge seems to have come at the expense of the suffering and death of non-human animals. I wonder if the day will come that our species will evolve to the point where we no longer consider this acceptable behaviour. But alas, that is another book.

Fabrizio Benedetti conducted an interesting study in 2003 that included both sufferers of Parkinson disease and healthy volunteers, who were both told that a drug (which was actually a saline solution placebo) would deliver pain relief and increase the production of growth hormone while inhibiting cortisol secretion. The verbal suggestion worked for pain relief but not for hormone secretion. However, the patients were then conditioned by replacing the placebo with sumatriptan, a drug that stimulates growth hormone while inhibiting cortisol. When this was later replaced by the placebo, the same pattern of growth hormone stimulation and cortisol inhibition was observed, suggesting that pre-conditioning, not suggestion, influences hormone secretion. In the case of pain relief, where the patient can observe the effect, the opposite was true (Benedetti 2003).

Frequency of use

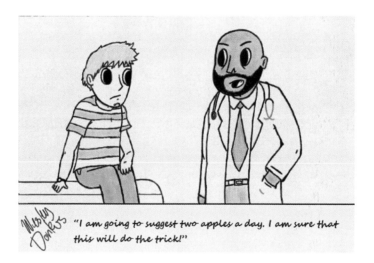

"I am going to suggest two apples a day. I am sure that this will do the trick!"

Fig. 2.2

One well-established conditioning principle is that increased frequency of use of either placebo leads to improved results. One duodenal ulcer study found that when placebos were taken four times a day, healing rates were better than in the group taking placebos twice per day (De Craen et al. 1999). What this means for you and your practice is that when you are assigning remedial exercises to your patient, there is justification for an increased frequency in the regimen of activities. Certainly doing an exercise twice per day is better than only once per day. The same principle applies to the number of repetitions within the exercise schedule. However if the exercise schedule becomes too onerous, then patient compliance will be reduced, so it is not advisable to increase the frequency of exercises beyond that which you believe there will be patient compliance.

Patient compliance

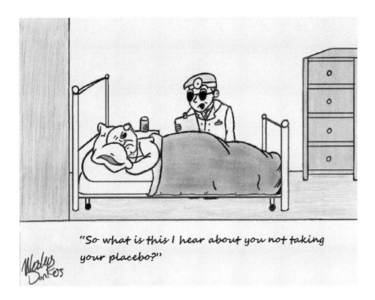

"So what is this I hear about you not taking your placebo?"

Fig. 2.3

An extremely well-established principle in medicine that applies equally to the placebo effect is that of patient compliance or adherence to their treatment regime, whether it might involve medications, lifestyle changes or homecare. While this might seem obvious, what is not so obvious is to find that in multiple studies, patients who took all their prescribed placebos did significantly better than those who took only 80% of them (these results mimicked those in the active treatment groups; this has been shown for studies of heart attack survivors, post-chemotherapy infections, treatment of schizophrenia, and others). Knowing this, it is important to know that no matter whatever technique you apply, whatever ritual you surround your treatment with, and whatever homecare you suggest to your patient, you (and your patient) should be cognizant of the fact that the more 'buy-in' or compliance that you get from your patient, the better the treatment outcomes will be. Every section in the second part of this book should help to increase patient compliance, but it is good to always remember the concept of compliance as a quantifiable aspect that will always improve treatment outcomes.

Frequency of visits to practitioner

As one might expect, there is an increased placebo response with increased frequency of visits to the doctor/practitioner (Ilnyckyj et al. 1997).While most aspects of the placebo effect are in line with best practices, the matter of frequency can cause some professional concern because a practitioner of low moral character could abuse the phenomenon by having the patient visit more frequently than necessary. However, playing devil's advocate for a moment, I have always struggled with suggesting a high frequency schedule of visits, even though I am aware that in the early stages of treatment, there is clear justification and benefit derived from this degree of frequency. The reason for my hesitancy is that I tend to put myself into the patient's shoes from a cost perspective and sometimes suggest a more conservative treatment schedule. However, realizing that increased frequency is associated with a stronger healing response would help to tip the scales for those of us struggling with suggesting an increased frequency of visits until improvement in the condition is seen.

Putting conditioning theory into practice

So we have established that the placebo effect can be a conditioned response. What does this mean for you and your patients? Well to begin, if you have a patient that has responded poorly in the past to a particular therapy (perhaps with a different practitioner) that you want to employ, then conditioning will work against you. Also if they may have had poor results from manual therapy in general, your manual therapy in particular, or the specific technique that you are using on them, then this cycle needs to be broken. You can approach these situations with the following phrases:

- **Altered or additional technique,** e.g. put a new twist on an old technique or add a different technique at the beginning or the end. You can say something such as: '*I have found that modality B is more effective if I combine with modality A.*'
- **Different technique,** e.g. '*I'd like to try a technique that I haven't used on you previously. I've had very good results using this modality on other patients with this same condition.*'
- **Linking techniques**. If they have responded poorly to a technique or an approach that you feel you need to use, determine what they have responded positively to and link your modality to it, e.g. '*You have responded well to muscle energy techniques in the past. I am now going to add ultrasound. While you may not have responded to ultrasound in the past, we have found ultrasound therapy to be more effective if it is followed by a manual therapy technique such as muscle energy.*'
- **Linking remedial exercises to clinical techniques.** We have all used techniques where the patient experiences either immediate reductions in pain, or increases in range of motion, or both. When we see these gains it is good to immediately suggest an exercise that they can do at home to reinforce the gains that the patient has just experienced. e.g. '*This is a phenomenal improvement in your shoulder. To maintain this pain-free range of motion I want you to_____ three times per day until your next appointment.*'

- **Different order**, e.g. *'Let's try a different approach this week. Instead of doing (A) first, we do (B) first instead, followed by (A). I have found this approach successful with other patients.'*
- **Change the intensity of your technique**, e.g. *'I have seen some improvements in your function, but I think that we can help with the pain if I work deeper/lighter.'*
- **Completely different approach**, e.g. *'Let's try something completely different this week. No one therapy works for everyone. This is normal. This week I'm going to suggest we try _____.'*
- **Hot new technique**, e.g. *'I have this new technique that I just learned at a workshop. I received my training from a leader in his/her field. (S)he has found it to be very effective in treating individuals with similar symptoms.'*

In these examples, you (as their practitioner) recognize that in some way both you and the patient are aware that a given modality has not worked for them. Be sure to play up the positive as they may still have had functional gains or improvements in their pain scales. Then use expectancy (the next concept that we will look at) to try to break negative conditioning that may be affecting their recovery.

Negative conditioning is something that you probably see every day to some extent in your practice. Sometimes it is previous negative conditioning that brings people to complementary/integrative therapies such as ours in the first place. If a patient has had no progress with traditional allopathic approaches then desperation may lead them to see us. In this case the patient may have negative conditioning around *any* progress with their condition i.e. hopelessness. The advantage is that we will typically be using a technique/modality/approach that the patient has not experienced. This will work well both from an expectation and conditioning viewpoint. The previous conditioning that we have as an obstacle was more of a generalized hopelessness around any success, but we have our manual therapy approach that they have not yet experienced as a new hope for their problem. This is clearly the point that we need to focus on. Consider employing one of the following statements:

- **Raising patient's hopes**, e.g. *'Your body has had to deal with this for quite a while, and I know that you have had some disappointments with previous therapies, but together, we can turn things around for you. The fact that you sought me out tells me that you haven't given up hope.'*
- **Highlighting previous successes that you have had with other patients**, e.g. *'I want you to keep an open mind as we try this therapy. I have had hundreds of success stories with other cases similar to yours.'*
- **Creating and focusing on realistic short-term goals**, e.g. *'I want you to keep focused on your range of motion in this area of your body over the next few days. You will begin to notice that you are feeling freer and looser. Do not focus on the pain. That will soon pass. First we need to focus on feeling freer and looser.'*

- **Focusing on quantifiable progress,** e.g. *'When you began treatment you had 60 degrees range of motion, now you have 75. This is excellent progress!* 'or *'At the beginning of your treatment you reported pain as being a six out of ten, and now it is a four out of ten. This is excellent progress!'*

Once again, expectancy and hope are being employed to try to break the negative conditioning.

On the other hand, conditioning can work in your favor if your patient has had previous positive associations with bodywork or with the technique that you are using, particularly if they have positive results with your personal touch. Examples of using positive conditioning are:

- **Reminding patient of previous success**, e.g. *'You will remember that the last time you had this symptom we used* e.g. ultrasound (insert appropriate modality) *with great success. I suggest that we follow a similar protocol this week.'*
- **Reminding patient of previous success and increasing its effect with another modality.** Following up on the previous suggestion you could also say, *'I suggest that we follow a similar protocol and augment it with _____ to increase its effectiveness.'*
- **Reminding patient of previous success and adding a homecare suggestion,** e.g. *'I suggest that we continue with a treatment identical to last week which worked so well but augment it with this homecare activity _____ to increase its effectiveness.'*
- **Reinforcing progress in a quantifiable manner,** e.g. *'When you first arrived your range of motion was only 50 degrees, we are now at 85 degrees'* or *'When you first came in you described your pain as eight on a scale of zero to ten, now it is a four. That is real progress!'*
- **Temporarily increase frequency of successful homecare,** e.g. *'I am going to suggest you follow up this treatment with the homecare that helped you so much last time. This time I want you to perform them not just once, but twice daily, for increased effectiveness.'*
- **Increase their frequency of treatments,** e.g. *'I am going to suggest two treatments this week and two next week to speed your recovery.'* Needless to say, the treatment frequency has to be justified and medically appropriate. This uses the principle that increased frequency leads to increased healing results.

If you have had positive results but want to change treatment directions, try the following strategy to ease the transition using previous conditioning:

- **Using previous successes to change treatment direction,** e.g. *'Previously we (or you) had success with _____. This time I want to try a slightly different technique/modality that uses the same principles and has been shown to be very effective with your condition.'*

Note that in human beings a second system of signals known as *language* increases the possibilities and complexities of conditioning. Words can function as powerfully as concrete stimuli, creating emotional reactions and potentially affecting the HPA axis. For example, if you consider each of the following words 'meditate', 'income tax', 'baby', or 'cancer'. Each of them carries a strong emotional charge. Sometimes the emotional value that someone else might assign to a given word may be somewhat predictable, sometimes not. Consider the word 'ocean'. For one person this might conjure up the idea of a Caribbean holiday, full of lots of fun and relaxation. For another person it might conjure up a fear of shark attacks, drowning or any number of unknown perils. For another it might bring about the thought of a great sailing adventure. The point being that you never know just what baggage your patient may have around a particular word or concept. So whether you think your language is quite benign or not, it is good to clarify and have your patient echo back what you have said, to clarify their interpretation. When they do, listen for any fears or negative language that they may use, indicating negative conditioning around a word or concept. Furthermore, you really want to avoid using emotionally charged words, such as 'pain' as much as possible. If you must, you need to diffuse the emotional charge of the word, in an attempt to break any negative conditioning that they may have around it. *'How'* you say something is extremely important and will typically vary with each patient. This requires the ability to 'read' your patient.

EXPECTANCY

Open your mind to the infinite possibilities that exist for you. Born through your dreams, crystallised into form by your desires, given impetus by your expectations, then made real through your beliefs.

Steven Redhead, from
Keys to the Laws of Creation
(Redhead 2010)

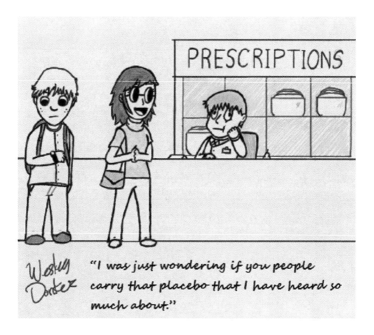

Fig. 2.4

A concept different from conditioning is expectancy. This involves patient's expectations of the outcome, but also involves yours as well, as you transmit all sorts of signals during the treatment about their potential prognosis. In this section, we will be looking at the patient's expectations. Conditioning is referential to the past whereas expectancy is future-oriented. Because of the nature of these two frames of reference, we can pretty much say that expectancy is therefore the more 'plastic' of the two concepts, though what has passed is not necessarily written in stone. We can actually rewrite our own stories. This will be discussed later in 'Enhancing meaning through stories'.

We have all heard the old adage, 'Bring about what you think about'. Now that you understand the placebo effect and the nocebo effect, this saying paraphrases the concept of 'expectation' quite well. The expectation model is one of the cornerstones of the placebo world. There are many studies substantiating the effects of expectations in placebo studies.

One pioneer in this area was Dr Stewart Wolf who began research into expectations in the late 1940s. One of his early experiments looked at the effects of contradictory cues when volunteers received ipecac, which causes vomiting (increasing smooth muscle contractions), and atropine, which calms the stomach, decreasing smooth muscle activity (Wolf 1950). He began by giving the participants ipecac and noticed the increase in smooth muscle activity. He then administered atropine – as might be expected, smooth muscle activity typically decreased. He then gave them a placebo but told volunteers that he had given them ipecac. Many of the subjects reported nausea and showed increased smooth muscle activity. He then gave them a placebo and told them that it was atropine. As you might expect, a large number of participants indicated that their stomachs felt better and Wolf measured reduced smooth muscle activity. This is one example of expectancy. What happens (to a large degree) is what the patient is expecting to happen. It is also fairly easy to see the important role that suggestion plays in expectancy.

Other participants in that same study were actually given ipecac, but told that it was atropine and had paradoxical reactions (smooth muscle activity and nausea decreased). The outcome of these studies was the recognition that a person's expectations could produce a bodily reaction, whether given a chemically inert or active agent. Wolf's work is considered groundbreaking in that he was the first to show objective changes as a result of placebos. His work also challenged the idea that placebo effects were only temporary when he measured effects that were as pronounced and as long lasting as the active medication (Brody 2000a). Another dramatic illustration of expectancy was the Japanese lacquer tree experiment (Ikema & Nakagawa 1962) mentioned under 'Nocebo' (see p. 53). This study of 57 blindfolded high school students, who were exposed to lacquer tree leaves on one arm and chestnut tree leaves on the other, but were deliberately misled, yielded very interesting results. In over 50% of cases, the arm rubbed with the benign chestnut leaves reacted within minutes by developing itching, redness, swelling and eventually urticaria. Interestingly enough, very few persons exposed to the lacquer tree leaves developed an allergic reaction, despite the fact that many of these boys had previously been sensitized to lacquer tree leaves. Once again, expectation has tremendous power, to the point of initiating or curbing an allergic reaction.

The sham mammary ligation surgery mentioned in 'A historical perspective' (see p. 23) is another dramatic illustration of the power of expectancy. In both the control group and the mammary ligation group, approximately 75% of *all* patients reported substantially lower pain levels, had greatly increased exercise tolerance, and had less need for vasodilation drugs. In some participants, the results lasted for years. There was, in fact, no statistical difference in the results of the surgery group or the control group. These results were probably so dramatic because patients had no idea that they might even receive a sham (placebo) surgery. As well, one principle that we will look at later is the effect of the perceived power of symbols. In the world of treatments, not surprisingly surgery is perceived as the most powerful symbol, so it induces the strongest placebo effect. In this case, researchers saw objective improvements in vast numbers of patients that lasted for the full length of the study.

A 2001 study looked at the effect of expectancy on a drug's efficacy using remifentanil, a very powerful opioid analgesic. Researchers used functional magnetic resonance imaging to record brain activity to corroborate the effects of expectations on the analgesic efficacy of the drug to reveal the underlying neural mechanisms. What researchers found was that positive treatment expectancy substantially enhanced (doubled) the analgesic benefit of this drug. In contrast, negative treatment expectancy abolished its effects. This is pretty amazing when you think of a powerful opioid's effect being doubled or negated by expectancy alone. It is worth noting that the subjective effects described were substantiated by significant changes in the neural activity in brain regions involved with the coding of pain intensity. On the basis of subjective and objective evidence, researchers contended that:

> … an individual's expectation of a drug's effect critically influences its therapeutic efficacy and that regulatory brain mechanisms differ as a function of expectancy. We propose that it may be necessary to integrate patients' beliefs and expectations into drug treatment regimens alongside traditional considerations in order to optimize treatment outcomes.

(Bingel et al. 2011)

In a study mentioned earlier, women who believed it was very likely that they would have severe nausea from chemotherapy were *five times more likely* to experience severe nausea than fellow patients who thought its occurrence would be very unlikely (Roscoe et al. 2004).

A very recent study of 134 US Marines with musculoskeletal injuries of the back, knee, or shoulder found that: *'the strongest predictor of injury recovery at the 1-year follow-up was recovery expectations '* (Booth-Kewley et al. 2014). The authors suggest applying the lessons learned from this study to military populations with interventions designed to modify recovery expectations with the aim of improving rates of return to duty and reducing rates of disability discharge.

A cohort study entitled, 'The relation between expectations and outcomes in surgery for sciatica' (Lutz et al. 1999) questioned 273 patients and their surgeons from the offices of orthopedic surgeons, neurosurgeons, and occupational medicine physicians in Maine. All patients had undergone discectomy surgery for sciatica. This study found that a patient's expectation was a strong predictor of surgical outcomes; even more so than surgeons' expectations. More patients with favorable expectations about surgery had good outcomes than patients with unfavorable expectations. Physicians' expectations were overly optimistic. This study reminds us of how important a patient's expectations really is. If our patient's expectation is poor, we really need to explore this subject with the patient and find ways to alter their expectation.

Several studies have shown that being put on a 'waiting list for treatment' has better therapeutic effectiveness than being put in a 'no-treatment' group, even though there is no formal treatment in both cases (Samueli Institute 2013). Expectation is clearly one component of this effect. People on the wait list are expecting to eventually receive treatment, while the no-treatment group have no expectation or hope of receiving treatment.

A 2015 University of Southampton study looking at patient expectations in relation to acupuncture treatments for lower back pain found strong correlations between expectations and outcomes (Bishop et al. 2015). This study of 485 patients recruited from 83 acupuncturists found that patients with low expectations of acupuncture before they start a course of treatment gained less benefit than those people who believe it would work. Studies in the areas of pain, anxiety and Parkinson's disease where the administration of active medications was hidden were shown to be less effective than when compared with an open administration in full view of the patient (Colloca et al. 2004). These studies show that the patient's expectation is extremely important if you want a therapy to be effective. It is not enough to simply administer a treatment and say, 'well, let's see how your body responds to this.' It is important to create a positive expectation, to maximize a treatment.

One very telling study was the analysis performed by Alan Roberts and his colleagues (Roberts et al. 1993). They studied five different treatment procedures for four different conditions, where expectations of participants were heightened by the fact that they were receiving 'the latest treatment.' When Roberts and his team analyzed the results of early trials they saw 30% poor outcomes, 30% good and 40% excellent outcomes. This is an overall 70% positive response rate. Years later these same procedures were all found to be inefficacious, so were abandoned. Once again, we see a very dramatic illustration of the effects of patient expectations on the outcomes of a treatment. These treatments were brand new, so people had high hopes for the treatment. These hopes or expectations manifested themselves as positive outcomes.

Hope is certainly an appropriate topic to bring up at this time. Even if the patient is not necessarily *expecting* a positive outcome, he/she may still be *hopeful*. Hope is certainly a future-focused concept but is perhaps a bit less loosely framed than expectation. It is, however, an extremely important human need. You will recall the perspective of psychotherapist Jerome D. Frank in the Preface (p. xi) when he said, *'hopelessness can retard recovery or even hasten death'* (Frank & Frank 1991, p. 132). In psychotherapy, a patient's hope is considered a primary starting place. To quote Jerome Frank again:

> *The task of the therapist – whatever his or her technique – is to clarify symptoms and problems, inspire hope, facilitate exercises of success or mastery, and stir the patient's emotions.*

(Frank & Frank 1991, p. xiii)

Hope versus expectation

An interesting study that attempted to separate hope from expectation was performed in an out-patient clinic (Park & Covi 1965). Patients were suffering from what was diagnosed, at the time, as a 'neurosis'. This was an extended portion of an existing study comparing a placebo with active drugs. A new and separate group of participants were told, quite frankly and outright, that they were being given sugar pills containing no active medication. They were also told that many patients had got better when taking one of these same pills three times daily for 1 week. Patients filled out a detailed symptom checklist before starting, and then again after 1 week of taking the pills. Fourteen of the 15 participants who agreed to the study returned 1 week later. Thirteen of the 14 saw improvements (including one suicidal patient). Participants were then queried about what they believed was going on. What they heard from participants were basically three different scenarios. In the first scenario, participants took the placebo to placate the researchers, *still believing that they had been given an inert pill*. In the second scenario, participants *believed that they were given an active drug*, not a placebo. Both of these groups were described in this study as seeing 'substantial' improvement. The third-reported scenario was that participants weren't really sure what was going on. They did not know if researchers were trying to trick them or what. Interestingly enough, this is the group that saw the least improvement. Now there are a number of holes in this study, not the least of which is the sample size. The other problem is that these people were told that they would be receiving other forms of treatment in the future if needed. Either fact could easily skew the results. What is very interesting indeed, however, is that one group of people were sure that they were being given placebos, but still got better. Presumably, this group had *hope* of improvement but did not necessarily have high expectations. Certainly we want our patient's expectations to be realistic, but it is very important to remember that they must *always* have hope of improvement, no matter how dire the circumstance. Even in the case of palliative care, the patient still needs hope. Hope of peace after death and an end to their suffering, and hope for peace for all those left behind. We can curb people's expectations if we feel a very strong professional need to do so, but we should never rob *anyone* of hope.

Another area that we need to consider in the area of expectations is the general statement of informed consent. You most certainly need to inform your patients of the risks of any given treatment, but be cautious how you frame your informed consent. It should be clear to you by now that the risk statement within informed consent can plant the seeds of the nocebo effect, so reading a long list of side-effects in a rote manner to your patients is probably not the best route. You have to be honest, but it is important to present the information in such a manner so as not to create negative expectations in their minds concerning side-effects. An example of what not to say might be: 'I'm working really deep here, so you are probably going to hurt like heck tomorrow'. Instead, you might want to say: 'This area is tight, I can release it over several treatments with little or no pain, or we can work deeper today if you would prefer that we work this issue out in one treatment. Deep work does run the risk of (delayed onset) muscle soreness the next day. However, there are steps that you can take to minimize that soreness that I can show you. How would you like me to proceed?' Here you have given the patient control and you have offered solutions to potential side-effects, empowering the patient. In 'Establishment of a feeling of control' (p. 128), we will look at the importance of that concept and how you can help your patient achieve a feeling of control.

Another interesting finding of placebo trials is that it clearly appears that the more powerful the symbol, the more marked the placebo effect is. For example, injections work better than drugs taken by mouth. Injections that sting work better than injections that don't. The more powerful the symbol, the more powerful the effects are (Evans 1974) with surgery scoring at the top end of this scale. What this means is that if you are working with very subtle therapies, you will want to make sure that your other signals are such as to maximize the placebo effect. It is very common for practitioners to be more interested in subtle therapies as they mature in their profession. My personal sense is that these same practitioners are convinced of the efficacy of these modalities and this confidence is then projected onto the patient. Confidence is an incredibly potent placebo cue, as we will see in sections ahead. Either way, my suggestion is that if you are working with subtle therapies, then you should probably compensate in another placebo area, since expectancy can sometimes be impaired in the beginning. Certainly if you get a positive response from your first treatment, you then have conditioning on your side.

Expectancy and conditioning are not mutually exclusive concepts; rather they are typically both interwoven in some manner into the placebo effect. It can happen, but it is rare indeed that the patient has no conditioning whatsoever. However, even in the case of a new patient that has never met you, nor experienced your therapy, there will be cues in the waiting or treatment room, smells in your office, diploma and certificates on your wall, their personal history of the ailment that brought them to you, and even your personality type, all of which have some degree of conditioning attached to them. Numerous complex experiments have been designed to determine whether conditioning or expectancy win out when the two notions are pitted against one another (i.e. one message is positive and one message is negative). These studies have produced conflicting results. In some case experience (conditioning) wins out (Voudouris et al. 1989). In others, expectancy has won out (Montgomery & Kirsh 1997). What is of interest is that in these studies the effects of these two signals, when opposed, have not cancelled one another out. A positive placebo effect was always seen in a percentage of participants. When the two signals are sending the same positive message, the effects appear to be cumulative (Price et al. 1999). So it could be stated, then, that expectancy and conditioning overlap and complement one another. This will be found to be true of virtually all concepts put forth in Part 2. What this tells you in your practice is the more cues you can give your patient to stimulate inner healing, the stronger the healing response is likely to be.

One study that was mentioned earlier deals exclusively with expectancy. In this study doctors successfully eliminated warts by painting them with a brightly colored, inert dye and promising patients the warts would be gone when the color wore off (Frank & Frank 1991). It is highly unlikely that these patients had experienced previous conditioning around their warts and dye.

This would be a good time for us to revisit some aspects that were touched upon earlier.

1. **The effects of a placebo increase if the pill is physically larger.** Effects will decrease if it is smaller. This might be relevant to a particular modality in your practice; for example, a hand-held TENS machine will not be as powerful a symbol as a clinic version of TENS or, for instance, an interferential current therapy machine.
2. **As placebos go:**
    *   Tablets are better than pills
    *   Capsules surpass tablets
    *   Injections are seen to be more effective than drugs administered orally
    *   Injections that sting work better than injections that do not
    *   Medical treatment machines surpass injections
    *   Sham surgeries surpass machines.

There are several lessons to be learned here even though most of my audience cannot prescribe medications. Subtle therapies will have less placebo effect than other modalities. Also we all know the patient who strongly believes 'no pain–no gain'. This information unfortunately supports that sort of thinking. It is not to say that you need to work deeply, but if you are using subtle, gentle therapies then you need to explain what you are doing and why you are doing it. There will be a tendency among a percentage of your patient base to think that they need you to work deep, and if you don't they will think that the therapy was useless. You need to spend time convincing this type of patient that the therapy needs to be subtle, and you have to get their buy-in.

The other lesson here is use of machines. Depending upon your background and profession you may or may not use machines to deliver your therapies.

The group of manual practitioners least likely to use external devices is massage therapists, in that they tend to trust our own hands over any device or machine. That being said, many massage therapists employ such devices as interferential current therapy, therapeutic ultrasound, cold laser, and ionic footbaths to augment their manual therapies. Other practitioners are less reticent to use machines and devices to augment their therapies. These devices exist as symbols in your treatment room, whether you are actually employing them in a particular treatment or not. Even something such as an electric table has a potential placebo effect. Patients who are visiting me for the first time always remark on my electric table. Not only does it help with the ergonomics of my work, but it also has a symbolic value to the patient. For example, the patient sees me lower the table so that I can employ a specific modality on their hip or leg for example, allowing me to more effectively work on that particular body part.

3. **New or novel treatments (or drugs) often out-perform older ones.** This is an important aspect of the placebo effect to capitalize upon. If you have just been on a new course or learned a new modality, it is good to let the patient know that you are employing a new modality that has been shown to have been successful in treating conditions such as theirs. Rather than quietly going about your work, let the patient know about the therapy that you are employing, especially if it is a new therapy or a new way of approaching the body.

4. **Brand name placebos work better than generic placebos.** We have all been witness to this in many areas of our lives. Branding makes a difference in the consumer or patient's eyes. You might be employing a therapy/modality that follows the same principles as a highly branded system. If you choose not to get the certification and training of the system, then you need to do some explaining about your modality in comparison to the branded modality to get your patient's belief system on board. We have all seen this many times when a patient asks about another modality that they are wondering about. An obvious approach is to tell them what you know about it and how it compares with the methods that you are presently employing. If the modality uses a sufficiently different approach you could suggest that they try it, but if it is pretty much what you are doing but with a new fancy name, then this gives you an opportunity to explain exactly what you are doing and how it compares with the branded name.

5. **The more expensive the placebo is (within reason), the better it works.** This is another one of the aspects of the placebo effect that one hates to bring up for fear that persons of low moral character may want to exploit the phenomenon. I can certainly attest to this aspect of the placebo effect personally. At one point in my career I worked in a high-end spa that charged almost twice what my clinic rate was for a 1-hour

therapeutic massage. Many people walked out of the treatment room of the spa and told me that they just got the 'best massage of their life'. Of course they did...they just paid twice as much for it! This is also a basic business psychology. It has to do with the valuing of your services. Undervaluing your services allows accessibility to your practice to a larger demographic; but other challenges ensue when you are not charging enough. As you increase the price of your services, you experience a shift in the demographics that you treat, as well as your patients' perspective of your competency and professionalism. The concept here is that if one charges well for one's services, you can expect improved clinical outcomes. The challenge is that there is a large (and growing) sector of society that cannot afford our services, and increasing our rates makes our services even further out of reach for that demographic. This is probably a good topic for another publication, so the author will leave it with you to wrestle with at this point, and to find your own comfort zone with the complicated ethics of this aspect of the placebo effect.

Let us now consider some actual examples of other ways that you can manage expectancy in your practice. What the patient expects to happen will shape the outcome of your treatment. So, knowing this, what could you do differently to positively affect your patient's expectations?

- **Always offer hope.** Always keep in mind those personal stories that you have either witnessed or heard where someone refused to accept the limitations of their diagnosis in chronic or even terminal conditions and returned to a full life with full function. Use this mindset to offer genuine 'from the heart' hope to your patient. In no way is this offering false hope or misleading if you have personally witnessed these events or express it as a genuine belief. Let me reiterate; do not confuse realistic expectations with hope. If you feel the need to curb expectations, never put limits on the patient's hope. e.g. *'It looks as though you have returned to 80% function Jane. Please keep in mind that while the last gains may be gradual, I have seen many patients return to full function after an injury such as yours.'*
- **Always keep the door open to full recovery**. Always remember that there are vast numbers of asymptomatic people walking around with herniated disks, degenerative discs and arthritic joints operating at full function without pain. Diagnosed structural pathology doesn't equal pain and loss of function. The connection between structural issue and pain/function is more tenuous than you might think. In his heavily referenced article, entitled 'Your back is not out of alignment', science writer Paul Ingraham points out that not only are structural explanations for pain generally unsupported by any scientific evidence, the last 25 years of research results mostly undermines them, often impressively (Ingraham, 2014).

e.g. *'While the range of motion in your shoulder appears to have plateaued, I have personally witnessed many complete recoveries. My suggestion is that you continue with your exercises and keep an open mind.'*

- **Emphasize positive self-talk,** e.g. *'Mrs Jones, the mind is incredibly powerful. Studies show that positive mindset yields much better outcomes for patients. I encourage you strongly to keep a positive outlook for your own sake and for the sake of your body.'*

- **Project a positive outcome to the patient,** e.g. *'I am sure that we are going to see improvement from this treatment Mr Johnson.'* or *'I see no reason not to expect a full recovery here.'*

- **Tout your other successes,** e.g. *'I just treated someone last week with the same condition and they have bounced right back. I am sure we will have you back to full function in no time.'*

- **'Create a reality' for your patient.** This is especially important for patients with a pessimistic outlook, or a complicated health history. e.g. *'This is how I see things progressing Ms Johnson…'*

- **Set easily attainable goals at first,** e.g. *'I want you to just get out for a five minute walk every day,'* or *'Do this simple exercise twice daily and we will measure the progress on your next visit'* or *'I just want you to focus on things feeling freer and looser; pain will decrease over time.'*

- **Informed consent**. As mentioned earlier, remember that the seeds of the nocebo effect can be sown in the risk statement of informed consent, so be cautious of how you frame risks/side-effects and always offer solutions to those side-effects.

- **Informed consent around expectancy of increased short-term pain**. *'Mr Jones, be aware that some people do experience some discomfort the day after a treatment of this type. This does not happen to everyone; however, if it should happen to you, I suggest _____ to minimize and shorten the time frame of the discomfort.'*

- **Offering alternatives.** If you cannot get around the matter of expectancy concerning discomfort, be sure and offer an alternative where the patient is less likely to experience side-effects. Just knowing this can free the person from the fear of expecting side-effects. e.g. *'If you do experience any discomfort from this treatment, we will try a different approach next time.'*

- **Hot new technique**, e.g. *'I have this new technique that I just learned at a workshop. I received my training from a leader in his/her field. (S)he has found it to be very effective in treating individuals with similar symptoms.'*

Please note that there is research which supports the notion that expectation is enhanced when the treatment offered is consistent with the patient's belief system (Brown 2013). This is another reason for involving the patient in the proposed treatment plan, querying them on their opinions on what they believe gives them relief of symptoms, and to adequately explain if the proposed treatment falls outside of patient expectations. With this idea in mind, one might employ the following lines of dialogue:

- **Query.** Ask open-ended questions to determine the patient's expectations concerning their issue. This could include causes, exacerbating factors, potential treatments. The purpose of this line of questioning is to attempt to either attempt to align the treatment with their belief system, or align their belief system with the treatment. Dialogue might go as such:
  - *'What do you feel is causing (or exacerbating) your symptoms Mrs. Brown?'*
  - *'What are your thoughts on exercise as a method to reduce pain?'*
  - *'What do you feel would improve your arm movement?'*
  - *'I am considering employing therapeutic laser to treat this condition. Do you have any experience with this particular modality?'*
  - *'I realize that you are hesitant about this particular treatment, but I am convinced that this is the best line of treatment for us to follow. I would like you to try it for 3 weeks. I am sure that we will see progress at that time. If we do not see substantial improvement, we will reassess at that time.'*

MOTIVATION AND DESIRE

If you're going through hell, keep going.

Winston Churchill

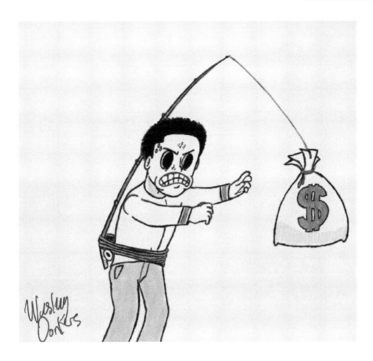

Fig. 2.5

Something that is related to expectancy, but has definite differences, is desire. You can expect a certain outcome without desiring it and vice versa, so we need to consider these as two separate factors. In the early 1990s an important study by Jensen and Karoly (1991) teased out desire (motivation) from expectancy. Their study looked at the effects of placebo stimulation and also placebo sedation on four groups of participants:

1. High expectancy with high desire
2. High expectancy with low desire
3. Low expectancy with high desire and
4. Low expectancy with low desire.

Their study actually concluded that desire was more important than expectancy. Further studies have shown the importance of desire in the healing process. One study of placebo analgesia in IBS concluded that 'Expected pain levels and desire for pain relief accounted for large amounts of the variance in visceral pain intensity…(up to 81%)'. While the word 'desire' shows up in the research literature, the term 'motivation' seems to be largely interchangeable. While there is a difference between desire and motivation, from a research construct they are considered to be the same thing. This is just as well, because while our patient may (for whatever reason) not have a strong desire to get to a specific goal, we can certainly help to motivate them, or get them motivated toward a specific goal. Anyone who has raised children or been a stepparent knows that the universe does not hand out equal doses of motivation to all individuals.

Motivation need not be a higher concept or a long-term goal. Oft times more immediate needs, such as return to work or improved ability to perform activities of daily living, serve as excellent motivators. As practitioners, we might like to see our patients motivated for higher reasons, but ultimately if they are motivated to get better, then that alone should be enough. If they are not motivated and we are playing a cheerleading role then we are more likely to try to steer them along a more 'righteous' road, or we are going to feel some guilt that they have traded a problem for a vice, but alas in the end the patient will determine what that carrot will be. One example of a short-term 'righteous carrot' for a poor exercise or eating habit might be to ask the patient how they want to feel in 1 hour. This is not very long to wait to feel better, and while one's long-term goals might be further off in the future, often there is a short-term payoff for many healthy decisions and habits in the immediate future. This is an important point to drive home to your patients.

If your patient has little motivation or desire, then the road to healing is likely to be a long one. How can you motivate another individual? It is possible in some cases that there may be complex reasons why patients lack motivation. If this matter falls beyond your scope of practice, then you may want to suggest a referral to a qualified psychotherapist or social worker/therapist. If so then you will need to handle the matter gingerly; however, if you phrase it in non-judgmental pragmatic terms you can explain that their internal healing process may be stalled by internal motivational factors and this is a matter where other health professionals can intervene to kick-start healing processes within their own body.

Many of my patients pay out of their own pockets to see me. This is a great motivator. We have all had experience with patients who feel that they are owed something either by their insurer or their employer etc. and they are trying to extract every cent possible out of them. This is difficult demographic to work with. My most motivated patients have been self-employed with very little extra money and who need to get back to work as quickly as possible. That's motivation! Stretching out an automobile accident claim over several years is possibly the other end of the spectrum. We will talk more about the issue of victimology in the section entitled The Narrative: how we make sense of the world.

If the patient is motivated, then you may find that acting in somewhat of a 'cheerleader' role may help to increase or redirect the patient's desire. While there is little information available on desire per se, there is a wealth of information on motivation. Motivation has been a tremendous growth industry in the past few decades, so there is an abundance of self-proclaimed 'professionals' or 'experts' out there speaking about and making money on this topic. There are certainly many people making money in motivational speaking but it is ultimately buyer-beware when it comes to spending money on their approaches. The fact that so many people do well making money in this area speaks to the power of the placebo effect. What follows is one approach to motivation. This is a generic approach that has been adapted to apply to a health goal.

1. **Set a major health goal, but follow a specific path**. Any path has small goals along the way. As the patient succeeds at the minor goals, they will have increased motivation to challenge larger goals.
2. **Finish what you start**. Quitting can be a habit just as much as completing a goal can be a habit. Highly motivated people are by nature not quitters. If your patient is a quitter by nature then he/she may need some prodding to stick to a regime. For this type of individual have them set tinier goals (road marks along the way to their goal) and tick them off as they complete them.
3. **Socialize with others with similar goals**. Mutual support is motivating. Experts believe that we are likely to develop the attitudes of our five best friends. If they are losers, we will be a loser. If they are winners, we will be a winner. To be a triathlon runner one must associate with triathlon runners. Your patient may need to be encouraged to seek out like-minded people to achieve their health goal. Everything is harder to do on your own, and you can often feed off the enthusiasm of others.
4. **State the goal publicly**. No one wants to feel shamed so if your patient makes a statement about his or her goals to their friends and family, they are more apt to follow through on the stated goal. This works if your patient had a desire to be viewed as someone who sticks to his or her word.
5. **Continue lifelong self-learning**. We all have the ability to learn without instructors. It is built into all of us. Encouraging your patient to progress along their own individual learning path will evoke the child in them, which is the source of abundant energy. Encourage them to learn what they can about their condition. You can give them an information handout, but they can also be encouraged to empower themselves by learning all that they can about their issue (see point 7).
6. **Harmonize natural talent with interest that motivates**. Everyone has his or her own unique strengths, weaknesses and talents. Exercising one's own natural talent actually fosters motivation. Often, we suggest a specific regime for our patient forgetting that this may not be the best way for them to approach the activity. If we listen to the patient, we can often hear clues as to how to better approach their therapy, homecare or their exercise regime.

7. **Increase knowledge of the subject matter**. Beginning the education process of your patient and then encouraging them to become more educated in that area can often create an inner motivation. The more we know about a subject, the more we typically want to learn about it. A self-propelled upward spiral develops. If they are using the Internet you can suggest reliable sources such as The Mayo Clinic (http://www.mayoclinic.com/), The Centers for Disease Control and Prevention (http://www.cdc.gov/), Health Canada (http://www.hc-sc.gc.ca/index-eng.php), OSHA (http://www.osha.gov/). As well there are excellent sites to go to for specific conditions such as the Canadian Cancer Society, The Canadian Heart and Stroke Foundation etc. You can help to guide your patient to reputable sites so that they are getting accurate information.

8. **Finally take risk.** Failure and bouncing back are elements of life, health and motivation. Failure is not an endpoint in therapy or health, it is a learning tool. Remind your patients of this. It is unrealistic to expect a nice straight upward trajectory to perfect health. No one has ever succeeded at anything worthwhile without a string of failures. Health is no different in this matter.

TRUST

Trust is the glue of life. It's the most essential ingredient in effective communication.
It's the foundational principle that holds all relationships.

Stephen R. Covey

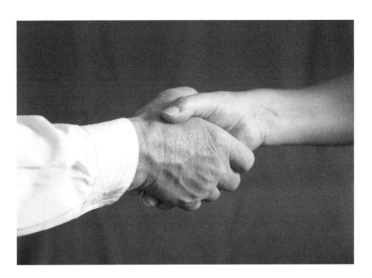

Fig. 2.6

Mulling this book over in my head and bouncing ideas off other people, I heard the word 'trust' come up repeatedly. Pouring over the literature, I did find recent studies on trust, which we will examine. Linking trust to the placebo effect in research yielded few results but clearly having trust in a professional healer is implicit in each of the concepts presented in this section of the book. Researchers have long identified the importance of trust in the physician–patient relationship, so fortunately this topic has been at least looked at and studied. Trust is important in any relationship, but is even more of a factor when someone is surrendering control to someone else. The placebo effect involves surrender of power and control. When a patient surrenders power, they need to know that you have their best interests at heart. For example, if you are suggesting a treatment schedule of three visits per week, they need to feel that this frequency is essential for their recovery, and not to create a steady cash flow for your business. It is critically important that your patient trusts you, your motives, and your abilities as a healer. This is absolutely essential. Anything that undermines trust in the practitioner–patient relationship will be extremely detrimental to your ability to access and turn on their inner healer. It would be reasonable to assume that the more trust your patient has in you, the greater the chance there will be of you being able to facilitate the placebo effect and help to turn on their healer within.

In a recent study entitled, 'Do patients trust their physician?'(Holwerda et al. 2013), researchers related *attachment theory* scale as directly relating to the degree of trust that cancer patients formed with their physician, rather than the distress that the patient was experiencing. Attachment theory sees adults as fitting onto one of four styles of attachment: secure, anxious-preoccupied, dismissive-avoidant and fearful-avoidant.

- Securely attached adults tend to have positive views of themselves, their partners and their relationships. They feel comfortable with intimacy and independence, balancing the two.
- Anxious-preoccupied adults seek high levels of intimacy, approval and responsiveness from partners, becoming overly dependent. They tend to be less trusting, have less positive views about themselves and their partners, and may exhibit high levels of emotional expressiveness, worry and impulsiveness in their relationships.
- Dismissive-avoidant adults desire a high level of independence, often appearing to avoid attachment altogether. They view themselves as self-sufficient, invulnerable to attachment feelings and not needing close relationships. They tend to suppress their feelings, dealing with rejection by distancing themselves from partners of whom they often have a poor opinion.
- Fearful-avoidant adults have mixed feelings about close relationships, both desiring and feeling uncomfortable with emotional closeness. They tend to mistrust their partners and view themselves as unworthy. Like dismissive-avoidant adults, fearful-avoidant adults tend to seek less intimacy, suppressing their feelings.

This study found that, 'Insecurely attached patients trusted their physician less than securely attached patients, and in turn were less satisfied with their physician. Their higher levels of general distress were not related to their lower levels of trust' (Holwerda et al. 2013). What this study indicates is probably what your instinct tells you, and that there are some patients that need to be 'handled' more delicately and who are higher maintenance, for which you might still anticipate a poorer prognosis as a group because of their personal challenges in the area of attachment. According to this theory, these issues developed at a very young age, so these are deep-seated issues.

Another recent paper also looked at the issue of patient–doctor trust with cancer patients. It analyzed 11 studies that drew attention to the conceptualization of trust. Patients' trust appeared to be enhanced by:

- The physician's perceived technical competence
- Honesty
- Patient-centred behaviour.

A trusting relationship between patient and physician resulted in:

- Facilitated communication and medical decision-making
- Decrease of patient fear, and
- Better treatment adherence (Hillen et al. 2011).

Another study on trust in the doctor–patient relationship, by Thom and colleagues (2004), identified physician behavior associated with increased or decreased trust, based on patient focus groups; and interviews and patient survey found that physician behavior identified by patients as increasing trust generally falls into the categories of:

- Competency
- Communication
- Caring
- Honesty
- Partnering.

This study also mentions, in addition, that investigators in psychology and sociology have identified factors that promote interpersonal trust in experimental settings. In a medical setting application of these principles would include:

- Emphasizing mutual interests (i.e. the patient's health)
- Checking patients' understanding of communication
- Taking opportunities to fulfill trust (e.g. phoning with test results)
- Reducing power differences (e.g. sharing information)
- Responding to patients' self-disclosures in a supportive and non-judgmental way, and
- Promoting continuity of care.

Whether or not you are perceived as trustworthy by your patient is largely in your hands. There is a lot that you can do to build a trusting relationship and to be perceived as trustworthy. Anything that you do to undermine that trust will adversely affect your relationship with your patient and, ultimately, their desire to work with you on their health goals. Some obvious things and not so obvious things that help build trust include the following:

1. **Keep your appointments and all other agreement with your patients**. If you book your patient in at 3:00 on a particular day, ensure that you are ready to begin the appointment at that time. Each time you break an agreement with a patient, you break a trust.
2. **Create realistic expectations**. Don't promise them the world. It is good to project positive expectations on to them to employ their inner healer but be realistic in your projections.
3. **Help your patient to understand the healing process**. This is basically a communication issue. If your patient understands for example that a disease-healing trajectory is not a straight line then they will be less frustrated by setbacks.

4. **Explain your plan and strategy**. Once again this is basic communication. Let your patient know not just what you plan on doing today, but what your longer term strategy is (within reason) recognizing that each case is unique. This will help the patient know what to expect and when to expect it. Trust comes when the patient feels confident and comfortable with the plan and the strategy. Your patient may be silently wondering if he or she can afford the whole treatment plan if it lasts for an extended period of time. This issue needs to be addressed. You need to develop a plan that is within their financial means and they need to know that you are not just looking at them with dollar signs in your eyes. If you have ever felt pressure from a health professional to see them at a higher frequency than you felt was necessary, you will know what I am alluding to here. Many of us have stories relayed to us by our patients where they were talked into a frequency of treatments with another health professional that resembled a business plan more than a health plan.

5. **Carefully explain the patient's role**. It is important to communicate the fact that the patient needs to take ownership of his or her health. You can do only so much as a health professional and the rest is up to the patients and his/her inner healer. This allows you to work better as a team and build trust.

6. **Avoid making the patient feel diminished in any way**. No one likes to feel stupid. You have spent your entire life learning about the body and this is why they have come to see you. They, on the other hand, are the experts where their own body is concerned. They live in their body 24 hours a day. If they are made to feel any less because of something that they said, they will begin to clam-up and now your relationship is moving in the wrong direction. Health professionals undoubtedly do not set out to make a patient feel diminished. In fact it may be an attitude, an inadvertent comment, or a look that gives the patient that impression. Even be aware of your inner thoughts because your thoughts if not expressed as words will become expressed as body language.

7. **Don't allow interruptions during treatments**. This will make patients feel as if they are not important to you. This habit will erode the good will and trust that you worked so hard to build.

8. **Don't be afraid to admit that you don't know something**. There are limits to anyone's knowledge and ability to predict the future. Don't fear being perceived as having feet of clay. Your patient is not perfect and doesn't expect you to be perfect. Admit it when you don't know something.

Finally, keep in mind the results of the first study that we looked at, i.e. it is easier to develop trust relationships with some patients than with others. Recognize individuals that have an attachment issue and work extra hard to build trust with these patients. If you follow the many points raised in this section, you will find yourself developing strong trust relationships with even the most difficult of patients.

THE POWER OF LISTENING

Listen to your patient – they have inside information.

Old adage

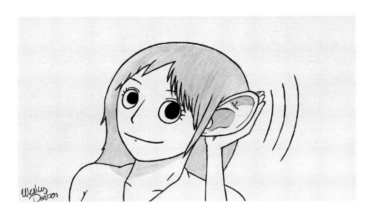

Fig. 2.7

Feeling heard or listened to is a basic human social need. Have you met many people that do not want to tell their story? Even people that are very socially withholding are typically doing so as a defense mechanism, secretly hoping that someone will find their life interesting and their stories worth a good listen. The best way to engage anyone is to ask the person about his or her life. This is true, whether it is a patient, friend or casual acquaintance. We all secretly love to talk about ourselves – *some of us not so secretly.*

Rebecca Zandbergen, host of CBC Radio West, has this great curiosity about intriguing classified ads. She makes a habit of calling the numbers on ads that she finds interesting and chatting to the people who have placed the ads, typically getting all sorts of personal details about their life. She claims that almost everyone shares all sorts of details to a complete stranger. Why do people do this? Undoubtedly, she makes them feel safe, but one reason for sure is that she is a good listener. As health practitioners, we always need to be good listeners, whether it comes natural or not.

An interesting study looked at the physiologic measurements of the Holocaust survivors with those of the student listeners. What researchers found was that the more individual survivors talked about the horror, the greater the reduction they experienced in these stress indicators. However, the opposite was true for the listeners. Their stress indicators increased as they listened. It appeared that experience seemed to cause a shift in the physiology of the speaker and the listener toward a convergence. A follow-up study 14 months later revealed that the degree of disclosure during the interview was positively correlated with the subsequent health of the speaker (Pennebaker et al. 1989). This speaks strongly to the power of listening. It also warns us that there is a temporary cost involved. The listener carries some of the burden of the speaker for a time as a function of the therapeutic exchange.

Part of the basis of narrative therapy (a well-established psychotherapeutic modality) is simply allowing the patient to be heard. Most of us have been told anecdotal stories from fellow practitioners who made tremendous progress with someone by simply taking the time to hear their detailed life/health story, because they were the first health professional that ever took the time to actually listen to them. As powerful as anecdote may be, we need to examine the evidence on this topic. Some very interesting studies in this matter have been performed in Canada.

Dr Martin Bass and his team at University of Western Ontario have conducted a few very enlightening studies of family physicians' practices. The goal of their study was to find the strongest predictor of a patient's reported progress. In the first study they looked at a wide array of common symptoms and looked at such factors as original intake interview and assessment, lab tests ordered, radiographs performed, medications prescribed etc. After a month's time, patients were questioned concerning their improvement (subjective). Surprisingly the strongest factor linked to patient's improvement was not the thoroughness of the medical history nor the physical assessment or tests ordered, nor drugs prescribed. The single most important factor was whether or not the patient indicated that the doctor had carefully listened to their description of their condition on the first visit (Bass et al. 1986a). This study speaks volumes about how to conduct yourself with your patients, and is considered seminal in the area of physician–patient agreement about the nature of the patient's problem. The physician-patient agreement is not likely to happen unless you really listen to your patient.

Bass and his colleagues conducted another study, but this time focusing on headaches, following patients for 1 full year. The results were the same. The strongest indicator was whether or not the patients felt that they had a chance to discuss their problem fully and that their physician was able to appreciate what it meant to them (Bass et al. 1986b). A similar study was conducted at Johns Hopkins University of public health clinic patients (Starfield et al. 1981). Its conclusions were the same – as a health professional, listening to your patient is the single most powerful tool that you have in your arsenal.

Patient surveys indicate that patients are most satisfied with their medical encounters when the clinician discusses the patient's personal lives (Brown 2013) and how their symptoms make them 'feel'. Asking open-ended questions give the patient the space required to explore the issue more broadly, allowing the patient to share matters that they feel are important. Asking open-ended questions and really listening to what the patient is saying, not only about the malady in particular but also about the contributing life issues, allows you to be a much better listener than to just ask yes-or-no questions.

Hopefully I have convinced you of the importance of listening. So let's talk a little about listening. In a therapeutic environment, how do you go about this? Admittedly, the best way to learn how to listen is to take an active listening course, or at least read a little on the subject. Listening is a learnable skill. Some of us are naturally good at it, and some of us (like the author for example) have to work at it. Most of us could use some improvement in this area. Keep in mind that listening isn't a passive process. It is an active process on your part where you engage the patient in a non-judgmental manner and gently steer the conversation with appropriate questions. What follows is simply a short primer on the topic. To make real progress in area, I highly recommend adding an active listening course to your continued education studies list. However, this will not stop me from giving you a quick introduction to the subject. Consider focusing on one of the following 15 points during your next workday. The following day, focus on another point; and so on, until you have covered all of the following suggestions. In this way, you will see a dramatic shift in your listening abilities.

1. **Before you even begin**, prepare yourself with a positive and engaged attitude. Effective listening is an active process. As a practitioner, you need to be aware that this is your activity of the moment. Like all activities, the more personal focus, the more energy and the more training you put into it, the better your skill and level of performance will be.
2. As with your treatment, you need to be '**in the moment**'. One effective way to practice and hone this skill is to practice meditation.
3. **Focus all of your attention on your patient**. Stop all non-relevant activities beforehand and orient yourself to your patient with solid eye contact.
4. **Avoid all distractions** (period).
5. **Seat yourself appropriately close** to your patient during the interview, to give them your full attention. This will also help to avoid distractions.
6. Acknowledge any emotional state that you experience, but try not to drift 'into' the emotion. Instead, practice **emotional detachment**. This is your opportunity to practice therapeutic empathy (more on this later). If necessary there will be ample opportunity after the appointment when you can delve into your emotional reactions, but it is of no benefit to the patient if you react emotionally.
7. **Set aside your prejudices** and your opinions. You are there to learn what your patient has to say, not the other way around. There will be a time when the patient will be looking to you for advice and guidance; however, the first thing that you need to do is to listen thoroughly, attentively and dispassionately. This will not happen if you carry your prejudices, opinions and judgments into the treatment room. The environment must be completely non-judgmental. This sort of attitude

and approach on the part of the practitioner requires one to be very vigilant and self-aware.

8. **Be truly 'patient-focused'**. Follow and understand your patient as if you were walking in their shoes. Listen not only with your ears, but also with your eyes, hands and other senses.

9. **Be aware**: Acknowledge points non-verbally through body language. Let your patient's story or description run its course. Don't agree or disagree, but encourage the train of thought. If the patient wanders truly off topic you can gently steer him or her back on topic.

10. **Be involved**: Actively respond to questions. Use your body position (e.g. lean forward) and attention to encourage your patient and signal your interest.

11. **Express appreciation** for the sharing to build trust and encourage dialogue – especially with new patients.

12. **Paraphrase** what you have just heard by restating their story more concisely. Paraphrasing is a very important tool and will lead you down an important communication road. Paraphrasing **clarifies your own understanding** of what you have just heard and **will communicate that you have understood the information and the message**. This reduces the chance of miscommunication between patient and practitioner.

13. **Clarification** is a technique that you should employ when paraphrasing. Clarification is the process of bringing vague material into sharper focus, by weeding out excess information, untangling the essential information, and distilling it into one clear message. Clarification, more than anything else, will help to avoid wrong interpretations on your part. It also typically leads to your patient revealing more information and often has the added benefit of allowing your patient to see other points of view.

14. **Questions** will need to be asked for clarification. When doing so, ask questions in a non-threatening manner, allowing pauses before asking questions; be patient.

15. After you have both had a chance to speak and clarify the issues, check to see that you have understood by **restating key points, summarizing** the message.

Don'ts:

- Don't judge
- Don't react
- Don't interrupt
- Don't show disapproval
- Don't jump to conclusions
- Don't rush the process of listening
- Don't allow yourself to become distracted
- Don't spend your time 'preparing your response'.

Now is a good time to introduce the topic of empathy. **Empathy** in the patient–practitioner relationship could be most easily and succinctly described as the ability to put yourself in your patient's shoes. Empathy is not to be confused with sympathy, or even pity. To begin with let's start by understanding these three terms as H.A. Wilmer (1968) describes them:

- Pity describes a relationship, which separates physician and patient. Pity is often condescending and may entail feelings of contempt and rejection.
- Sympathy is when the physician experiences feelings as if he or she were the sufferer. Sympathy is thus shared suffering.
- Empathy is the feeling relationship in which the physician understands the patient's plight as if the physician were the patient. The physician identifies with the patient and at the same time maintains a distance. Empathetic communication enhances the therapeutic effectiveness of the clinician–patient relationship.

Empathy can be used effectively by a skilled practitioner to enhance communication, but sympathy can be burdensome, emotionally exhausting, and as you might expect, a factor in professional burnout. Empathy could also be described as engaged detachment. In empathy, we 'borrow' our patient's feelings to observe, feel and understand them; but not to take them onto ourselves. In this detached role we can succeed in understanding how our patient feels. Now you might be saying that empathy is a gift that some people are born with, and some are not. While there might be some truth in that, there is now sufficient evidence to show that empathetic communication is a teachable, learnable skill (Platt & Keller 1994, Spiro 1992) and that it has very real benefits for both practitioner and patient. It is an important part of 'active therapeutic listening'. Appropriate use of empathic listening will improve all exchanges with your patients and will also increase the efficiency of information gathering. But, above anything else, empathetic listening honours the patient. By placing the patient first, you can always expect better health outcomes. Empathy is a cornerstone concept in several communication models, including 'the four habits' model (invest in the beginning, elicit the patient's perspective, demonstrate empathy, invest in the end) developed by The Permanente Medical Group's Terry Stein with Richard Frankel (Frankel & Stein 1999); 'the four Es' (engage, empathize, educate, enlist) model used by the Bayer Institute for Health Care Communication (Keller & Carroll 1994); and the 'PEARLS' (partnership, empathy, apology, respect, legitimization, support) framework adopted by the American Academy on Physician and Patient (Barrier & Jensen 2003).

Practicing empathetic listening/communication can help to balance your emotional stance as a clinician. For example, if you feel yourself taking on emotional weight from your patient, you can use empathetic communication to develop the emotional distance necessary to maintain a professional, therapeutic relationship. If you find yourself saying, 'I have no sympathy for this person' then remind yourself that you are not supposed to have sympathy; you are, however, supposed to have empathy. Using the proper techniques you can have an empathetic exchange with your patient, rather than a dismissive, judgmental, non-sympathetic position.

So, how do you employ empathy? The six key steps outlined by Frederic Platt (Platt 1992) include:

1. Recognizing the presence of strong feelings in the clinical setting (e.g. fear, anger, grief, disappointment)
2. Pausing to imagine how the patient might be feeling
3. Stating our perception of the patient's feeling (e.g. *'It sounds like you're upset about…'* or *'I can imagine that that must feel'*)
4. Legitimizing that feeling (e.g. *'I understand your frustration under the circumstances'*)
5. Respecting the patient's effort to cope with the predicament
6. Offering support and partnership (e.g. *'I promise to work with you until the resolution of this issue'* or *'Let's see what we can do together on this matter.'*).

You don't have to be a mental health expert to employ empathetic communication, you only need to be aware of the opportunities for empathy as they arise during your exchanges with your patient. This type of opportunity arises from a patient's expressed emotion. It may be expressed directly or it may simply be implied. Once their emotion has been expressed, you have the opportunity to pick up the ball or to drop it. After a situation such as this arises, you should consider offering a gesture or statement of empathy. Statements that facilitate empathy have been categorized as queries, clarifications, and responses (Coulehan et al. 2001). Examples of each are as follows:

Queries:

- *'Would you (or could you) tell me a little more about that?'*
- *'What has this been like for you?'*
- *'Is there anything else?'*
- *'Are you OK with that?'*

Clarifications

- *'Let me see if I have this right'*
- *'I want to make sure I really understand what you're telling me. I am hearing that…'*
- *'Tell me more about that'*
- *'I don't want us to go further until I'm sure I've gotten it right'*
- *'When I'm done, if I've gone astray, I'd appreciate it if you would correct me, OK?'*

Responses

- *'That sounds very difficult'*
- *'It sounds like…'*
- *'That's great! I bet you're feeling pretty good about that'*

- *'I can imagine that this might feel…'*
- *'I can see that you are…'*

Ideally, after your response, your patient will express agreement or confirmation. If not then clarification is in order. Allow your patient to correct your perception.

Conclusion

One important communication tool in medical interviews is empathy. Empathy builds patient trust and extends your understanding of the patient, well beyond the history and symptoms to include such things as values, ideas, and feelings. Empathetic listening and communication produces tangible benefits for both practitioner and patient.

As you undoubtedly now recognize, listening is not even remotely a passive experience. You must be actively engaged whether you are purely listening, echoing back information, clarifying issues, responding to questions or summarizing what has just been said. Listening, like all of your professional actions, is most effective when you are there truly 'in the moment'. During the listening process, you must be aware of both your own body language and the body language of your patient as well. In the end the patient has to 'feel' listened to, and it is up to you to make sure that he or she feels that way at the end of their session with you. The best way to achieve this is to follow the steps of active listening by focusing intently on your patient, paraphrasing what he or she has said, clarifying issues and details, summarizing and getting confirmation that your patient has felt, heard and understood. In so doing you will be maximizing your exchange with your patient and helping them to employ their own healing systems.

FEELINGS OF CARE AND CONCERN FROM THE PRACTITIONER

No human interaction is neutral. It is either healing or wounding.

Dr Balfour Mount

Balfour Mount MD has spent his life working with the sick and dying. In 1985 he was made a Member of the Order of Canada in recognition for having founded the first Palliative Care Service at Montreal's Royal Victoria Hospital. He is considered the father of palliative care. The preceding quote of his is very important to keep in mind as you walk around the planet, 'creating your world'. It is also important to keep in mind when interacting with your patients, because they will unconsciously assign either a positive or a negative value to everything that you say or do. As it turns out, neurologists now believe that the brain assigns a positive or a negative value to all its processes before they reach the cortical (conscious) areas of consciousness. As we saw in Biological Pathways and Theories, our immune system is affected by our emotions via the limbic system. It is important to keep this idea of positive and negative associations in mind when interacting with your patient.

One study which delineates care and concern from the practitioner was performed by Kaptchuk and colleagues at Harvard Medical School. This 6-week study (Kaptchuk 2008b) looked at 262 adults diagnosed with IBS and was designed to investigate whether placebo effects can experimentally be separated into three components:

1. **Assessment and observation**. Participants in this group were put on a waiting list for the duration of the study.
2. **Placebo only**. This group received a placebo in the form of sham acupuncture (the shaft of the sham device does not actually pierce the skin but creates the illusion of doing so because it retracts into a hollow handle). The limited patient–practitioner relationship was established at the initial visit during which practitioners introduced themselves and stated they had reviewed the patient's questionnaire and 'knew what to do'. They then explained that this was 'a scientific study' for which they had been 'instructed not to converse with patients'. The placebo needles were then placed and the patient left alone in a quiet room for 20 minutes – a common acupuncture practice – after which the practitioner returned to remove the 'needles'.
3. **Placebo plus a supportive patient–practitioner relationship**. This group also received the same sham acupuncture but this time from a practitioner instructed to exude warmth, empathy and confidence. Specifically, the practitioner incorporated at least five primary behaviours

including: a warm, friendly manner; active listening; empathy; 20 seconds of thoughtful silence while feeling the pulse or pondering the treatment plan; and communication of confidence and positive expectation. Kaptchuk chose these qualities because previous studies indicated that these were important factors in the practitioner–patient relationship.

Participants of the three groups were evaluated at the 3-week period for adequate relief of symptoms and for symptom severity. Group 1 showed 28% improvement at that time. Group 2 showed 44% improvement and Group 3 showed 63% improvement! Assessment at the 6-week period showed similar findings. The findings of this study clearly indicate the importance of the therapeutic relationship. It does not tease out caring and compassion from other important aspects of the practitioner–patient relationship but it clearly shows that administration of a placebo is powerful on its own. It further shows that the quality of the practitioner–patient relationship greatly enhances that placebo effect.

A systematic review on this topic by Di Blasi and colleagues (2001) looked at 25 RCTs which examined different aspects of the doctor–patient relationship. The authors noted that enhancing patients' expectations through positive information about the treatment or the illness, while providing support or reassurance, significantly influenced health outcomes. Furthermore, there was a relatively consistent finding that physicians who adopt a warm, friendly and reassuring manner are more effective than those who keep consultations formal and do not offer reassurance. Although this might seem obvious to you, the whole point of doing studies is to test a hypothesis. Also, it is surprising how often any given study of human interaction turns up some gem or another. Whether a particular gem gets picked up on or not by the study authors is another matter.

At the very least, you are observing your patient, and your patients are aware that you are observing them. This leads to a very interesting area of study. There is a term that you may have heard around the topic of observing the behaviour of others, the Hawthorne effect. This refers to a series of studies performed in a Hawthorn Works factory in the late 1920s and early 1930s which yielded some rather interesting and beguiling results. Hawthorne Works had originally commissioned a study to see the effects of different light levels on workers' productivity. The workers' productivity seemed to improve when changes were made and slumped when the study was concluded. Other changes were also made, such as pay rate, relocating workstations, improving cleanliness of work stations and clearing floors of obstacles. Each change seemed to increase productivity for a short period of time, after which productivity returned to normal. This was true of each of the individual workers as well as of the group mean. It was suggested that the productivity gain was due to the motivational effect of the interest being shown in them. Many interpretations have been made of these results and other experiments have followed. What is generally agreed is that when persons are observed, their behaviour changes and the more that they feel they are being observed, the more behaviour seems to change (up to a point). The lesson here is that your patients are more likely to be working on their own health issues if they feel that you are observing or showing concern for them, as opposed to just having them show up at your office for their treatment.

The topic of care and concern is not rocket science. We all want to feel special, that we are not just a number, so when someone shows interest in us or our health we perk up and bask in their attention. It makes us feel better, and we are more likely to follow homecare regimes if we feel that our practitioner is interested in our well-being and will be asking us about our progress. Keeping the focus on your patient may or may not be natural for you. If it is not then be sure to pull the focus away from anything else that may be diverting your attention, whether it be other distractions from your office, from your day, your surroundings or your own home life. These things can only take you away from your task of focusing on your patient.*

Once you are in that place of giving them your full attention, then you need to relay your concern for their situation during the whole treatment, not just when greeting them. If you work with large blocks of time, as massage therapists do, this can be quite a challenge. Over the course of a 1-hour treatment, conversation will naturally drift off in different directions, but it is your job to always direct the conversation and the focus back to the patient.

Care and concern for the patient cannot really be faked; it has to be genuine. However, following the exercises laid out in the previous section on active listening will help you on your road if you are having trouble with this area. The great thing about following the exercises is that you really do not have to admit to anyone else that you are not a natural at this. You only need to admit it to yourself and then take steps to improve your professional focus. Improvements in this area will make you a better practitioner/therapist/health professional/person and your patient will benefit with improved therapeutic outcomes.

As mentioned earlier, the exercises that will help you in this endeavour are outlined in the previous section. The concept of listening is different from feelings of care and concern, but as you can see, if you are performing the exercises of active, *empathetic listening* with authenticity, then you will necessarily be transmitting feelings of care and concern for your patient. You can work on developing more empathetic skills. Caring will have to come within you, from your heart and all of your actions and words will indicate that you do indeed care for your patient's well-being and health.

Take-home points

- The quality of your relationship with your patient directly affects their health outcome.

---

*I have worked in more than one therapeutic setting in my life and I have observed a wide range of natural abilities of therapists in the area of being patient-focused. Some therapists naturally focus on their patient's health and life, others seem to have endless personal stories to tell. It is fine to occasionally reveal a bit about yourself to help establish a trust relationship, but this does not require a large degree of self-revelation.

- Know that patients consciously and unconsciously assign a positive or negative value to everything that you say or do.
- Simply observing your patient's progress and making them aware that you are observing it by asking questions can produce a positive 'Hawthorne effect'.
- Practice active listening to convey that you care and are involved in your patient's progress.
- Always keep your focus on the patient during the treatment. If you offer an anecdote, quickly return your focus to the patient.
- Making your patient feel special conveys that the quality of their health is important to you.
- Provide a commitment to stick with them until their condition has improved to the patient's own level of satisfaction.

The practitioner/patient relationship is probably more important than ever these days because 'time' is such an issue in modern medicine. Often, patients are feeling rushed in and out of procedures because time is so precious. Medicine can also be very dehumanizing as people are hooked up to machines, having a barrage of tests performed, waiting to see specialists. When you stop and show your patient that you genuinely care, a very important message is communicated and an important bond is formed, which is an essential element in the therapeutic relationship that allows the placebo response to manifest to its fullest.

I would like to finish this section with a quote from Francis Peabody. In 1927 Peabody wrote the medical landmark article, 'The care of the patient'. Peabody affected medicine so greatly that Harvard Medical School has a Francis W. Peabody Society to this day. Peabody was known for many great contributions to the field of medicine, not the least of which was recognizing the paramount importance of the health provider–patient relationship. In the following quote (Peabody 1984) he reveals the remarkably simple secret of caring for the patient:

The good physician knows his patients through and through, and his knowledge is sought dearly. Time, sympathy and understanding must be lavishly dispensed, but the reward is to be found in that personal bond which forms the greatest satisfaction of the practice of medicine. One of the essential qualities of the clinician is interest in humanity, for the secret of the care of the patient is in caring for the patient.

ESTABLISHMENT OF A FEELING OF CONTROL

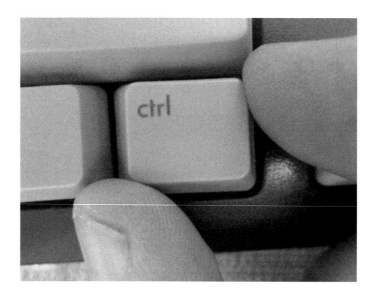

Fig. 2.8

Control certainly seems to be a very large and multifaceted area that both allopathic medicine and complementary therapies see as being very important to therapeutic outcomes. Most people need to feel as though they are in control of their own life and situation. While, admittedly, there are an immense number of things that can radically affect our lives in a positive or negative way, there is much peace of mind that comes from 'feeling' in control. As we learned previously, the HPA axis appears to be involved in the placebo effect, and clearly, one's anxiety levels will be elevated if you feel that you are becoming more ill and you have no control over your situation. This will clearly ramp up the HPA axis. Our patients look to us for expertise and for guidance throughout their illness, and anything that we can do to lower their anxiety levels will help to enhance their inner healer. Helping them to feel more in control of their situation is one way of doing this.

> *The task of the therapist – whatever his or her technique – is to clarify symptoms and problems, inspire hope, facilitate experiences of success or mastery, and stir the patient's emotions. The second theme is that the main effect of such activity is to alleviate the patients' sense of powerlessness to change themselves or their environment.*

Jerome Frank
(Frank & Frank 1991, p. xiii–xiv)

The previous quote is from Jerome Frank's book *Persuasion and Healing.* This is considered to be a seminal exploration of the topic of the healer/patient psychotherapeutic relationship. In the preface, Frank lays the recurring themes in his book. We can see here how important Frank viewed the need for the patient to feel 'in control'. Two of the three themes that run through his book involve the patient's need to achieve control (what he terms mastery) over their situation.

Whether your patient tends to be highly control-based or very relaxed, this person will benefit from a sense of control over their pain, loss of function, etc. That being said, I am sure that most manual practitioners have encountered patients that they felt would honestly benefit more from psychotherapy than manual therapy. We have all encountered patients who feel that they need to control every aspect of their life and the lives of those around them. Dealing with a patient like this is very challenging. While this is typically stemming from some internal sense of being out of control, we are not psychotherapists. Likewise, it is a very sensitive professional call in trying to decide how to help a patient who is hanging on to themselves much too tightly, and it takes a skilled health professional and a special therapeutic environment for a practitioner to be able to suggest a psychotherapeutic referral for this (or any other) issue without offending the patient. We all have patients that are just a bit too control-oriented for their own good, and it is this group in particular that will benefit most from the techniques discussed in this section. Paradoxically, these same patients would probably benefit from relaxing their own need for control.

Much research has been done in the area of patient control. As you might expect, the majority shows that improved therapeutic outcomes (less perceived pain, less depression, decreased healing times etc.) are linked to patients' increased feelings of control over decision-making surrounding their treatment. For example, a study of 90 first-time pregnant women in Hong Kong shows a direct relationship between their involvement in decision-making surrounding medical intervention, increased feelings of control and reduced anxiety levels (Cheung et al. 2007). A British study found a similar correlation (Gibbins & Thomson 2001). A study by Nancy Lowe (Lowe 1989) found that maternal confidence was the most significant predictor of feelings of control and reduced anxiety levels inpatients. Lowe then went on to develop standards for measuring these concepts and outcomes in maternal settings. As far as she is concerned, confidence is primarily obtained by achieving a sense of control. Quoting directly from her section (Lowe 2003) in Barbara Redman's book *Measurement Tools inPatient Education*:

The importance of confidence to the perception of pain during labor is supported by data from clinical studies, which indicate that more than one half of the variance in early labor pain and about one third of the variance in active labor pain can be explained by the single variable of maternal confidence in ability to cope.

She goes on the say that confidence can be significantly increased by maternal education, including observation of others performing successful labor.

One interesting study of 884 older adults hypothesized that high levels of role-specific control were likely to develop a deep sense of personal meaning and subsequently enjoy better health than older adults who are unable to find meaning in life. Data from this nationwide survey (Krause & Shaw 2003) supports this theory and yields some interesting results, most interesting of which was that older adults who feel they have control over the role they most valued (e.g. father, grandparent, caregiver, mentor) live longer than those who do not. The data tends to suggest that control over one's role was even more important than the sense of control over one's life. This is perhaps the 'wisdom of the years' that recognizes that much of life is beyond our control, so if you establish control over one important area, such as what you see as your primary role, you can relax about other aspects of your life. The participants in this study scored higher on having a sense of control over the role that was most important to them and were more likely to be alive at the 6- and 7-year follow-ups. Those adults who scored lower were more likely to engage in unhealthy behaviours such as drinking alcohol, smoking or they were obese; all of which are risk factors for premature death.

A study by David Brody helped to get the ball rolling on the issue of patient involvement in their healthcare delivery. In his study of 117 patients, 47% reported playing an active role; 53% reported playing a passive role. After adjusting for age, sex, baseline illness ratings, and physician-rated prognosis, 'active' patients reported less discomfort, greater alleviation of symptoms and more improvement in their general medical condition than did 'passive' patients. These differences were not influenced by the roles patients desired to play. Active patients also reported less concern with their illnesses, a greater sense of control of their illnesses and more satisfaction with their physicians (Brody et al. 1989).

A 2015 study at University of Southampton in the UK looked at psychological factors involved with therapeutic outcomes inpatients with back-related disability undergoing acupuncture (Bishop et al. 2015). This study found strong association patient expectations and outcome as mentioned in the section on Expectancy, but it also found that those people who have a positive view of back pain and who feel in control of their condition experience less back-related disability over the course of acupuncture treatment. Study author Dr Bishop stated (University of Southampton 2015):

When individual patients came to see their back pain more positively they went on to experience less back-related disability. In particular, they experienced less disability over the course of treatment when they came to see their back pain as more controllable; when they felt they had better understanding of their back pain; when they felt better able to cope with it; were less emotional about it; and when they felt their back pain was going to have less of an impact on their lives.

As one might expect, most things in life exist on a continuum and patient control is no different. Just as a powerless patient with no feeling of control leads to poorer outcomes, the same has been found for patients who want complete control. A massive study by Catherine Breach and colleagues (2007) of 1027 HIV patients receiving highly active antiretroviral treatment (HAART) looked at patient involvement in decision-making, their subsequent adherence to their antiretroviral program and their subsequent HIV RNA blood analysis. Patients were asked how they preferred to be involved in decisions (doctor makes most or all decisions; doctor and patient share decisions; patient makes all decisions). Overall, 23% patients preferred that their doctor make all or most decisions, 63% preferred to share decisions with their doctor, and 13% preferred to make all final decisions alone. Compared to patients who prefer to share decisions with their health provider, patients who prefer that their provider make all/most decisions were significantly less likely to adhere to their HAART and patients who preferred to make decisions alone were significantly less likely to receive HAART or to have undetectable HIV RNA in unadjusted blood analyses.

Several things about this study strike me. Firstly, the patient who surrenders control has a poorer health outcome. Often as a healthcare provider, you tend to assume that perhaps a patient who wants you to make all of the decisions is just a more passive personality, so you are delivering healthcare appropriate to their comfort level with the assumption that you are providing them with the best of care. It turns out that it is perhaps in their best interest that you push them out of their comfort zone a little and remind them that it is actually for their own good. Secondly, the 13% who make their own decisions exclusively could be perhaps viewed as being highly involved in their own healthcare, but are in fact making poor choices on what is, in the case of this study, a life and death matter. The important point to note here is that as healthcare providers we are trying to accommodate for each patient, but we must do so armed with the knowledge that as patients move out to either end of the 'control spectrum' that they will typically have poorer health outcomes. One example of the 'control' end is where a patient asks you to work deep in an area where your own instinct and good judgment tell you otherwise. Accommodating this patient's request will leave them quite sore the next day. You have undoubtedly encountered patients who want you to continue working on an area that in your opinion has already had enough soft tissue work for one session. Once again, it is good that they are communicating their concern that the area still needs loosening up, but that does not mean that you should overwork and inflame the area. It is important for the patient to be involved in the decision-making, but this doesn't mean that you should surrender your professional responsibility.

In Canada, the concept of patient decision-making has come of age. We actually have an acronym for it, SDM (shared decision-making). There is considerable interest in SDM within the Canadian healthcare system. SDM has reached a higher profile through increased research funding, medical training and some initiatives embedding patient decision aids within the process of care. Due to informed consent, the legal obligation for doctors to fully disclose information enabling patients' participation in decisions has spawned professional codes and guidelines with a vision of patient's empowerment through the use of patient decision aid and SDM. That being said, a survey of general practitioners in 2002 indicated that they perceived their role as relieving anxiety induced in patients rather than engaging them in informed decision-making. The main point being that our own patients' need for a sense of control over their medical treatment now covers the whole gambit from theory, to research to practice, and even to institutionalization. The question here isn't really if you should be employing SDM in your practice, it is really more a matter of how you are going to implement it.

In two different studies by Greenfield and co-workers (1985, 1988), patients were trained to be more effective at the task of eliciting information from their physicians (by asking questions) and compared against a control group. The patients trained to ask more questions had improved functional status and were more satisfied with care than the control group. Some of us may not want to encourage our patients to ask more questions as it might lead to 'more work' for us, but let's face it, it's not about us, it's about the patient. Encouraging the patient to ask more questions will lead to an increased sense of control on their part, and this will lead to improved outcomes.

There is much that we can say or do to give our patients a sense of more or less control over their situation. It is not just about the delivery of the treatment itself, but this is a good place to begin. Admittedly there are some patients that want to give little input into their treatment, but according to information and research presented in this section we should encourage passive patients to become more involved in their own healthcare. However, we need to keep in mind that our patients are not medical experts and they do not want to feel overwhelmed by complicated choices. Pushing people to make too many choices could backfire and lead to a patient feeling that they have too much responsibility and these people can feel a sense of loss of control (Green et al. 1990); the exact opposite of what we actually want. This has been shown to lead to poorer health outcomes. In fact, there are many times when patients find reassurance from being told what to do by health professionals. There are times when being told what to do does not mean losing control to professionals. This is a line that you need to walk as a health professional, but you must walk that line favoring patient control.

Modern healthcare has moved toward empowerment of the patient, but there are still many patients who still want you to 'fix' them. In a study by Avis at Queen's Medical Centre in Nottingham, UK, where day surgery patients were asked in-depth questions about their views on participation in their surgery, the overwhelming conclusions of the research was, 'Their expectations of participation can be summarized as 'being told' and 'going in to get it fixed'(Avis 1994). This may be something that you run up against in your practice. Even though you want your patients to take a more active role in their health and their health care decisions, they still keep handing the reins of control back to you.

So with all of these caveats aside, let's look into ways that you can reduce your patients' anxiety levels and either allow or encourage them to a position of more control over their health delivery. The previous midwifery studies mentioned that the patient's sense of control was or could be achieved through:

- Support from partners
- The positive attitudes of the midwives caring for them during pregnancy and labor
- Information giving during pregnancy and labor
- Being able to make and be included in decision-making during labor
- Education including observation of others performing successful labor.

- **Reassuring statements**, e.g. *'We will do whatever it takes here to get you better. I'm not going to abandon you. We will both work on this until we have figured out what is going on here.'*
- **Provide information on their condition**. As mentioned earlier, being well-informed leads to an improved sense of control. You can do this verbally, but it is best backed up with handout material. It is also good to suggest quality sources where patients can find additional information if they are so motivated.
- **Keep two-way lines of communication open,** e.g. *'How do you feel things are progressing at your end?'*
- **Empower them to speak up if they have any concerns,** e.g. *'If you feel any discomfort let me know and I will alter my pressure'.*
- **Offering alternatives.** If you cannot get around the matter of expectancy of discomfort, be sure and offer an alternative where they are less likely to experience side-effects. Just knowing this can free them from the fear of expecting side-effects, e.g. *'If you do experience any discomfort from this treatment, we will try a different approach next time.'*
- **Be available to their concerns.** Just letting them know that you are available should they have any issues will alleviate a lot of potential anxiety. e.g. *'Do not hesitate to call me if you have any questions or discomfort.'*
- **When empowering the patient, give them some specific options to choose from,** e.g. *'You had some short-term discomfort after the last treatment. If you would like, I can alter my treatment today or we can use a similar approach. How would you like me to proceed?'*

- **Sometimes some 'steerage' is required on your part.** Many of us tend to have small comfort zones and even when given an option, will still tend to stay in that comfort zone. This human tendency can work against you giving the patient options. Although it is good to give them options, be aware that you may have to steer them in a certain direction to avoid a stalled healing scenario. e.g. *'I know that you are more comfortable with X because this is what you have been exposed to for the past few months, but I feel that if you were to try Y that we would see quicker progress.'*

Box 2.1

REDUCING YOUR PATIENTS' ANXIETY LEVELS

Man is not worried by real problems so much as by his imagined anxieties about real problems

Epictetus

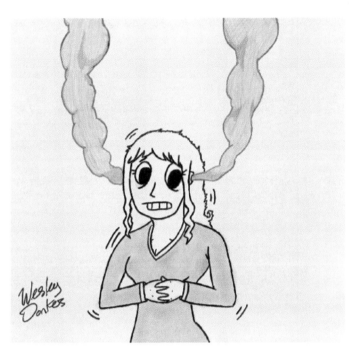

Fig. 2.9

One thing that we learned in the section Biological pathways and theories is that the sympathetic–parasympathetic pathway is clearly one powerful pathway that comes in to play with the placebo effect via the hypothalamo–pituitary–adrenal axis or HPA. Put quite simply, the more that you can allay your patients' fears, the stronger the placebo effect will be. The link between overstimulation and disease is well established. The list involves, at the very least, hypertension, arteriosclerosis, cardiac distress, cardiac arrest, osteoporosis, memory loss, accelerated aging, stomach ulcers, fibromyalgia and chronic pain syndromes, eczema, and vulnerability to infections. Helping to reduce your patients' anxiety levels will help their bodies heal themselves. There is a multitude of ways to achieve this as we will see in the following paragraphs.

Anticipatory anxiety versus real-life coping mechanisms

One tool that you can use to help allay fears of a patient headed toward loss of function is to apply what we understand about human coping mechanisms.

We are all more adept at coping than we often realize. Most humans peak physically in their mid-20s. I have reached the ripe old age of 60 and like most people my age, my eyesight has dwindled to the point where I now need corrective eyewear for distance as well as up close. My hearing is far from optimal and most of my other senses short of touch are operating at about 60–70% of optimum and are not getting better. Arthritis in many of my joints flares up regularly, interfering with my activities of daily living and causing pain at those times. I have a torn left anterior cruciate ligament from 30 years ago and subsequent knee issues that now limit the activities that I can partake in. My hair is thinning and grey! I don't have a single tooth in my mouth that hasn't had a filling in it or that hasn't been crowned. I have two spinal segments that 30 years after herniation are all but naturally fused due to osteophyte growth. I could go on, but I think that you get the idea. The point is that if you ask me about my quality of life, you will get the response that in fact I have an extremely high quality of life. It is every bit as high as it was when I was 21 when I was acutely aware that I was at the physical peak of my life. I may not be able jump as high, run as far and as fast, but life has this habit of giving you another gift every time that it takes something from you. These are what are termed 'coping mechanisms', and we seem to do much better at dealing with problems when immersed in them than we do when we are anticipating the adversity. Another example of this is the following quote from Margaret Somerville, Director of the Centre for Medicine, Ethics and Law at McGill University who has spent some time studying this phenomenon. She says (Somerville 2013):

> *If you ask people where they would place, for example, blindness on a scale of zero to minus ten, with minus ten being the worst thing that could ever happen to them, most sighted people put it at minus seven to minus eight. On the other hand, blind people put it at around minus two. Likewise, recent research shows that although others judge the quality of life of a group of old people to be very low, those same old people do not judge the quality of their own life nearly so negatively. In other words, the anticipation of a dread event can be much worse than the experience of that event.*

This sort of information can help to allay the fears of someone who feels that they are going to lose all quality of life, due to a physical limitation that they are beginning to face. This is not an empty platitude; this is what we have learned about human nature from years of study and research.

Commitment from a knowledgeable authority figure

Another way to allay fears is with your personal commitment to your patient's health. One story relayed earlier spoke of the professional engineering consultant who had been called into a few situations where anxiety levels were running very high due to the complex nature of the problems, the time pressures involved and the ever-present economic constraints. His response in these situations is to say, 'Okay everybody, I'm here. This may not be an easy problem to solve, but it is doable. This is my area of expertise, and *I will not leave until we have solved this problem.'* He said that you can see the anxiety level drop immediately, and suddenly big impossible problems become bite-sized manageable problems. There are several elements to this story that strike me as factors that reduce anxiety levels of participants:

- The commitment shown by the professional who intervenes and make a promise to not abandon the person(s) involved.
- The expertise that the professional brings to the table. This person (substitute you) has been at this place before and helped others through the problem that they are facing.
- The problem gets broken down into bite-sized pieces. This is important for many reasons. It usually makes the problem more manageable, more measureable in terms of success or failure, and reducing the size of any problem will necessarily reduce the anxiety levels.

Breaking problems into bite-sized pieces

Each one of us has experienced that feeling of being overwhelmed by a task or a problem that we face. One strategy, faced with an intimidating task is to break it up in manageable sized pieces. As was just mentioned, not only does this lower your patient's anxiety levels, but if you work with your patient on this problem, you will both end up with concrete measurable goals.

Use of touch

Those of us working in the manual therapy profession are all blessed for many reasons. One of these reasons is that patients recognize human touch as a signal of caring. Medicine is creating some massive machines that do some amazing things, but remember this: *machines don't comfort people.*

There is plenty of research out there to support the use of touch to reduce anxiety levels. (To access research on touch therapy, including massage go to http://www6.miami.edu/touch-research/. There you will find a plethora of research connecting touch therapies with among other things, anxiety reduction.) The Touch Institute in Florida has spent decades researching the positive effects of touch and reduced anxiety levels is a common finding among the studies performed. Never underestimate the power of your touch, when properly used to reduce anxiety levels. If you work in manual therapy, but do not perform massage therapy, perhaps there is a way to incorporate a relaxing touch therapy into your practice for patients in need of anxiety reduction, or you could refer your patient to a massage therapist for treatment and stress reduction.

You will remember from the section, Biological theories and pathways, under the heading 'Sympathetic/parasympathetic pathway' that continued stressful circumstances can potentiate amygdala(e) functioning in the brain, allowing it to become more powerful, even wilful over time, sometimes exerting subcortical control over our human cortical reasoning. This is well worth remembering as a practitioner. Because of the neuroplasticity of the brain, any area that gets overstimulated will potentiate and undergo physical changes. The overstimulated HPA axis tends to feedback into itself. The important take-home message here is that unhealthy patterns in our patients can eventually be replaced with healthy patterns. An exaggerated sympathetic response can eventually be tamed, but the old habit needs to be broken.

In addition to things that you can say or do, you can also suggest to your patient anything appropriate from the list of stress-reduction techniques below.

Exercise

The benefits of exercise are well documented. This is not something that we really need to cover, but it is important at this time to remind ourselves also of the stress reduction capability of a good workout. At the very least, exercise can emotionally remove one temporarily from a stressful environment or situation, but it goes much further than that. Every one of us has experienced the lifting of the fog, a.k.a. 'cotton-brain' that develops when you have either been concentrating too long (you know ... like reading or writing a book), or you have been in a funk. There are many reasons for why exercise reduces stress, not the least of which is endorphin release. These endorphins give us a feeling of happiness and positively affect our overall sense of well-being. Our patients look to us for guidance in the area of exercise. It is commonplace for us to prescribe specific stretching or strengthening exercises for injury recovery, and it would be entirely appropriate for us to also prescribe a mild cardio regime for those patients that are sedentary. We are in as good a position as anyone to assess their general health and to suggest types of exercise that they should avoid. This will also have the benefit of reducing anxiety somewhat for patients for whom this might be indicated.

Guided or auto relaxation techniques

Meditation

Meditation's powerful effect on the parasympathetic system has been well researched (Garland 2007, Shapiro et al. 2006, Tang et al. 2009). The link between meditation and relaxation is irrefutable. Its use in a medical setting has also been well established (Shapiro et al. 2005, Kabat-Zinni et al. 1985). There are many ways for your patient to approach meditation. If you are experienced then you could choose to do basic instruction in this area or you could suggest classes, books, websites or audio files to help them get started with meditation. Any one of these approaches should help your patient to control their stress levels by evoking the body's relaxation response. Regularly practicing these techniques will build their emotional resilience, heal their body, and boost their overall feelings of joy and equanimity. There are many secular meditation practices, so one doesn't need to worry about it being aligned with religion. The meditative state is one in which there is a deep centering and focusing upon the core of one's being; there is a quieting of the mind, emotions, and body. The meditative state can be achieved through structured (as in a daily practice of a routine) or unstructured (for example, while being alone outdoors) activities.

One generic form of meditation, which was popularized several decades ago by Harvard physician Herbert Benson, is termed the relaxation response. Benson went to great lengths to make this form of meditation simple, accessible, medically-based and secular (non-religious). It is designed to evoke the parasympathetic body response. Its value has been documented in the reduction of blood pressure and other bodily stress responses. Like other forms of meditation, it can be learned on one's own, but time and practice are required to elicit the desired relaxation state.

Autogenic training

Autogenic training is a relaxation technique developed by the German psychiatrist Johannes Schultz in the late 1920s. The technique involves the daily practice of three sessions that last around 15 minutes (morning, noon and night). During each session, the practitioner repeats a set of visualizations that induce a state of relaxation. Each session can be practiced in one of variance postural positions (for example, lying down, sitting meditation, sitting like a rag doll). Schultz emphasized parallels to techniques in yoga and meditation and has many parallels to progressive relaxation. The practitioner focuses on different body sensations, such as warmth or heaviness, in different regions of the body.

Autogenic training has been used by physicians as a part of therapy for many conditions. In 2002 a meta-analysis was done on autogenic research (Stetter & Kupper 2002). Autogenic training appeared to perform similarly to other relaxation techniques. The literature in this study found efficacy for autogenic training was effective in treating tension headache/migraine, mild to moderate essential hypertension, coronary heart disease, bronchial asthma, somatoform pain disorder (unspecified type), Raynaud's disease, anxiety disorders, mild-to-moderate depression/dysthymia, and functional sleep disorders. In Europe it is extremely well accepted and is even covered by some insurance plans. No particular physical skills or exercises are involved; however, just like most other forms of structured relaxation, people desiring to learn this technique must be prepared to invest time and patience. Once again, if you are qualified in autogenic training you can guide your patient through the process. If not then you can suggest autogenic training classes for your patient.

Example of an autogenic training session

1. Sit in the meditative posture and scan the body
2. 'My right arm is heavy'
3. 'My arms and legs are heavy and warm' (repeat 3 or more times)

4. 'My heartbeat is calm and regular' (repeat 3 times)
5. 'My solar plexus is warm' (repeat 3 times)
6. 'My forehead is cool'
7. 'My neck and shoulders are heavy' (repeat 3 times)
8. 'I am at peace' (repeat 3 times)
9. Repeat steps 2 through 8
10. Repeat steps 2 through 8 again.

Biofeedback

Biofeedback is used by many practitioners for a variety of psychological and physical conditions. It is based upon the principle first advanced in the early 1960s that the autonomic nervous system is trainable. Instruments are used to measure heart rate, blood pressure, brain activity, stomach acidity, muscle tension, or other parameters while your patient experiments with postural changes, breathing techniques or thinking patterns. By receiving this feedback, your patient learns to identify the processes that achieve the desired result such as blood pressure reduction or decreased heart rate. While biofeedback is an interesting and effective way of achieving relaxation and controlling stress responses, it requires equipment that few of us have in our clinics. Hopefully you have someone in your region to whom you can refer patients.

The Association for Applied Psychophysiology and Biofeedback (AAPB), the Biofeedback Certification Institution of America (BCIA) and the International Society for Neurofeedback and Research (ISNR) jointly approved a Task Force on Nomenclature definition of biofeedback, as follows:

> *Biofeedback is a process that enables an individual to learn how to change physiological activity for the purposes of improving health and performance. Precise instruments measure physiological activity such as brainwaves, heart function, breathing, muscle activity, and skin temperature. These instruments rapidly and accurately 'feed-back' information to the user. The presentation of this information – often in conjunction with changes in thinking, emotions, and behaviour – supports desired physiological changes. Over time, these changes can endure without continued use of an instrument.*

Certification for Biofeedback can be done through The BCIA, a non-profit organization that is a member of the Institute for Credentialing Excellence (ICE). The BCIA education requirement includes a 48-hour course from a regionally-accredited academic institution.

Guided imagery

Imagery is a very basic mental language that we all use. The mind processes everything that we do through images. When we recall events from our past we think of pictures, images, sounds, pain, etc. It is hardly ever through words. Imagery in this sense isn't necessarily limited to visual images, but can be sounds, tastes, smells or a combination of sensations. Guided imagery in this application is the use of pleasant or relaxing images to calm the mind and body. By controlling breathing and visualizing a soothing image, a state of deep relaxation can occur. This method can be learned by anyone and is relatively easy to try out. Advocates of imagery contend that the imagination is a powerful healing technique that has been largely overlooked by practitioners of Western medicine. Imagery is said to relieve pain, speed healing and help the body subdue ailments such as depression, impotence, allergies and asthma.

Guided imagery is not simply an esoteric notion, it is a safe powerful tool and its efficacy has been shown in several clinical trials. To help bring you on board with this idea, close your eyes and think of some very stressful experience in your life and spend half a minute recalling this event. You will quickly find that not only do a whole series of images come into your mind, but your whole body will begin to go into sympathetic mode. Likewise, if you now close your eyes and conjure up an image of a perfect moment of relaxation that you have experienced, whether a beautiful beach paradise or just a wonderful peaceful Sunday morning listening to birds, drinking your favorite morning beverage. Once again not only do a series of images appear in your mind, but your whole body will begin to relax, and your parasympathetic nervous system is allowed to surface.

Imagery is the language that the mind uses to communicate with the body. Proponents of guided imagery would say that, for example, you can't really talk to an illness and say 'go away,' because this is not the language that the brain uses to communicate with the body. However, if you picture yourself in perfect health, or you visualize the injury healing etc., the body may be nudged toward a healthier state. Imagery could be said to be the biological connection between the mind and body. Visualization is extremely useful in mind–body healing. It is estimated that an average person has over 10 000 thoughts or images flashing through their mind each day. At least half of those thoughts are considered to be negative, such as anxiety surrounding a deadline, personal finances or job related anxiety, etc. Unharnessed, a steady dose of negative images can alter your physiology and make you more susceptible to a variety of ailments. Guided imagery attempts to move your patient out of the state of negative images and replace those images with images of healing.

Affirmations and visualizations are an important tool used by most high level athletes. Imagery has been taught by top coaches for several decades now to improve athletes' performance, to help give them the winning edge. Steven Covey, in his best seller, *Seven Habits of the Most Effective People*, suggested that we can use our right brain power of visualization to write an affirmation that will help us become more congruent with our deeper values in our daily life. According to Covey, a good affirmation has five basic ingredients:

- It's personal
- It's positive

- It's present tense
- It's visual, and
- It's emotional.

Using these principles, a medical affirmation may look like the following: 'When I [personal] feel [emotional] pain, I will visualize [visual] the area as being [present tense] in a healing state, and I will relax, knowing that my body has the wisdom to heal itself [positive].' It is then recommended that your patient use this affirmation for a few minutes each day, feeling every physical process in the affected region and then visualize the area as being fully healed.

Imagery is very effective in treating stress. It is used extensively in relaxation techniques which have been shown to release gamma-aminobutyric acid (GABA) and other natural body tranquilizers that lower blood pressure, heart rate and anxiety levels. Guided imagery has traditionally been used for stress-related conditions such as headaches, chronic pain in the neck and back, high blood pressure, spastic colon and cramping from premenstrual syndrome. Recent studies are showing powerful effects in treating everything from allergies, to psychiatric disorders to cancer.

A 2010 study at the Department of Psychosomatic Medicine at Munich Technical University (Lahmann et al. 2010) studied the effects of guided imagery on immunoglobulin E (serum indicator of type I hypersensitivity allergies) in dust-mite allergic asthmatics. Their conclusions found, 'Our study confirmed a positive and clinically relevant effect of functional relaxation and guided imagery on total serum IgE levels.'

Guided imagery has also been found helpful in treating some psychiatric disorders. A 2009 study (Apóstolo & Kolcaba 2009) at Coimbra Nursing School, Coimbra, Portugal on the effects of guided imagery on psychiatric inpatients with depressive disorders found that 'repeated measures revealed that the treatment group had significantly improved comfort and decreased depression, anxiety, and stress over time.'

Recent studies have shown extremely powerful effects using guided imagery in cancer patients. A 2009 study (Eremin et al. 2009) of 80 women at United Lincolnshire Hospitals in the UK undergoing drug therapy, chemotherapy and radiation therapy had the following findings:

Significant between-group differences were found in the number of CD25+ (activated T cells) and CD56+ (LAK cell) (lymphokine-activated killer cell) subsets. The number of CD3+ (mature) T cells was significantly higher following chemotherapy and radiotherapy, inpatients randomized to relaxation and guided imagery. Using a median split, women who rated their imagery ratings highly had elevated levels of NK (natural killer) cell activity at the end of chemotherapy and at follow-up. Significant correlations were obtained between imagery ratings and baseline corrected values for NK and LAK cell activity, and IL1beta. Relaxation frequency correlated with the number of CD4+ (T helper) cells, the CD4+:8+ (helper:cytotoxic) ratio, and Interleukin 1beta levels. Relaxation training and guided imagery beneficially altered putative anti-cancer host defences during and after multimodality therapy. Such changes, to the best of our knowledge, have not been previously documented in a random controlled trial.

Guided imagery is now such a widely recognized tool that it is being used by major health care institutions, such as Kaiser Permanente, Blue Shield of California, the US Department of Veterans Affairs and hundreds of US hospitals, including Mayo, Columbia Presbyterian, the Cleveland Clinic and Bethesda Naval Hospital. Several major pharmaceutical companies even recognize the power of imagery and have distributed over half a million CDs to chemotherapy and radiation patients.

Virtually everyone can successfully use imagery. It's just a matter of basic training and then patience and persistence. Most proponents suggest practicing your imagery for 15–20 minutes a day initially, and then as skill level increases one just needs to invest a few minutes at a time as needed throughout the day. The most effective images seem to be ones that have meaning to the participant. For example, when battling tumors, people might imagine that their healthy cells are plump, juicy berries, while their cancerous cells are dried, shrivelled pieces of fruit. They might picture their immune system as birds that fly in, pick up, and carry away the raisin-like cancer cells, while the rest of the cells flourish. However, for another personality type, these images might not click. Guided imagery is most effective if you create images that fit with your outlook and approach.

Studies indicate that imagery works best when it is used in conjunction with a relaxation technique. When your physical body is relaxed, you don't need to be in such conscious control of your mind, and you can give it the freedom to daydream. Meditation, progressive relaxation or yoga are the most common relaxation techniques used with imagery. A guided relaxation imagery session might go as follows:

- Dim the lights, and ask your patient to take off their shoes, loosen their clothing a bit, and sit comfortably on a soft chair.
- Have them take in a few deep breaths, then picture themselves descending a wonderful staircase.
- Suggest that with each step, they notice that they are feeling more and more relaxed.
- When they are feeling relaxed, imagine a favorite scene. It could be a beach, a nature retreat or a particularly enjoyable moment with friends or family.
- Have them go into this same scene each time they practice their imagery. Repetition will increase the power of this image. Once they have created their own safe place, they will feel more secure and it will make them more receptive to other images.

- Once they feel comfortable in their favorite scene, gradually direct their mind toward the ache, injury or illness in question.
- As the practitioner you would now suggest an appropriate image such as a tumor shrinking, a joint moving more freely and injury healing, etc.
- Tell them to let the image become more vivid, and then focus in on it. Don't worry if it seems to fade in and out.
- If several images come to mind, choose one and stick with it for that session.
- Have them repeat this same exercise several times each day at home. Each time have them imagine that at the end of the session their ailment is completely cured.
- At the end of their session have them take a few slow deep breaths and picture them self-ascending the staircase and gradually becoming aware of their surroundings.
- Have them open their eyes, stretch, and welcome them back and assure them that the healing process has already begun. Just like a muscle, each time that they repeat this exercise it will help more and more with their ailment.

Progressive muscle relaxation

Progressive muscle relaxation (PMR) is a technique that was developed for reducing anxiety by American physician Edmund Jacobson in the early 1920s. It involves alternately tensing and relaxing the muscles of the body, first locally, then regionally then globally. Jacobson argued that since muscular tension accompanies anxiety, one can reduce anxiety by learning how to relax the muscular tension; sort of horse and cart thing. If you can't slow down the horse, then you put brakes on the cart. PMR has established itself as an efficacious treatment for several nervous disorders. To quote one recent study, (Chen et al. 2009) 'Progressive muscle relaxation training is a useful intervention as it is proven to reduce anxiety levels across a spectrum of psychiatric disorders.' PMR is so powerful that one recent critical review (Pluess et al. 2009) of literature on the topic found, 'muscle relaxation therapies have been as effective as cognitive interventions directly addressing the defining symptom . . . worry.' Interestingly enough, a pilot study (Campos de Carvalho et al. 2007) of PMR for management of nausea and vomiting inpatients receiving cancer chemotherapy, found that, 'The results indicated that progressive muscle relaxation lead to statistically significant changes in physiological and muscle conditions and in nausea and vomiting levels.' As you might expect, PMR has been found to be an effective treatment for tension headaches. As well, a recent meta-analysis (Palermo et al. 2010) found PMR to be effective in treating chronic pain stating that, 'cognitive-behavioral therapy, relaxation therapy, and biofeedback all produced significant and positive effects on pain reduction.'

A typical PMR session might go as follows. Make sure that your patient is comfortably supported in a quiet place, then:

- To begin with have them take three deep abdominal breaths, exhaling slowly each time. As they exhale, have them visualize tension flowing out of their body.
- Next have them clench both of their fists. Hold that position for 7–10 seconds and then release for 15–20 seconds.
- As they tense their muscles in each and every area of their body have them notice all of the sensations of tension in that region.
- As they relax, likewise have them explore the wonderful feeling of relaxation throughout that area of their body.
- Use a phrase such as 'feel the tension in your forearm, leg, etc.' for each and for every area that you have them create tension.
- Likewise, as you ask them to relax an area, say something like 'now notice the wonderful feeling of relaxation. Feel how wonderful it is to experience the feeling of relaxation in every cell of your body.'
- Use these same time intervals for all other muscle groups.
- Next have them tighten their forearm muscles, hold and then relax.
- Have them tighten their biceps by drawing their forearms up toward their shoulders and 'make a muscle' with both arms. Hold … and then relax.
- Have them tighten up their shoulders, then hold … and then relax.
- Then have them tighten muscles in the whole region, fists, forearms, biceps and shoulders at the same time.
- Have them tighten all of the muscles in their feet, then hold and relax.
- Then follow through the whole body and don't forget anything, even muscles of the face, each time doing individual areas, then the whole region.
- Then have them tense up their entire body, holding tension in every imaginable muscle. Then have them relax their entire body and enjoy the feeling of relaxation.
- Then have them scan their body for any residual tension. If a particular area remains tense, repeat one or two tense–relax cycles for that group of muscles.
- Now have them imagine a wave of relaxation slowly spreading throughout their entire body, starting at their head and gradually penetrating every muscle group, all the way down to their toes.

The entire PMR sequence should take about 20 minutes. Once your patient learns to do the process on their own they may find that it takes less time but by no means do they want to rush through it. That will completely destroy the positive effects of this modality. Your patients can also purchase a CD or download MP3 files that are readily available to guide them through the whole process. As with the relaxation response, practice and patience are required for maximum benefits.

Movement therapies

Movement therapies all require instruction for proficient instructors. Many manual practitioners pursue accreditation in these areas, while most will suggest that their patients attend nearby classes. All movement therapies have multiple benefits including relaxation. There are many other movement therapies that are not listed here, but these ones in particular have relaxation components to them. Each and every movement therapy is in effect an endless journey. There is really no limit to the eventual growth that one can achieve once one decides to commit to any one of these disciplines. By the same token your patient can simply attend weekly classes in one of the following therapies, getting whatever they wish out of the modality.

Qigong

The martial art qigong is an ancient Chinese health care system that combines physical training (such as isometrics, isotonics, and aerobic conditioning) with Eastern philosophy and relaxation techniques. Like most oriental disciplines, there are many different varieties including medical qigong. There are more than 10 000 styles of qigong and almost 200 million people practicing these methods! Some forms are practiced while standing, sitting, or lying down while most involve slow graceful structured movements and controlled breathing techniques to promote the circulation of qi or chi within the human body to enhance the practitioner's overall health. Qigong has been used for centuries in China for the treatment of a variety of medical conditions. Learning qigong involves time, commitment, patience and determination. Learning from a master or group is the recommended method. Persons generally study qigong to gain strength, improve their health or reverse a disease; however, if you pursue it long enough, gaining skill working with qi, you can actually become a healer.

Tai chi

The Westernized version of Tai chi is a series of 19 movements and one pose that together make up a meditative form of exercise to which practitioners attribute physical and spiritual health benefits. Some studies have found the practice to reduce stress and relieve certain ailments. Like qigong, Tai chi is a Chinese martial art. It has been termed a kind of 'meditation in motion' and is characterized by soft, flowing movements that stress precision and force. As with qigong, training from a master is necessary to properly learn the art. Tai chi has recently been studied for its health effects. A 2009 York University workplace study (Tamim et al. 2009) found that, 'Significant improvements in physiological and psychological measures were observed, even at the large class sizes tested here, suggesting that TC has considerable potential as an economic, effective and convenient workplace intervention.' Quoting again from the same study, 'There were significant positive results in several areas including resting heart rate, waist circumference and hand grip strength.' Most urban areas have Tai chi classes. This would be the suggested route if you felt that your patient would benefit from this discipline.

Yoga

If Tai chi and qigong are to be viewed as expressions of eastern philosophy, then likewise yoga can be viewed as an expression of East Indian Hindu philosophy. Like most religious practices, there are hundreds of different schools or approaches. The practice of yoga is believed to be over 5000 years old. Outside India, the term yoga is typically associated with Hatha yoga and its asanas (postures) as a form of exercise. One goal of Hatha yoga is to restore balance and harmony to the body and emotions through numerous postural and breathing exercises. While I have recommended yoga for many of my patients who seem either restricted in motion or just generally out of touch with their bodies, I am always cognizant of the fact that more than any other form of exercise there is a small degree of what some would call 'cultism' or 'religiosity' surrounding the practice of yoga. That being said, there are many instructors out there who attempt to make yoga accessible to Westerners by keeping it as secular as possible and who do not 'sell' the philosophy too strongly. With those caveats aside, yoga is an excellent discipline which aids in relaxation, keeps people more flexible and in touch with their bodies.

- A recent meta-analysis (Ross & Thomas 2010) at the School of Nursing, University of Maryland, Baltimore looked at 10 studies which compared yoga with traditional forms of exercise. This paper concluded that, 'The studies comparing the effects of yoga and exercise seem to indicate that, in both healthy and diseased populations, yoga may be as effective as or better than exercise at improving a variety of health-related outcome measures.'
- A Medline search study by Balaji and colleagues in 2012 reviewed relevant articles in English literature on evaluation of physiological effects of yogic practices and Transcendental Meditation. They found that 'there were considerable health benefits, including improved cognition, respiration, reduced cardiovascular risk, body mass index, blood pressure, and diabetes. Yoga also influenced immunity and ameliorated joint disorders' (Balaji et al. 2012).

Other stress reduction techniques

If you are fortunate enough like me to work as a massage therapist you have an amazing opportunity to reduce your patients' stress in a very real and measurable manner. It is also advisable to remind your patients to recall the stress-free moment that they experience during their massage whenever they feel stressed.

Stress reduction is a big topic these days. While admittedly, there are many stressors in today's world, I am equally sure that our early ancestors also had lots of concerns about where their next meal was coming from and about whether or not they themselves were being hunted by another tribe, or another predator.

The point here is that stress has always been with us as a species. As a matter of fact we are so good at dealing with stress that faced with no challenges or stressors, most of us are very good at creating our own stress. In the end, most stress is created and dwells between our ears and within our own bodies. Learning to deal with stress effectively is definitely an important life skill that we can assist patients with, without moving too far out of our scope of practice. Undoubtedly, the bulk of the regulated health professionals that are reading this book walk the line between allopathic medicine and holistic-alternative-complementary-integrative medicine. As well, most of our patients view manual practitioners as alternative practitioners, and stress management is an important focus within alternative medicine. For this reason, I have included a section at the end of this section entitled 'Getting patients to maximize their own healing response'. There you will find many stress management strategies for your patients.

RECEIVING ADEQUATE EXPLANATION OF THE PATHOLOGY

A positive placebo response is most likely to occur when the meaning of the illness experience is altered in a positive direction. A positive change in meaning occurs when one or more of three things happens: the patient feels listened to and receives a satisfactory, coherent explanation of his illness: the patient feels care and concern from those around him and the patient feels an enhanced sense of mastery and control over his symptoms. Because the meaning that we attach to events in our lives often hinges on the stories we construct about those events, this model helps explain the importance of narrative in medicine.

Howard Brody MD
(Brody 2000b)

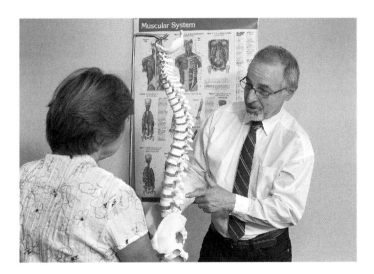

Fig. 2.10.

As this quote indicates, few sections in this book are conceptual islands. This quote actually has relevance to many sections in Part 2. Adequate explanation definitely overlaps with sections on Trust, Establishing a feeling of control, Time spent by the practitioner, The power of listening, and Enhancing meaning through stories. But this is the nature of the holistic approach. Everything is connected to everything else, but for the purposes of study and presentation they are being broken down into separate concepts. Once you apply these ideas, you will blend them into one seamless approach.

The relative nature of explanation

Receiving adequate explanation is an interesting topic. As you might imagine, there is no universal approach here that will work for everyone. This is an area where you really have to know your patient. Some people are the take-charge type when it comes to their health as well as most other aspects of their life. These people typically want detailed explanations of their condition, what your treatment plan will consist of and, often, what they can do for themselves. They are highly motivated, they want logical medical explanations, and they follow through with their homecare because they really want to get back to their activities of daily living as soon as possible. However, this is only one type of patient. When we talk about 'adequate explanation', this is very much a relative term.

In massage therapy, for example, it is not unusual to see a sector of patients who think largely in terms of 'energy'. This type of patient will likely get a glazed look in their eyes if you give them an explanation based on the Western model of medicine, because this is not how their mind thinks. Some patients, even if logically minded, have limited capacity for understanding details of their condition. However, what is universal is that your patient needs to understand, on their own terms, what is going on with their body. We all need to make sense of our world. This is a theme of the previous section on feeling control of their illness as well as the next section on enhancing meaning through stories. We all need to make sense of our world and narrative is the universal way we do that as humans, but the key here is to get to know your patient and appeal to their inner narrative.

Using explanation to allay fears

One of the most basic, even primal human fears is *the unknown*. Some of the most basic universal human fears (Seaward 2006) include the unknown, rejection, failure, isolation, loss of self-dominance and death. Helping our patients with their anxieties around their pathology is an important part of the therapeutic exchange. Anxiety is something that we all experience. We are all actually hardwired for it. The state of anxiety is a part of our survival instinct. The amygdala, a part of our limbic system, plays a primary role in the processing of memory of emotional reactions, particularly fear. Part of the placebo process, as we saw in earlier sections, is the calming of anxieties, allowing the parasympathetic nervous system to do its job of recharging and healing. Sometimes just the naming of a fear can cause it to lose its power over us. You have undoubtedly heard the expression '*name it and claim it*'. This is particularly useful around fears. Once you give a fear a name, it loses some of its power over us. This is probably due, in part, to the fact that the fear is no longer in that realm of the subconscious. Naming it causes it to enter the land of the living, the conscious realm, where we can begin to wrestle it to the ground. Explanation of the pathology to the patient does this. It names the enemy, allowing the patient to move from victim to someone who can develop power over his or her body.

There are many aspects to the topic of giving your patients explanations. For example, you can explain to a patient who is apprehensive about their pain that pain is a signal from their body, that it is a process that will run its course, and that as their therapist/practitioner, you will guide them through this process. This is employing explanation along with your pledge of commitment, both of which will help to alleviate their anxieties surrounding their situation.

Another thing worth mentioning is that based on the information presented in this book, we can see that when projecting a future course of your patient's pathology it is wise to err on the side of a positive projection. It is in fact ethical and in the patient's best interest to do so. This is perhaps a difficult line to walk for many of us. We do not want to deceive the patient, nor do we want to produce false expectations; however, studies consistently show the power of positive thinking on people's conditions. Your job is to help them with a positive mind-frame, no matter what their condition, whether chronic or acute. Acute conditions are perhaps easier, because they are typically self-limiting. There is usually a more predictable time course for the illness, and you can relay the typical course and suggest that many people's symptoms resolve on the lesser side of the suggested timeframe. Chronic illnesses are somewhat different. Hopefully for all parties concerned, you are being presented with a condition with which you have had reasonable success in the past. This puts you in the best position to confidently project a positive prognosis, and a projected time frame for their condition.

Shared decision-making

A study of 102 women and 73 men at Royal Prince Alfred Hospital in Camperdown, Australia entitled, 'A matter of trust' (Salkeld et al. 2004) revealed the wide diversity of attitudes mentioned previously among patients. Persons in this study were all receiving treatment for colorectal cancer. Interestingly enough, 58% of women preferred a SDM role in their healthcare compared with 36% of men. Older patients, not surprisingly, were significantly more likely to prefer that their surgeon decide upon treatment when compared with younger patients. But the conclusion drawn by the researchers was very interesting, and it led to the renaming of the study to 'A matter of trust'. In Glen Salkeld's words:

> *Regardless of whether a patient prefers an active or more passive role in decision-making, having a surgeon explain treatment options in a clear, unhurried and open manner is vital to how patients feel about their treatment. Whilst acknowledging that individual patients will have different needs for information and preferences for treatment, there are several factors amongst many in the process of decision-making which are considered very important by patients with CRC. A surgeon who adopts a consultation style that is open and informative, that offers patients the chance to participate in the process of decision-making and **clearly** explains treatment options and outcomes will engender trust with their patient.*

Trust is a theme that we see surfacing constantly when it comes to improving patient outcomes. Anything that you can do to build trust with your patient will improve your relationship with them, and increase your chances of turning on their inner healing systems. Explaining the pathology, the treatment plan and the homecare to your patient is one important way to build trust with your patient.

Explanation: the most important aspect of treatment, after clinical competence

I am, by calling, a dealer in words; and words are, of course, the most powerful drug used by mankind.

Rudyard Kipling

Words that we use with our patients are extremely powerful, whether it is words to provide information, words to explain the illness or the treatment, or simply words to put the patient at ease. One study which was effectively a comparison of patients' and physicians' opinions found that both parties agreed that (as you might guess) clinical skill is most important; however, patients ranked provision of information second in importance whereas physicians ranked it sixth (Laine et al. 1996). This is an important piece of information to keep in mind as you interact with your patient. Whether time is limited or not, it is important to take the time to explain the following:

- What is going on with their body to the best of your understanding
- What you plan to do about it
- What the patient can do about it
- And how the recovery is likely to progress.

One very good reason for adequate explanation is to achieve a high degree of patient adherence. A 2009 meta-analysis of the exact subject of physician communication and patient adherence to treatment (Haskard-Zolnierek & DiMatteo 2009) contains the following quote:

Communication in medical care is highly correlated with better patient adherence, and training physicians to communicate better enhances their patients' adherence. Findings can contribute to medical education and to interventions to improve adherence, supporting arguments that communication is important and resources devoted to improving it are worth investing in. Communication is thus an important factor over which physicians have some control in helping their patients to adhere.

Open versus hidden trials

One more good reason for explaining what you are doing as you conduct your treatment is that several studies have shown (as you might expect) that when participants were either made aware that they were receiving a placebo with basic standard care versus participants receiving standard care without the placebo, there is found to be substantial improvement in the placebo group. The 2010 Harvard study by Kaptchuk and co-workers entitled 'Placebos without deception: a randomized controlled trial in irritable bowel syndrome' (Kaptchuk et al. 2010) mentioned earlier in the section 'Ethics and informed consent' provides useful insight into explaining your treatment. This study involved 80 participants diagnosed with IBS, a condition known to respond to placebos. The study was designed to test whether open-label placebo (non-deceptive and non-concealed administration) is superior to a no-treatment control. Patients were randomized to receive either open-label placebo pills presented as 'placebo pills made of an inert substance, like sugar pills, that have been shown in clinical studies to produce significant improvement in IBS symptoms through mind–body self-healing processes' or no-treatment controls with the same quality of interaction with providers. What they found was that the open-label placebo produced significantly higher improvement scores both in subjective and objective measurement scores than the no-treatment group. Note that the researchers did not just say, 'We are going to give you a sugar pill.' They presented the context of the placebo so that a) there was no deception about the fact that it was a placebo and b) they were informed that clinical studies showed that there had been significant improvement in others with the same condition who had taken the same pills (or followed that same course of treatment) through mind–body self-healing processes. This directly applies to what those of us in the manual therapy profession do. If we explain what we are doing as we apply our treatment, there will be an improvement in the outcome.

Another trial, performed at University of Turin in Italy, speaks directly to the importance of explaining the treatment (Benedetti et al. 2003a). The researchers begin by explaining that any medical treatment has two components, with the first being the specific effects of the treatment itself, and the second being the knowledge that the treatment is being performed (the placebo effect). The researchers created an analgesia study, in which post-surgical patients were randomized to receive their analgesics in the ordinary fashion from a clinician, or secretly by computer-controlled infusion through an intravenous line. The results show that the hidden administrations of pharmacological and non-pharmacological therapies are less effective than the open ones. It is also worth noting that while it is not the topic of this section, but the clinicians' presence in these studies increased the effectiveness of the treatment (as reported on a standard 10-point pain scale) by about a third. This in itself is a significant finding, that the same analgesic is 33% more effective if administered by a clinician. Apart from the important take-home point of explaining your treatment, it is important to remember that you are always a walking placebo pill yourself!

Encouraging questions from your patient

Explanation implies of course that you are trying to increase your patient's understanding of their condition. One of the best ways to ensure their understanding is to encourage questions from them. When explaining, take your time and be sure to look for body language and words from your patient that would indicate that they have a question about their condition. During the explanation or particularly at the end, be sure and ask them if they have any questions at all about their situation. For more on this important topic please consult the section on listening.

Examples of adequate explanation

1. Take the time to explain your patient's pathology in terms that are understandable to them. Meet them at their level. Examples are:
   - '*Mr J, your tests indicate that you have thoracic outlet syndrome. Thoracic outlet is…*'
   - '*Mrs G, your symptoms indicate to me that your heart meridian indicates a deficiency and is blocked in these areas.*'
   - '*Mr H, the body has its own energy field. At times this field gets blocked.*'
2. Remember that even if your patient tends to be the non-engaged type that you still take the time to give them an adequate explanation.
3. Explanation includes the treatment plan that you will jointly agree to:
   - '*This condition responds well to manual therapy. I would suggest two 20 minute treatments per week for 2 weeks, and then we can assess your situation. How do you feel about that?*'
4. Explanation involves not only what has happened to date, but also what the future course of their condition is likely to take, for example:
   - '*In my experience, with manual therapy and homecare, this condition will usually resolve itself in 4–6 weeks.*'
5. It is in the patient's interest to err on the side of a positive prognosis:
   - '*In my experience, with manual therapy and homecare, this condition will usually resolve itself in 4–6 weeks, but I have seen many people back to work in as little as 2 weeks.*'
6. A good explanation will allow and even encourage questions from the patient, so that their understanding is as complete as possible, for example:
   - '*My assessment of your condition is…(adequate explanation). Do you have any questions at all?*'
   - '*If you have any questions at any time, feel free to interrupt me during the treatment.*'

Conclusion

Depending upon your medical model, you may or may not have an abundance of time with your patients. In many manual therapy professions, we often have large blocks of time with our patients and, as a result, can give them as much background information and explanation as needed, without feeling pressed for time. If your model is different from this, then it is even more important to remember the importance of listening and explanation. It is very important to make time for these matters. If you run out of time during an appointment, then it is important to schedule a new appointment so that you have the time to listen and to provide an adequate explanation and address any concerns that your patient might have.

THE NARRATIVE: HOW WE MAKE SENSE OF THE WORLD

There have been great societies that did not use the wheel, but there have been no societies that did not tell stories.

Ursula K. Le Guin

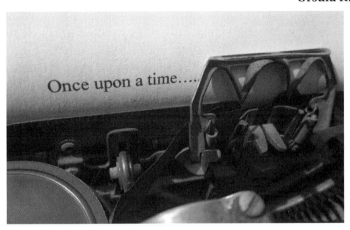

Fig. 2.11

One of the things about writing this book that I have enjoyed is the many roads, avenues and side streets that it has taken me on (you know... kind of like the Internet). The narrative is one such side street, but it is in fact a very interesting and important side street. I am not an expert on the topic of narrative, or maybe we are all, in fact, experts in this area without even realizing it. Many experts argue that the narrative (the story that we use to describe virtually every experience of our life) is a fundamental organizing principle of human experience. In the 1970s and early 1980s, there was a substantial amount of interest in the Artificial Intelligence (AI) field in story understanding and, in particular, story generation. Since the meaning of any given sentence is rarely determinable in isolation, because it requires relating the sentence to other sentences around it, to prior experience, and to some larger context, it seemed to make sense to bring narrative into AI. Eventually this was abandoned; not because narrative is not important, but because the models were intensely knowledge-based, which meant that these early AI models functioned only in very limited domains and could be made more general only by an intensive and likely infeasible knowledge engineering process. This basically changed AI forever because after that AI researchers moved toward making it more like engineering than a craft or an art. This requires that models focus on specific problems with discrete measurable outcomes.

So, it would seem that robots of the present and immediate future will live in the world of facts and figures, tasks and solutions. They will not live in the world that you and I live in; that is the world of a narrative. Without a story, few of us can give meaning to most experiences. Within storytelling, there is also a degree of plasticity. Undoubtedly, you have experienced a situation where you were next to someone whose version of events was quite different from yours.

Reaching a personal understanding of the power of the narrative is a way of giving meaning to our lives that is, in my opinion, literally life changing. For me, it was a real epiphany, or 'ah-hah' moment when I realized that I was writing the story of my own life. We all get to be author of our own life story, and in this story there are heroes and villains, winners and losers, love and loss. It is important for all of us to realize that as we write the story of our life, we alone get to decide whether we or others are victim or a hero. This is the point in anyone's life when the penny drops. In other words, this is an extremely significant realization in one's personal journey.

Writing about trauma

Let's look at some studies that elucidate things about storytelling. In one interesting study psychologist James Pennebaker, at the University of Texas, asked two groups of volunteers with chronic pain to sit down daily and write. The first group were asked to write stories about trauma (either their own or of others) for 15 minutes per day for 4 consecutive days. Those in the second (control) group also had four 15-minute sessions but were asked to write about anything that was non-narrative such as their plans for the day, shopping lists or aspects of the room that they were in. Would you expect a different outcome in these two groups? Researchers were shocked to find that as they followed the students' illness visits to the university health centre in the months before and after the experiment that those who had written about their thoughts and feelings drastically reduced their doctor-visit rates after the study when compared with the control participants who had written about trivial topics. Confronting traumatic experiences had a salutary effect on the physical health of the participants (Pennebaker & Seagal 1999).

So my doctor said to me, write a short story and call me in the morning!

Anonymous

During the 1990s, more than two dozen studies confirmed and extended those findings. A 1999 paper by James Pennebaker and Janel Seagal entitled, 'Forming a story: the health benefits of narrative', gathered the findings from these studies and combined with their student study and found the following surprising benefits from storytelling exercises. Benefits were found across different populations including maximum-security prisoners, medical students, distressed crime victims, arthritis and chronic pain sufferers, men laid off from their jobs, and women who had recently given birth to their first child. These effects have been found in all social classes and major racial ethnic groups. Writing influenced more than just physician visits. Documented benefits included positive effects on blood markers of immune function (T-helper cell growth, antibody response to the Epstein–Barr virus and antibody response to hepatitis B vaccinations), lower pain, decreased medication use and lower levels of depression. Additional experiments even demonstrated that the exercise of writing (that is to say, constructing a series of events into a narrative format) is linked to higher grades in college and reduced unemployment periods among senior-level engineers who have been laid off from their jobs (Pennebaker & Seagal 1999). There were no clear connections between personality types and benefits conferred from writing. Anyone engaging in this activity was potentially able to receive health benefits.

Just what is happening here? It is not possible from these studies to understand why writing stories appears to have health benefits, but researchers have working theories. The thinking is that the act of constructing stories is a natural human process that helps people to understand their experiences and themselves. As long as people have been around, they have told stories. In cultures that did not have written language, stories were passed down through an oral tradition. The process of writing first involves remembering. It then requires one to organize in a coherent fashion while simultaneously integrating thoughts and feelings. You could say that process gives individuals a sense of predictability and control over their lives. Constructing a story can lead to a sense of resolution about events which hopefully leads to less need to keep reliving the event and make sense of it.

Disclosure is unequivocally at the core of psychotherapy (and confession). The area of narrative psychology has long held that it is important for people to make sense of events in their lives by putting them into a story-like format (Gergen & Gergen 1988). So, when we write in a narrative format, we are engaging in self-therapy. Interestingly enough despite the clear health benefits, writing about traumatic experiences typically tends to make participants more unhappy and distressed during and for several hours after writing. Many people were in tears as they wrote about their experiences.*

Computer analysis of stories was also quite telling. Stories were first analyzed for use of positive and negative words. Then frequency was categorized as 'few', 'moderate' or 'many words' having positive and negative context. People who tended to use many words in the positive category and a moderate amount in the negative category had the greatest health improvements. The stories were also analyzed for words deemed insightful or causal. The analyses showed

---

*It is worth noting here that the process of writing about trauma is a painful process that can leave patients feeling sad and in pain as they relive the trauma. The payoff here is short-term pain for long-term gain. The benefits of this exercise appear to be well established.

strong and consistent effects for changes in insight and causal words over the course of writing. That is to say that people whose health improved, who got higher grades and who found jobs after writing went from using relatively few causal and insight words to using a high rate of them by the last day of writing (Pennebaker & Seagal 1999).

An interesting twist on this theory was presented when a study by Greenberg and colleagues asked previously traumatized students to write about an imaginary trauma rather than something they had experienced directly (Greenberg et al. 1996). Results of this study indicated that writing about someone else's trauma as though they had lived through it produced health benefits comparable to a separate group who wrote about their own traumas. Many of the findings in these studies appear counterintuitive at first, but on reflection, they all tend to indicate that organizing one's thoughts and making sense of traumatic events appears to confer health benefits. There is not a soul walking this planet that does not need to make sense of the world. I cannot tell you how many times I have heard people say 'everything happens for a reason'. I personally do not subscribe to the destiny school of thought, but it clearly demonstrates people's need to make sense of the chaos of the world that we live in. The philosophy of destiny is clearly rooted in this need to make sense of a disordered world. Whether one uses destiny, or any other vehicle to understand and make sense of the world, one has to use some vehicle, or else you are left floating around aimlessly in a chaotic world, and that is not a pleasant experience for anyone.

A constructed story, therefore, is a type of knowledge that helps to organize the emotional effects of an experience as well as the experience itself in your mind so that it makes sense to you. You can see from this discussion that if you encourage your challenging patients who have had a long and difficult journey (health or otherwise) to keep a 'narrative journal', it may help them to make sense of their struggle, reinforce progress and support more positive behaviour patterns. Don't just have them write measurements, facts and figures. They need to actually write in a narrative format. No one ever need see anything that they write. Once the story has been written, it can be deleted or ritually burned. We are not psychotherapists, and it is certainly not our role to analyze or to read their story, but only to convey the fact that numerous studies show many benefits from journaling about one's illness.

Active listening revisited

The giving and listening to the testimony of the ill is an important social practice by which, in the end, all of us are healed.

Arthur Frank

Something else to keep in mind as you have patients with either chronic or intense pain is that suffering is not the same as pain. Suffering happens in context.

Two persons can have the same pain but very different amounts of suffering. The difference is the story that each constructs around their pain. For example, if you hit your thumb with a hammer (as I have been known to do) it is excruciatingly painful. But you know that this pain will pass fairly quickly and the body will heal itself, so you put up with the throbbing thumb. Conversely, if you are diagnosed with cancer while simultaneously being pain-free, clearly the cancer diagnosis will induce more suffering. Suffering happens, as was said, in the context of a narrative; the story that you have built around your pain. Howard Brody says, 'A story of suffering is a story of meaninglessness, isolation and hopelessness. Suffering may persist even though the patient gets extensive medical treatment, so long as the story does not change.' If the patient cannot change their own story then we need to help them to change their story. One way of doing this is with 'active listening.' If you skipped that section, then now would be a good time to look at it. Listening is not a passive process. As you listen to your patient, you can actually help them to construct new stories around their pain and suffering with constructive input.

The hero's journey

Arthur Frank, a sociologist who survived cancer and a heart attack in his 30s spent a lot of time studying the stories of people's lives that had been irrevocably changed by illness. He found that people's stories fell into three basic categories: chaos, restitution, and the quest. **Chaos** is hopefully a temporary state; however, some patients do get stuck in this phase. This type of story is typically a tangle of emotion containing much confusion, with story and non-story elements within it. This narrative (and non-narrative) is difficult for others to listen to and often drives people away.

A **restitution** story, according to Frank, is either a short story with a doctor hero, or a longer story with a series of treatments with traditional and complementary practitioners with the last practitioner becoming the hero in the story. The patient eventually gets on with his or her life without the illness leaving a permanent mark on their identity. These are often great stories with a beginning, a middle and a happy ending; however, these stories are often a bit too simplistic, denying elements of the aging process and the temporal nature of life. They bear a similarity to long fairy tales.

Finally there is the **quest**. These stories often begin with an injury, and illness, a quest or a hardship (think Tolkien). There are adventures, suffering and foes along the way. Helpful strangers befriend the hero(ine) and bequeath various tools and magic spells. In the end the hero(ine) returns home, but has been deepened and toughened by the experiences. The hero(ine) also returns with new skills and wisdom, which are then shared with those to whom (s)he has returned. As fanciful as this story sounds, this is the story that all of us, according to Frank, need to create. We need to become the central hero in the story of our own lives. There are, as

indicated, very important figures that we encounter that are absolutely life changing for us, and we might well call them heroes, but if we are not the hero in the
story that we create, we end up becoming a victim in our life story.*

The world certainly is large and mysterious, and this is the magic in our story.
We explore this idea in a later section, 'Acceptance of the mystery of healing'.

In Arthur Frank's view, many people with chronic pain suffer terribly because
they are still clinging to restitution stories that do not work for them, and have not
yet figured how to tell a quest story. 'They are already well along on their journey,
but don't realize it, so have not yet created the hero's quest story'. Our task is to
encourage them to rewrite their personal story, not by deceiving themselves, but
by incorporating more positive and meaningful elements into their life/health
story. One of the ways that we can do this is by active listening with constructive
input at the appropriate moment. Another method involves encouraging them to
do private, confidential narrative exercises at home. A good book to guide them in
this process is *Writing to Heal* (Pennebaker 2004).

Final words from Dr Balfour Mount

Finally I would like to touch on something dear to my heart. What do you say to
someone who has more burden than they can carry? At times in the past I felt
as if I was at a loss for words when I encountered friends and relatives who were
overwrought with tragedy. Likewise, many of us have had patients who were facing a terminal diagnosis, or for whom life is/was highly limited, and their time on
earth was drawing near. Like all of life; we live it one day at a time, but we still need
a frame of reference (a narrative) to give the experience meaning, and to be able
to process it and accept the experience as an important part of one's life. A life
narrative attempts to explain where we are coming from and where we are going
to, and admittedly death's final door awaits us all at the end of this journey. Religious souls out there may find solace and comfort in the idea of an afterlife with
a place in heaven. But that is not where many patient's beliefs lie. What can you
say to these people when at times things seem hopeless, or they are at the end of
their physical life? What story can be constructed around their experience? It is at
this time that I find comfort in the words of Dr Balfour Mount, founding Director
of the Royal Victoria Hospital Palliative Care Service, the Palliative Care program

---

*If you happen to find the theme of the hero interesting, then I highly recommend reading just about anything
by the late, great Joseph Campbell. Frank has undoubtedly borrowed heavily from Campbell's work and I guess
that you could say 'medicalized' the message. Joseph Campbell studied cultures from around the world and
found one theme constantly ran though the stories of every culture, the hero's journey. Campbell's ideas about
mythology, mythological stories and the importance of the hero are truly timeless and they greatly affected my
life and rang a very strong chord with me as I was developing my own ideas about what was really important
in life; why humans seek religion and just what the enduring things in life really are. His book The Hero with
a Thousand Faces is particularly relevant to this chapter. There is also an excellent video entitled 'Finding Joe'
(2011) that explores various quotes of Joseph Campbell and uses them to tell the story of the hero's journey
through several peoples' eyes. This movie is 80 minutes long, but I highly recommend it for you as a therapist
and for any patient who is stuck, or who shows interest in the narrative format.

at McGill University and the McGill Programs in Integrated Whole Person Care. Balfour Mount has dedicated his life to end of life care. I extracted the following quote from an interview of him for the CBC program, 'Ideas', on the topic of pain. This quote is not borne out of idealism; it is borne out of a lifetime of experience working with terminally ill patients.

> *When I think of transcendence, I mean our capacity to see beyond the ego dominated self to see our connectedness…our part of the greater whole. I don't have a romantic perception of death. I've seen too much, for too long a time to romanticize death and illness, and I've experienced too much personally to be talking out of theory. I'm talking out of experience, and the experience that I'm talking of encourages me that life need not get the best of us, that the best of us is within us to bring to life, and that we need never be beaten, whatever the situation.*

Balfour Mount

I found this passage to be so inspiring that it still affects me deeply when I read it. I have always kept a copy of it on file for inspiration in difficult times. Our final story is undoubtedly the most important story that any one of us constructs. Whether religious or not, we need to understand and create a story that connects us to the whole world. We already are intimately connected to everything; we just need to be reminded at times. My sense is that this is an important realization to come to, both as a human being and as a health practitioner.

ACCEPTANCE OF THE MYSTERY OF HEALING

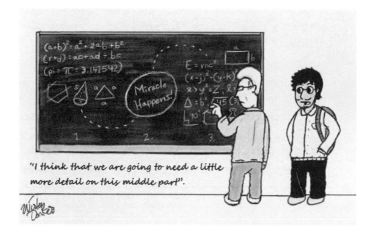

Fig. 2.12

Acceptance of the mystery of healing is discussed in Howard Brody's book, *The Placebo Response*. The mystery of healing is not a popular scientific notion since we are talking about what is not yet understood. It is not evidence-based largely because these modes of healing have not been systematically pursued by the regulated health professions. Still, there are some research papers on the topic. If this topic gets too far-fetched for you, then simply move on to the next chapter. The material that is available on PubMed had such titles as, 'Esoteric healing traditions: a conceptual overview', 'Shamanism as a healing paradigm for complementary therapy', and 'What is esoteric healing? 'Overall, scientific papers do not appear to dismiss the possibility that this type of healing is taking place. There seems to be recognition that there are some very mysterious and unexplained things happening in the area of healing and healers. Shamanism and other esoteric forms of healing are not the subject matter of this book, but what it is important to address is the fact that even as extremely competent health professionals, we can at best 'affect' the healing process. The rest we leave up to the patient's own healing system, the universe, or what some would call God. Most of us in the manual therapy professions sense that while we are working at one level with the body, that there are untold things happening at many (perhaps countless) other levels. If you think for one minute that we understand the body or healing, or the mysteries of the universe, then perhaps it is time to let go of that notion. If you somehow had the magical opportunity to return to this planet in 1000 years, you would not even recognize the medical system and your profession or mine would undoubtedly not even exist. Our mistake, which is a mistake of pride, is to assume that because we have made apparent progress in our understanding of the body and that we have built fancy machines and developed amazing technologies that we now know most of what is going on with the world and our bodies. A quote from Einstein, one of the smartest men in the last century saying, 'We still do not know one thousandth of one percent of what nature has revealed to us', reinforces this idea. In massage therapy school studying pathology, I was shocked to see the phrase 'etiology unknown' describing so many of the diseases that we studied. Even if you look at the diseases where the origin is known, there are often variants deemed idiopathic because the original trigger is not known. This is all to emphasize the point that there is so much that we do not yet understand.

Once you accept the notion that you only have a partial handle on what is happening, it is rather easy to entertain the concept of the mystery of healing. Even something as simple as a cut finger, for example; it is quite amazing to watch it heal without the medical professional or the patient doing anything. There is a whole cascade of chemicals and events that bring the healing from the acute phase to complete resolution. This simple process is actually quite complicated on a biochemical level. If you just look at the acute phase, several cells get in on the action including macrophages, dendritic cells, histiocytes, Kupffer cells and mastocytes. A biochemical cascade involving cytokines, tumor necrosis factor, interlukin-1 and interlukin-6 come into play. There are acute phase proteins involved such as C-reactive protein, serum amyloid A, and haptoglobin. This is just part of what is happening with a simple paper cut. The good news is that neither you nor your patient really needs to know this information. This all happens automatically thanks to the wisdom of the body, a cooperative community of over 30 trillion cells (Bianconi et al. 2013). To me there is an amazing mystery in what we already know, let alone what we do not know. It is the unknown to which the chapter title refers. You can only understand and control so much, and likewise your patient can only understand and control so much of what is happening in their body. The rest we have to give up to the wisdom of the body and the mystery of healing.

Perhaps we are talking about faith here, but this word arrives with a copious share of religious baggage, which may or may not be welcome by the patient. We could be talking about a case where your patient might be frustrated because she is eating right, exercising and following all of your homecare advice and still does not understand why her healing is stalled. At some point, after the patient has done everything possible and all options have been exhausted but full function is not restored, or pain is not reduced to a background level, then it may be time to accept that like almost everything else in life, much of it is beyond your control, and what will be will be. This still does not preclude miracles, though. They do happen, and they actually happen all the time all over the world. Acceptance of the mystery of healing also involves being open to these sort of possibilities as well.

One of the images concerning the mystery of healing that arises in my mind is the wonder of a child. Most of us sadly tend to lose that child-like sense of wonder as we get older, and I'm not really sure that it serves us well. On the one hand, it is good to understand processes so that we don't fall prey to snake oil salesmen.

On the other hand, something is truly lost when one loses one's sense of wonder. You can find pleasure in the simplest of things and you can believe that anything is possible if you keep your sense of wonder intact. With this in mind, it seems to me that our sense of wonder can serve us well, not only in our youth but also through-out our entire life. It is not a requirement that we have this sense of wonder, but there is actually a greater chance of something happening if we are open to the idea of something happening. With the acceptance of the mystery of healing there is not only an acceptance of the wisdom of the body and the universe, there is also an opening up to the possibility of a miracle, or miracles.

So what is the take-home message of this section?

This is a concept that you cannot use on every patient, but is perhaps useful for patients at both ends of the spectrum of wonder. For the frustrated, jaded patient, it is good to accept the fact that much is beyond our control and that nature will run its course as it sees fit. This, in effect, is putting trust in the universe, or God, or the wisdom of their body. For the patient who is open to the wonder of the world, it is a way for you to relate to them on a new level and encourage a mindset that allows and encourages miracles to happen.

Box 2.2

CERTAINTY OF THE PATIENT

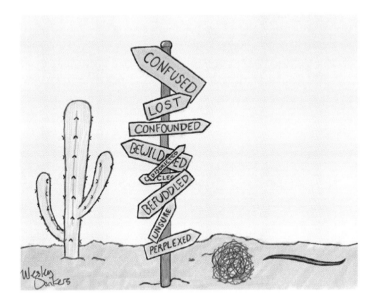

Fig. 2.13

You may recall the study at an out-patient clinic (Park & Covi 1965) discussed in the section on expectations. In this study, 15 patients diagnosed with a 'neurosis' were given a placebo with full disclosure that it was in fact an inert pill. Although they were all told that they were being given a placebo, not everyone was sure that they were actually receiving one. Patients filled out a detailed symptom checklist before taking pills, and then again after 1 week of pill taking. All but one of the 15 participants who agreed to the study returned 1 week later. Thirteen of these saw improvements. Participants where then queried about what they believed was going on. What they heard from participants were basically three different scenarios. In the first scenario participants took the placebo to placate the researchers, still *believing that they had been given an inert pill*. In the second scenario, participants *believed that they were given an active drug*, not a placebo. Both of these groups were described in this study as seeing 'substantial' improvement. The third-reported scenario was that participants weren't really sure what was going on. They did not know if researchers were trying to trick them or what. Interestingly enough, this is the group that saw the least improvement. The study points to the importance of certainty within the patient's mind as an important factor. This brings to mind the famous song by The Clash, 'Should I stay or should I go?'. The cognitive dissonance and psychoemotional stress that is created by indecision definitely robs us of much of our healing powers. We all recognize that in the final analysis, there is rarely if ever a path that leads to entirely positive consequences or that leads to only negative outcomes. Life is always much more complicated than that. In the end, however, after weighing out the merits of any decision, it is to our advantage to commit to it and see it through.

If we see this type of fence-sitting behaviour that is robbing our patients of their healing ability, we need to encourage them to make a decision and move ahead with their life. No decision will yield entirely positive or negative outcomes, because life is never that simple. What is important is that they get off the fence, accept all of the good and bad that comes with it, and get on with their life.

In the study of patients hospitalized with peptic ulcers mentioned earlier, 70% showed excellent results, lasting over a period of 1 year when given an injection of distilled water and told that it was a new medication that would definitely cure them. The second group were given an injection of distilled water and told that it was an experimental medication yet to be proven. This group saw only 25% improvement (Volgyesi 1954). We can clearly see here the benefits of patient certainty. As a practitioner, you play an important role in planting the seeds of certainty or uncertainty.

Benefits of a clear diagnosis

One interesting study (Thomas 1987) that elucidates the concept of certainty selected 200 patients who had presented in general practice with symptoms but no abnormal physical signs and for whom no clear diagnosis was determined. Thomas then devised an interesting experiment dividing them into four random groups:

- Those in A1 were given a firm diagnosis and were told that the symptoms would resolve in a few days. No medication was given and patients were told that medication was not necessary for this condition.
- Those in A2 were given a firm diagnosis and were told that the symptoms would resolve in a few days. Patients were told that administered medication (a placebo) would definitely make them better.
- Those in B1 were told, *'I cannot be certain what is wrong with you.'* This group was administered a medication and told, *'I am not sure that this treatment will have an effect. If you are no better in a few days then return for follow-up.'*
- Those in B2 were told *'I cannot be certain what is wrong with you and therefore I will not prescribe anything for you at this time. If you are no better in a few days then return for follow-up.'*

Analysis of the results revealed the biggest statistical difference was found between groups A and B. The patients with a clear diagnosis group were on the whole twice as satisfied with their visit and 63% of them improved versus 3% of the two groups with no clear diagnosis. There was no statistical difference in health improvement between A1 and A2, or between B1 and B2. That is to say that in this study it did not seem to matter whether a treatment was given or not, but it did make a substantial difference that a diagnosis was made.

There are two lessons to be learned from this study. Firstly, a better health outcome can be expected if the patient has some degree of certainty about their symptoms and their prognosis. What that means from our perspective is that it is best to give a clear diagnosis (or in the case of some professions, give the patient a clear assessment if you do not have the medical authority to diagnose). This is the best way to help our patients with minor and vague symptoms that we feel could be idiopathic or psychosomatic in nature. Secondly, if there is no clear diagnosis that you feel that you can make, there are several things that you could say so that the patient is not left in the lurch, and yet not deceived. For example:

- *'This area appears inflamed (if you do indeed think that there is some inflammation),'* then give them a prescription or suggest a short-term homecare regimen for the inflammation. As we have learned from other sections, the homecare regimen is best given as a prescription or handout rather than just as a verbal suggestion.
- *'This is what we term idiopathic pain. I have seen this many times before in a number of my patients. This issue typically resolves within 2 weeks.'* You can then suggest a homecare regimen that they can follow.

The importance of thorough testing

One important aspect of treatment is doing all necessary tests to determine exactly what condition one is treating. As it turns out, these tests are not only for our benefit as practitioners, but they also affect the psychology of the patient. A study at Stanford University School of Medicine tested this hypothesis by measuring clinical outcomes of 176 patients with non-specific chest pain (Sox et al. 1981). Patients were randomly allocated either to have a routine electrocardiogram and serum creatine phosphokinase tests or, in the case of the second group, to have all diagnostic tests withheld. Fewer patients in the group receiving tests reported short-term disability than patients in the no-test group. Statistical analysis confirmed that the use of diagnostic tests was an independent predictor of recovery. Patients in the test group felt that care was 'better than usual', more often than patients in the no-test group. What this tells us is that it is extremely important to perform appropriate tests on our patients, both to increase our certainty, and theirs as well. If you have any doubt whether to perform any given orthopedic test then definitely perform it. Most orthopedic tests can be performed in less than a minute, and these tests will not only increase your certainty, but they will increase the certainty and confidence of your patients as well. If ordering radiological tests are beyond your scope of practice and you feel that a test is warranted then definitely suggest to your patient that they urge their primary care physician to consider ordering a test. If you are fortunate enough to have a relationship with the doctor, you could advocate on the patient's behalf, or perhaps write a letter for the patient to give to their doctor.

The power of certainty

Another example of certainty is the study of hotel workers, mentioned previously (see p. 13), which looked at the relationship between exercise and health being moderated by one's mindset (Crum & Langer 2007). The participants who could be described as more 'certain' that their jobs gave them adequate exercise showed a decrease in weight, blood pressure, body fat, waist-to-hip ratio and body mass index. The group that did not adopt this belief system saw none of these changes. What is pertinent is that the activity level in neither group had changed. What changed was their belief system.

Another illustration of the power of certainty is when one tries to quit smoking, tackle a large task, make a life change or any other life decision that requires discipline. There is a definite and clear power that comes from mental certainty. I have used the concept of certainty more than once in my life to achieve both major and minor goals and have witnessed it countless times in others. Although this counts only as anecdotal evidence, undoubtedly you can think of many examples in your own life which certainly generated a power that allowed you to achieve a personal goal. People that tackle difficult tasks are at a much higher risk of failure if they lack certainty about the outcome. This is not about positive thinking. Positive thinking is an entirely different matter altogether. Certainty is more along the idea of single-mindedness and the power that comes from certainty. There are many anecdotal examples to be found where patients were completely cured from a neurosis, depression or pain when given a sugar pill that they were certain would 'cure' them. This happened with reasonable regularity before the establishment of patient rights and informed consent in 1962. Before then it was not uncommon for a doctor to prescribe or dispense a placebo to their patients and there are undoubtedly hundreds of thousands of clinical cases where patients improved after being given a placebo that they were certain would cure or help them.

The body language of certainty

What is also recognized about certainty is that there is a specific body language associated with that particular state of mind, just as there is unique body language associated with say anxiety, depression or shame. The body language of certainty is a more upright posture than the other three postures, conveying vitality and health. Patients will subconsciously read your body language and it would serve you well to school yourself in reading their body language. It will go a long way toward helping you gather more information about them and their condition as well as to guide them along a healthier path.

Clinical application

How can you address this matter in your own clinical environment?

This falls very much under the heading of expectations and much of the advice in that section addresses the matter of patient certainty. The focus here is not only creating expectations of outcomes, but rather helping your patients realize that if they increase their certainty of an outcome, the outcome is more likely to manifest, whether the goal is medical or otherwise. Helping them (and yourself) arrive at this realization will help reduce the cognitive dissonance that robs energy from our body's own ability to heal itself.

Other things to keep in mind are:
- When in doubt, perform appropriate orthopedic testing.
- If at all possible, try to give a clear diagnosis of the condition.
- Be aware of the patient's body language around certainty. If you sense uncertainty, then broach the subject with your patient; then be sure to listen to and address their concerns.

Box 2.3

TIME SPENT BY THE PRACTITIONER

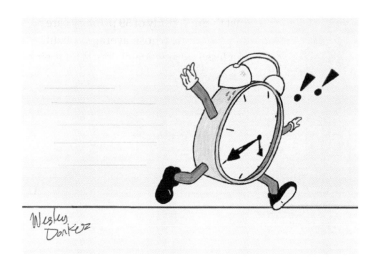

Fig. 2.14

I hope that you have found some interesting counterintuitive surprises in this book, as I have in researching various topics. However, much of the information concerning placebo response and improved clinical outcomes is common sense. In the 21st century, common sense is not enough; practitioners always need evidence to back up their procedures and methods. Einstein once said, 'Common sense is the collection of prejudices acquired by age 18'. With that in mind, it is always good to make sure that your common sense is based on fact, and not a preconceived notion. Literature surrounding the notion of time spent with the patient makes basic intuitive sense. If the patient feels as if they are rushed in and out quickly they will not feel satisfied with the treatment, but interestingly enough as the treatment time increases one sees diminishing returns. What becomes more important then, is what you do with your time. Let's look at some of the data.

Less time equals less patient satisfaction

Like and Zyzanski performed a patient survey in a university-based family practice in Cleveland to discover the determinants of patient satisfaction (Like & Zyzanski 1987). They found that patients who stated they wished they had spent more time with the physician were less satisfied with their medical encounter. One British study showed that by just adding 1 minute to medical consultations improved doctor–patient communication in multiple areas (Wilson et al. 1992). Two other studies from Britain found a greater likelihood of patients feeling they had inadequate time with their physician if visits lasted 5 minutes compared with visits lasting 10 and 15 minutes (Dugdale 1999).

Less time increases frequency of malpractice claims

Research also shows a definite link between time spent with the patient and the number of malpractice claims against them. A study of 59 primary care physicians in Oregon and Colorado found that physicians whose average consultation time was 18.3 minutes were experiencing less malpractice claims than their counterparts whose average consultation time was 15 minutes (Dugdale 1999). This is in keeping with the logic of the previous paragraph. If you feel that your treatment time didn't allow you or your physician enough time to address you issues, you will be dissatisfied. Malpractice would, of course, be at the extreme end of dissatisfaction.

Quality of time versus quantity of time: training patients to ask questions

Other studies demonstrate that, for visits between 16 and 30 minutes in length, it is not the actual time spent with the physician that affects outcome, but rather what happens during that time. In two different studies by Greenfield and co-workers (Greenfield et al. 1985, Greenfield et al. 1988) patients were trained to be more effective at the task of eliciting information from their physicians (by asking questions) and compared against a control group. The length of the appointment remained the same for both groups but the patients trained to ask more questions had improved functional status and were more satisfied with care than the control group. Time spent with the patient is important because it allows time for patient and practitioner questions, time for listening, for giving adequate explanations, for the development of trust, and for the time to address the many other concepts discussed in Part 2 of this book. Once these issues have been addressed, additional time appears to deliver diminishing returns.

Take-home message

Some data does suggest that shorter appointment times are linked to poorer health outcomes and decreased patient satisfaction; however, time spent with the patient is about quality and not quantity. For the patient, time is not about minutes, it is about their perception of whether you were listening to them and you were thorough. If you are taking the adequate amount of time to properly applying the critical concepts of Part 2 around active listening, giving adequate explanations along with your treatment, then the patient is not going to feel that they have been rushed.

From your perspective, time is about having the proper amount of time for assessment, treatment and explanation of homecare and remedial exercises. The patient's perspective is not terribly different. They want to feel that their condition was properly assessed, that they were given the adequate treatment, and that they know what self-care to do once they leave your office. Where things are likely to break down is in communication. As you are assessing, you will want to explain the basics of what you are doing. In this way, they understand that their condition was properly assessed. If the condition warranted a short treatment time, then it is best to explain this to the patient, so that he or she does not feel as if you were just in a hurry. If you do not personally instruct the patient in the area of home-care and remedial exercises, then be sure that he or she is given a printout of clear instructions on these matters.

Another point to remember is that there is a clear link between patients taking an active approach to asking questions and health outcomes. Therefore, you should actively encourage questions from your patients during your treatments. If patients are encouraged to ask questions, the chance of them feeling that their concerns were met during the treatment is much higher. Also, if more interaction is encouraged from patients, they will feel more involved in the process, and feel that the treatment was brought to a natural conclusion.

As far as treatment length is concerned, every manual therapy professional works from a different time model so there is no hard and fast rule as to treatment length. In the end, it appears to be about whether your patients 'feel' that they had enough time with you. Once way to determine if the patient feels that you have spent enough time on their condition is to ask a question at the end of the treatment such as:

- *'Do you have any more questions Mrs Johnson?'*
- *'How do things feel to you now?'*
- *'We only have a few minutes left. Is there any area that still hurts, or that you feel I have not properly addressed?'*

It is also helpful to clarify that the treatment has reached the end because of reasons such as:

- *'I think that we should stop now. If I continue to work this area any more, you will be very sore tomorrow.'*
- *'We have reached the end of our time now, but we will continue treatment next week.'*
- *'Unfortunately we have run out of time, but let's get you back in a few days and I will continue with this treatment. In the meantime, here are some exercises/stretches that you can do at home.'*

It is probably not necessary to mention, but just as a reminder; if you are in a hurry the patient will know. They will know because everything about your body language, your actions and your words will convey this message to the patient. You cannot fake being relaxed in your approach to treatment. We all have different temperaments and you have to be yourself. If you are high energy and enthusiastic, then by all means, continue to be high energy and enthusiastic. This is a good thing. However, do not be in a rush. If you ever feel like you are rushing through a treatment, then you are rushing, and your patient will know. Period!

If this was an area where you wanted to get feedback from your patients you could create an online survey that patients could complete anonymously. This allows them to give you information that they might feel uncomfortable delivering in person. It is also a good tool for getting a more balanced perspective on patient satisfaction. Companies such as http://www.surveymonkey.com/ allow easy and cost-effective collection of data from your patients.

USE OF RITUAL

Verbal suggestions are not the only means to induce expectations. The whole therapeutic setting (health professionals, medical instruments, hospital environment) represents what can be called the ritual of the therapeutic act. Indeed, drugs are less effective without therapeutic rituals.

Fabrizio Benedetti MD,
Professor of Physiology and Neuroscience,
University of Turin Medical School (Benedetti 2012)

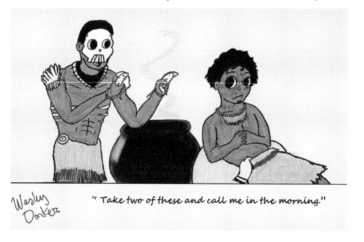

" Take two of these and call me in the morning."

Fig. 2.15

We will look at ritual from two perspectives in this section. One perspective is extremely pragmatic and involves components of conditioning and expectation. The second involves notions of 'the sacred' and transcendence. Both perspectives contain important concepts, but it is likely a percentage of the readers might gloss over the section on ritual as it relates to the notion of transcendence. For those who are strictly analytical and empirical in their thinking, feel free to move to another section once things get too abstract. I happen to think that ritual involves some very intriguing ideas, whereas you may not be inclined to think in the same way. However, before you decide to skip over this section, please read the next few paragraphs and then check out the text below on centering yourself before each treatment. This is an important exercise for all practitioners to practice before each treatment.

Practical components of treatment ritual

On the pragmatic or practical side of ritual, we can consider all the repeating events that the patient either experiences directly or sees you doing from the time he/she arrives until they leave. This could include any of, but is certainly not limited to, the following rituals:

- Patient's arrival and greeting by staff at the clinic.
- Shaking the patient's hand on arrival and departure.
- The type of music that is playing in the clinic.
- Your apparel.
- Taking the patient's BP and pulse.
- Performing basic orthopedic tests.
- Checking the patient's eyes, ears, nails.
- **Taking time to listen to the patient at the beginning of each treatment**.
- The many aspects of the treatment that you perform.
- Enquiring at the end of each treatment about the abatement of symptoms.
- Asking your patient how they feel at end of the treatment.
- Take-home material given to the patient (remedial exercises, patient education, pain or progress diary etc.).
- Giving the patient a glass of water at the end of each treatment.
- Virtually any ritual that you choose to adopt. Some rituals can be unique to your clinic, and even unique to each patient.

The practical side of ritual involves elements of expectation and of conditioning. If we look at the expectation aspect, typically your patients will have visited many other medical offices, so will come with some degree of expectation. Working as a massage therapist, I have seen a good number of professional looking clinics; however, I have also seen some offices, particularly home offices, which are far from professional. What I think does not matter, but what your patient thinks is something else again. It is important to recognize that the further that you veer from the professional office look toward the 'cosy, candle-lit, incense burning look', the more you will tend to reduce the placebo effect for the average patient. It's not that there isn't validity in creating a relaxed cosy environment; there is. However, we are talking about expectations here; and with each element of professionalism you remove from your office, there is some loss in the placebo effect with the average patient.

The other aspect of ritual is conditioning. Several times, I have heard a patient say, 'You forgot to pull on my legs' (distraction of lower limbs) or some other maneuver near the end of a treatment. First off, sometimes I was not aware that I was ritually performing a certain move, such as a calf stretch or distraction on the lower limbs, as I finished a treatment on a given patient – but he or she had definitely noticed. Secondly, I was not performing the maneuver in this instance because, based upon my assessment, the stretch (or distraction) was not warranted. However, the patient was expecting this maneuver based upon prior conditioning. Therefore, if one wants to maximize the effect, one needs to follow the ritual. As you can see from the list above, ritual elements can be a whole host of things. I hope that when I workshop this book with professionals that we can augment the preceding list.

Note that the science that supports the use of rituals is the same science that supports conditioning theory; probably the most concrete aspect of the placebo effect. Any cue surrounding a treatment that occurs on a repeating basis reinforces previous outcomes and behaviours. Keep in mind that this can also work against you if you have had poor outcomes with a patient. If this is the case, not only do you want to change your treatment protocols, you want to change some of the conditioning cues or rituals surrounding the session. Just as the supporting science of conditioning theory applies to ritual, much of the practical treatment suggestions from the conditioning section apply here as well.

Another recent reference to the importance of ritual in manual therapy is the 2010 review of evidence, entitled Effectiveness of manual therapies: the UK evidence report, which looked at 49 recent relevant systematic reviews, 16 evidence-based clinical guidelines, plus an additional 46 RCT that had not yet been included in systematic reviews and guidelines. In their conclusions, the authors' state:

Additionally, there is substantial evidence to show that the ritual of the patient practitioner interaction has a therapeutic effect in itself separate from any specific effects of the treatment applied. This phenomenon is termed contextual effects.

(Bronfort et al. 2010)

Ritual, symbols and transcendence

There is one institution whose healing tradition probably goes back farther than medicine; that is of course the church, or broadly speaking…religion. The link between faith and healing is a very ancient notion. For example, the Ebers Papyrus dated at around 1552 BC shows evidence of the laying-on of hands, or faith healing at that time. Undoubtedly many cultures with oral histories before this also had healing interwoven into their religious traditions. What is typically interwoven into faith and healing is the sense that the sacred is intimately involved in the process. As soon as one conjures up the notion of the sacred, the practice will necessarily be a religious one. While religious healing is not the path that we are following as manual practitioners, we do need to have an awareness of the sacred honour that we have been given to enter the deeply personal space of each and every one of our patients.

A ritual is an opportunity to participate in a myth. You are in one way or another putting your consciousness, even the action of your body, into play in relation to a mythological theme, and, as I hope I've made clear, mythological themes are projections of the order of the psyche…by participating in a ritual occasion you are in a magical field, a field that is putting you in touch with your own great depth.

Joseph Campbell Audio Collection
(Campbell 2003)

Joseph Campbell spent his whole life studying rituals and mythology and he sees ritual as a mechanism which allows an individual member of a group to participate in a shared myth (in this context, myth denotes a larger truth, or ultimate truth), allowing them to experience transcendence. So, in this context, what is ritual in medicine? We all need to believe that there is hopefully more to life than just going through the motions. We all have the urge (and I would even say the need) to transcend this life at times, to rise above the mundane, and to be transported to a higher plane. Ritual has long been used to perform that function.

When it comes to managing symbols and ritual, one need look no further than your local church, synagogue or mosque. Churches have thousands of years of experience at this business and they do an amazing job of managing symbols and ritual specifically for the purpose of transcendence. My personal experience with religion was the Anglican Church that my parents took my siblings and me to every Sunday. In the (high) Anglican Church, there has always been extensive use of ritual. The priest would wear specific vestments (robes) for specific ceremonies. Servers (the Anglican version of altar boys) wore cassocks (a black and white robe) and performed various duties such as lighting of the candles, leading procession and aiding the priest in his various duties. Candles were lit after the congregation was seated, but before the service actually began. Lighting the candles signalled to the congregation that the service was about to begin and 'the magic was about to happen'. Then there was a procession into the church with the priest, servers and choir. There was often use of incense during the service. The choir led us in preces, responses, psalms and hymns. The Holy Gospel was read at intervals and the priest would always have a sermon for us. Central to most of the services was celebration of the Holy Eucharist where each member of the congregation that had undergone confirmation would consume a wafer of bread and drink administered by the priest, symbolically partaking in the body and blood of Christ, definitely the moment of magic for each parishioner (participant). At the end of the service there was a procession out of the church. Finally, all of the candles were extinguished, signalling the end of the ceremony or ritual.

Now, while I am no longer an Anglican nor a member of any organized religion, I still believe that this church and many churches do an amazing job of managing symbols and ritual. Right from the time that you walk into the church, all of the cues tell you that you have entered another plane; one with obvious religious context. The elements of these rituals evolved over hundreds and even thousands of years, like most good rituals. I only realized this years later as I encountered Joseph Campbell's theories on recurring mythological themes in cultures around the globe. Every society that has ever existed has had recurring themes in their central mythology (their core mystical beliefs), and ritual is the manner by which the individual society member partakes in the myth (i.e. in the divine). Central to this belief system is that the individual cannot access the myth directly. This is why a *ritual* is needed. A ritual is a means or a vehicle to facilitate the process of transcendence of this physical plane of existence and allows an individual to partake personally in the divine, or in the miracle. Each mythology has its own specific rituals that only work in context of that particular myth or truth.

The sacred act of healing

I hope that you are beginning to see why we are discussing rituals, symbols and transcendence. Our patients also want to transcend this plane, to partake in the sacred act of healing, of being healed, and we are the modern equivalent of the shaman that had all manner of healing rituals and practices at his disposal. This is the sacred role we as practitioners play in their lives.

Now there is a big difference between visiting a church and visiting one's doctor, but the point is that there are many cues that our patients are picking up on either consciously or unconsciously that tell them that they are in an environment where healing is about to take place. Healing is no doubt a sacred act, so while we are on the topic of sacred, now would be a good time to stop for a moment and look at what is sacred about what we do. We are, in fact, honoured in our profession to be in the privileged position of entering our patients' lives and personal space on so many levels.

- **Personal level** – some examples of this include our patient's health information and other personal disclosures brought forth.
- **Physical level** – this is obvious since we are using touch to effect change in their bodies to bring about healing.
- **Spiritual level** – this level is harder to quantify, but most therapists and practitioners recognize that there is a spiritual aspect to our existence. In my own practice, there have been deep transient spiritual connections with some of with my patients during a treatment that have been mutually acknowledged.
- **Other levels** – there are undoubtedly many other connections that happen simultaneously that are harder to quantify and describe, which go beyond the scope of this book.

The patient gives us permission to enter their personal space, to work in that space and then to exit the space, while holding all information from that exchange in confidence. We need to be clear in our mind that this is sacred space that we are entering. We need to remind ourselves constantly that we are honoured and privileged to be allowed to enter this space, and we always need to hold clearly in our minds that this is sacred work that we are performing. This was never once mentioned in my schooling, but it did not take me long while working as a massage therapist to realize that this is the case. In my opinion, this attitude, this approach, this belief will serve you well if you want to work in the profession for a long time, and if you want to affect people's lives in a positive manner.

Now let's get back to the sacred act of healing. Your patient has arrived with some expectations in your office. He or she may not be aware of it, but particularly if the patient has never been to your office before, he/she will have both spoken and unspoken expectations; both conscious and unconscious expectations that some magic is going to happen. It hasn't happened so far for them sitting at home, and they were really hoping that once they arrived in your office, the magic would start. I write this perhaps tongue in cheek, but at one level this is what they are really hoping will happen. For magic to happen, one has to be transported to a higher plane; that is to say that one has to transcend the human plane of existence for a short period of time. Far back in our history and in primitive cultures the shaman performed this function. We are the modern-day shamans that people go to for healing. Just like shamans of the past, and just like the church with the processions and the candles, we actually have rituals that are a part of our practice that guide the patient through the healing experience to give them the cues that 'the magic' aka the healing process is about to happen or is happening, or has happened.

Let me take a moment to get a doctor's perspective on use of ritual in medicine – Dr Abraham Verghese, Professor for the Theory and Practice of Medicine at Stanford University Medical School and Senior Associate Chair of the Department of Internal Medicine, said:

> *I find that patients from almost any culture have deep expectations of a ritual when a doctor sees them, and they are quick to perceive when he or she gives those procedures short shrift by, say, placing the stethoscope on top of the gown instead of the skin, doing a cursory prod of the belly and wrapping up in 30 seconds. Rituals are about transformation, the crossing of a threshold, and in the case of the bedside exam, the transformation is the cementing of the doctor-patient relationship, a way of saying: 'I will see you through this illness. I will be with you through thick and thin.' It is paramount that doctors not forget the importance of this ritual.*

(Verghese 2011)

The only thing to be added to this statement is that not just doctors, but actually anyone in the healing arts and healing profession should also take note of the importance of ritual.

Centering yourself

The first and most important ritual for you, and you alone, is a centering exercise. It is important that you be at your best for each treatment, to be present and in the moment. This means leaving all of your personal baggage at the door whether that is a negative experience from that day or a week or a month ago, the phone message that you just picked up, or even an earlier life experience that you have not yet worked through. It also means that you do not carry the last patient's issues forward to the next person. Centering is the best way to do this. It can be done in less than a minute but it requires that you take the time to do the exercise. It typically requires that you have a personal space to do this exercise. If you don't have that personal office space, then step into a treatment room or somewhere where you can shut the door and do a centering exercise. This is partly for your benefit, but real point of the exercise is actually to bring your focus and attention into the moment so that you can be well grounded and completely present for your next patient. There are various methods for centering yourself, but there are three basic elements to the exercise of centering:

1. **Leaving all of your problems at the door**. As when you go to sleep at night, this is not the time to work on your issues. Anything that pulls you away from the present will detract from the treatment that you are about to give. Worrying about the future or rehashing an experience from your past will only pull your focus away from the treatment that you are giving. You owe this to your patient to be there with them in that moment. Do these during your centering exercise so that when you enter the treatment room you are already at your best.
2. **Relax your body**. Learning progressive meditation exercises* and practicing them will condition you to be able to instantly relax your muscles and release tensions that you may be carrying in any area of your body.
3. **Relax your mind**. Making the mind quiet and entering the state where the brain can produce alpha waves allows you to decrease stress, increase intuition, as well as enhance creativity and healing (Jauk et al. 2012).If you train your mind by meditating, you will be able to relax 'on demand' and bring yourself into the present. Once your mind becomes trained, you will be able to center yourself in 30 seconds or less enhancing alpha wave activity in your own brain.

More than anything, this pre-treatment ritual needs to be done, as previously mentioned, to bring you and your focus into the moment at hand, leaving all other issues behind and allowing you to be the best that you can be for each and every patient.

The four elements of a healing ritual

What do the 'experts' say about the healing ritual? Well as you might guess, there are no hard and fast rules in this area; however, I would like to defer to Barbara Dossey, a pioneer in the holistic nursing movement. She notes that healing rituals typically have four characteristics:

- **Taking time to separate one's self from daily activities** – this involves centering yourself, which was previously discussed.
- **Creating a healing space** – the treatment room is the healing space by design. Actual design issues are covered in the section entitled Clinical/

---

*To read more on progressive relaxation techniques see the following non-profit site: http://www.helpguide.org/mental/stress_relief_meditation_yoga_relaxation.htm

healing environment. This would be a good time to mention that while you are in this space with your patient, that you try desperately to avoid any interruptions of any sort. Each interruption takes you and your intention out of the moment and leaves the patient feeling abandoned. An appropriate office policy can prevent this from happening. One related topic is out-calls, which some practitioners might occasionally perform. If we travel to our patients to perform treatments there are several challenges that arise such as distractions, confidentiality and patients who do not cease their daily activities during their treatment. These unique issues need to be addressed if the treatment is to achieve maximum potential.

- **Employing a health practitioner or team of practitioners** – this is reasonably self-explanatory. One point to keep in mind here is that if your patient is seeing other practitioners, it is important that you are all on the same page. This can be challenging. If this is the case then there needs to be some communication established between you and any other professionals to share what each has learned, to share what each believes is going on, and what needs to be done to correct the patient's health.

- **Intention** – this is one aspect that is not necessarily incorporated into the treatment by design. As the practitioner, you must focus on the science and the art of healing and on the patient's issues at hand. Centering yourself before each treatment will go a long way toward putting you into this mind state. Another aspect of intention is that the patient must also personally focus on their body if they want to maximize their treatment. This is a common theme in Buddhist healing, shamanism and many other types of ritual healing. The application in the medical environment would be that the patient should be reminded to focus their awareness on healing and to visualize their own recovery. Patients can be encouraged to follow whatever system of symbols appeals most to them whether that system is Christian, Buddhist, Ayurvedic, Traditional Chinese Medicine, Native North American or any other religion or belief system to which they happen to adhere. The label is not important; what is important is the powerful symbol that the healing ritual of each practice carries with it to the participant/believer.

The three phases of the healing ritual

Remember my church story at the beginning of this section? Well, as it turns out, I wasn't just rambling – I was actually going somewhere with that story. Just as there are clear markers about the beginning, middle and end of each ceremony, there also needs to be clear ritualized markers for the patient indicating where they are in the process. So what are the rituals and cues that we have in the manual therapy profession? Well, it will be different for each office and for each individual profession but some obvious ritual cues lie in the design, set-up and operation of your office; the medical environment itself. Most of this we will cover on the section entitled Clinical/healing environment, but what we need to discuss here is treatment itself. You could be working a one-person operation or in a much larger set-up. You may have complete control or limited control of the environment. If you are in a multi-person office, you may not do the initial greeting. Likewise, you may not actually handle the patients' rescheduling or payments, or you may not see them off as they physically leave the building. The good news is that these are not the central elements of the ritual, but if the wrong thing is said or done by office staff then it can detract from what you are doing. Therefore, this is an area where some training and education may be necessary. The time period where you should have autonomous control is from when you walk into the treatment room, until you leave the treatment room; this is where the three phases of the healing ritual all take place.

The treatment room contains a lot of items that are also symbols of healing, such as artwork, plants, scents, medical charts/posters, anatomical models, and therapeutic devices, such as ultrasound, laser or interferential current therapy machine, that signal to the patient that they are in a therapeutic/healing environment. The signals in that room might be slightly relaxation-oriented or they might be medically oriented depending on the message that you wish to convey to your patient. Any scent is a strong emotional trigger, but one must be cautious in the area of scent. If you have a scent that you use frequently, you will unknowingly experience neural adaptation. Your nervous system adjusts to the constant stimulus raising the sensory threshold and then you will find yourself using more of the essential oil to create the room scent. For example, you might think that it is wonderful to have bergamot or lavender, or whatever scent, in your clinic, but when you adapt to the scent, you will likely use it in higher concentration and you can easily overpower your patients' olfactory sense. As a result, essential oils should be used sparingly and intermittently for this and several other reasons.*

1. **The entrance or beginning** – this begins as you personally greet your patient (even though other office staff may have already greeted them and offered them seating in the waiting room). Presumably, you will be wearing a professional garment of some description to signal your training as a health professional. Whether this is a new or an ongoing patient, you will typically invite them into the treatment/examination room. If

---

*Scents have long been used to cover up other smells that are offensive. It is far better to clean the room thoroughly than to constantly mask the smell with a scent. Walking into any room with a detectable scent, the first thing that many people think is, 'What are they covering up?' The other issue around scent is stimulation of asthmatic symptoms and the effects of the chemicals involved on our health. There are no safe levels for airborne chemicals that are found in most perfumes and air fresheners whether spray, plug-in or passive. If you must use a scent, then only use a pure essential oil; but (as mentioned), use it sparingly. For more on this visit the CDC website: Healthy Housing Reference Manual, Section 5: Indoor Air Pollutants and Toxic Materials at: http://www.cdc.gov/nceh/publications/books/housing/cha05.htm

you use music then it should already be on. In large offices this music would typically be more tranquil that the upbeat waiting area music.

If this is a new patient, it is important to be as professional as possible while still being personable. This is your chance to give them all of the signals that symbolize that you are a trained professional who will guide them through the whole process. We don't want to veer too far off course here, but suffice it to say that this is your only chance to make a good first impression. If you follow all of your training on patient interviewing while keeping good eye contact, exuding confidence and following the concepts of all of the other sections in Part 2, then you will be off to a roaring start. For ongoing patients, ask them about the progress that they are making, what their chief complaint is today, and any other pertinent details or concerns that they might have. For both new and returning patients it is best to make notes in their presence, making measurements wherever possible to signal your focus on their condition and your competence as a health professional. Finally, you will instruct them on any garment changes or undressing that will be required on their part. At this point if garment alteration or undressing is required, you would close the door and give the patient a few minutes. This is probably a good time to do your personal centering, but if you are in a larger office that does not provide you with personal space then you may have already used the treatment room for this purpose.

2. **The body of the treatment** – use of the word 'body' is no accident. We are in fact treating the patient's body, which, as was mentioned earlier, is the sacred space that you are being given permission to enter. At this time you are conducting the laying-on of hands, probably the most powerful ritual symbol that we have in our possession. This is truly the time when, if all of our training and our symbols are aligned, the 'magic happens'. You know that there is more to it than that, and certainly healing will typically follow a course. However, from a ritualistic model of the experience, this is the sacred and magical moment where transformation takes place. Many patients do experience some instant relief during the treatment, and I cannot speak to the other manual therapy professions, but with all the sensory input that happens with massage, many patients are transported to another place, which may or may not be spiritual for them, but certainly is transformative. It is also worth mentioning at this time that static symbols within the treatment room, such as scents, medical posters, anatomical models and therapeutic devices, become ritualistic devices when you employ them in your therapy. For example, if you alter the room scent with aromatherapy, use the anatomical model or medical charts to educate the patient or to help them with visualization, or use an electrotherapeutic device; these devices have the capacity to become powerful ritualistic symbols at that time and conditioning symbols in the future.

3. **The exit and end** – everything in life comes to an end, as does the medical treatment. A typical ritual might involve making a statement that the treatment is now over, or that treatment is almost over if one is looking for clarification about where to devote one's energy during the remaining minutes of the treatment. For example, massage therapists work from a time-based medical model, so in this situation it is good to let the patient know that their treatment time is nearing the end. You can therefore clarify that you have addressed all the issues that the patient presented to you on that day. In other health models the practitioner might make a similar statement, just to clarify that patient expectations have been met. Then a statement might be made such as, *'Rise carefully and take all the time that you need. I will be in the office when you arrive there.'* At this point, the lighting in the room might be altered to provide another cue that the treatment is completed. All of these cues tell the patient in an unambiguous yet supportive manner that the treatment is finished. You have now signalled that a transformation has taken place. You have performed a manual intervention (or more likely multiple manual interventions) and this is the point where you signal that the process has come to its conclusion.

One other important message to communicate to the patient at this time is that the healing in their body will continue to take place over the next few hours, days or weeks depending upon the message that you are delivering. It is certainly important to communicate that a medical intervention has just happened, but that their body will actually continue to heal. Communicate that what is happening is in fact a healing 'process'. Their body will now take that information, adjustment or intervention and continue on its own healing path using the body's innate healing powers. It is very important that both you and the patient are aware, and reminded, that their body has amazing healing powers and that more healing will continue to happen after the appointment has ended.

THE CLINICIAN'S PERSONA

The doctor who fails to have a placebo effect on his patients should become a pathologist.

(Blau 1985)

This section is largely about the professional demeanour and image that you create around yourself as a health practitioner. This image may or may not actually be the true *you*. Your image might be a slightly more confident *you*, or a more controlled *you*. It might be a more positive *you*. Your professional image is not a complete transformation, but there are clearly attitudes, ideas and issues that we would discuss with friends that we would not discuss with patients. We might kick our shoes off and have a drink with a friend but we are not going to do this with a patient. Very few of us are our true relaxed selves once we don our professional image, and this is completely okay. The salient point here is that you are actually creating a professional image every moment that you are with your patient, and your patient sees that person(a) as their healer/therapist/health provider/practitioner etc. This persona is a construct, and as such, you can mold and build this image to maximize health outcomes in your patients. It is always important to remember that when we are talking about the placebo effect that your patient's perception of you and your ability to affect change in their health depends largely upon the image or persona that you have consistently constructed with all your interaction with that particular patient.

Cultural aspects of the placebo effect are also very interesting in that they are dynamic and highly variable depending upon where you live and the social sphere in which you practice. If the culturally dominant view of professionals and individuals is that they must be confident, it would be wise for you to adopt as much of that role into your professional image as you are comfortable with. This does not mean that you will not have private doubts, but much like other aspects of your persona, your professional image is not you; rather it is an image that you create. Likewise if the culturally dominant view is that a member of that society needs to be serious then a practitioner can only inject so much levity into a situation before running the risk of being perceived as a buffoon.*

The clinician's persona involves many aspects. Specifically we will look at a few aspects of that persona such as your professionalism, your belief system, the confidence that you project, your professional competence and your enthusiasm.

---

*Cultural variations in the placebo effect are actually a very interesting topic. If you are interested in this aspect of the placebo effect then I highly recommend Daniel Moerman's book, *Meaning Medicine and the Placebo Effect*. Moerman is an emeritus professor of anthropology at the University of Michigan-Dearborn. Most of his life has been spent looking at anthropological perspectives of medicine, which has necessarily brought him face to face with the placebo effect countless times. I find his perspective very refreshing. An internet search will generate a page with PDF files of much of his work.

Professionalism

There is a big push toward ensuring professionalism in many regulated health professions in North America. There are, of course, many aspects to professionalism and virtually every aspect aligns with improved clinical outcomes, because the foundation of professionalism is putting the patient's interests first. This is very interesting because we have now addressed some of the ethical questions concerning the placebo effect. As a health professional, your first and foremost commitment is to your patient. This commitment is always your guiding light toward making ethical and professional decisions. It is heartening to know that if you act professionally, you will be enhancing the placebo effect, thus improving clinical outcomes. Here is a sample working list of some of the defining principles, characteristics and behaviours of health professionals:

- As regulated healthcare professionals, operate within a framework of provincial, state or national regulations.
- Have undergone specific, detailed training and education.
- Have exhibited mastery in appropriate jurisdictional examinations.
- Have mastery of an uncommonly complex knowledge base.
- Have achieved the level of knowledge, skill and aptitude necessary to perform the task and skills required for your profession.
- Possess credentials indicating competence and licensing in area of expertise.
- Healthcare professionals are persons committed, first and foremost, to directly benefiting the people they serve. In fact, when someone says someone is acting unprofessionally, what they really mean to say is that person has placed their own personal best interests above those of his or her patient.
- In order to ensure professionalism, health professions enter into an agreement with society called the Social Contract. Within this contract, health professionals agree to serve and protect the well-being and best interests of their patients first and foremost. In exchange for this, society agrees to provide the health profession with the autonomy to govern itself and with the privileges and status afforded regulated healthcare professionals.
- We are committed to staying current with the latest research and current best practices.
- Maintain your commitment to continuing education.
- Follow your regulatory college's *Standards of Practice* document.
- Follow your regulatory college's *Code of Ethics* document. In the case of the College of Massage Therapists of Ontario, for example, there are four ethical principles:
  - Respect for persons
  - Responsible caring
  - Integrity in relationships
  - Responsibility to society.

- Exhibit and use professional judgment.
- Maintain competence in all aspects of professional duties.
- Provide and maintain accountability.
- Practice respect for persons.
- Maintain professional boundaries.
- Always practice informed consent.
- Maintain patient privacy and confidentiality.
- Maintain current and competent record keeping.

Striving towards excellence in professionalism is a major step on the road toward improving clinical outcomes. If you are acting professionally, you will be presenting an image of a person that your patient will respect and trust. This respect and trust the foundation of a professional relationship, and is fundamental to enhancing the placebo effect. This, in turn will improve clinical outcomes.

Clinician's belief system

One small double-blinded trial involved administration of a placebo inpatients with postoperative dental pain (Gracely et al. 1985). Patients were divided into two groups and were told that they would receive a drug which would do one of the following: 1) increase their pain (naloxone); 2) decrease their pain (fentanyl); or 3) have no effect (placebo). What was interesting about this study is that the clinicians were deliberately misled by being told that in one of the two groups there was no chance of administering an active analgesic drug. So here we have a study where the clinicians were manipulated but not the patients. The placebo response was dramatically less in the group where the clinicians believed that no analgesic therapy could be given, demonstrating that clinicians' beliefs can affect placebo effects.

There is little doubt that the clinician's beliefs come into play with any treatment. This was discovered very early on when clinical trials were first being conducted. Researchers were initially surprised to find that when a clinician was knowingly dispensing a placebo that it affected the outcome of the study. On one level it is hard to believe that such a subtle thing could skew results. It was doubtful that these individuals were saying anything different to the participant, but something was affecting the outcome. It has been suggested that it is a combination of placebo effect, observer effect* and/or experimenter/observer bias.[†]

---

*Observer Effect (aka Observer Expectancy Effect). This is much easier to explain than Observer Effect in quantum physics (thank goodness!). The simplest explanation of this concept is that people are likely to change their behaviour if they know that they are being observed. This, needless to say, poses a substantial threat to any study.

[†]Observer Bias occurs when the clinician or researcher know the goals of the study or the hypotheses and allows this knowledge to influence their observations during the study. One example of this is if an observer/researcher knows that the study hypothesized that a drug had a calming effect, they may observe and focus on calming cues, even though the drug is actually ineffective and has no calming effect. This is much akin to when you purchase a new vehicle and suddenly you notice the same model with increased frequency, even though the number of modes of this car has only increased by one.

Perhaps it was body language or something even more subtle than that, but clearly something affected the outcome. Either way it became immediately apparent that if studies were to produce accurate results they would need to be double-blinded. That is to say that neither the participant nor the clinician could actually know which treatment was the active treatment.

This speaks volumes about how we, as practitioners, must approach our daily work and how we approach our patients. If we are harboring negative thoughts about our patients or about the success of a treatment then we are affecting the outcome. This is not some new-age spiritual concept. This was established back in the 1950s when the clinical trial was evolving into what is now the gold standard of measurement, the double-blinded random controlled trial. Have you ever noticed on days when your mood is buoyant how many pleasant interactions you tend to have with complete strangers? Letting go of the many entanglements and anxieties that we carry around with us and just living in the moment creates an extremely different life experience. In much the same way, undoubtedly, you have noticed a very different exchange happening between you and your patients on the days when you are feeling especially 'light' happy and in the moment.

One obvious example of where your belief system comes in to play is with patients who arrive at your clinic with an obvious chip on their shoulder, feeling that they are owed something by the world or by their insurance company, or what have you. This type of patient can be very challenging to work with. If you let this affect your perception of them in a negative manner, then it will undoubtedly also affect the outcome of the treatment, and then subsequently their health outcome. Staying truly positive with this type of patient can challenge our ability to remain truly positive, non-judgmental and genuinely confident about their health outcome; but this is what we must endeavour to do.

- Examine your expectations and beliefs with your patients, especially the challenging cases or challenging patients.
- Be aware that if you harbor an unspoken negative belief, this will tend to create a negative outcome. For example, if you say to a patient, *'you will likely not get full use of this limb,'* or *'you may not get full range of motion back in this arm'*, you are in fact limiting the patient's belief system.
- Keep in mind that miracles happen every day and there are countless cases where a doctor tells a patient that they will never walk, skate, or play hockey etc. again and the patient with a strong will proves the doctor wrong. It is fine to be realistic in what you say, but always leave the door open to improved function or complete resolution of healing for your patient. The patient's belief system might be a limitation, but don't let your belief system be the limitation.

Confidence

Fresh out of school, most of us were intimidated by what we do not know and the experience we lack. In my early days, I tried to project confidence in my treatments but I actually had very little confidence in my ability to affect change (other than relaxation) through massage therapy. As my successes mounted, I developed a stronger inner confidence. The reason I use the words inner confidence is that I suspect very few patients saw me as someone troubled with doubts, because as a health practitioner it is in my nature to project a strong outer confidence. This confidence would in fact be part of the professional image that I don upon entering my clinic to work each day. There is an old adage, 'with experience comes competence, and with competence comes confidence.' This was probably a theme in most people's first years working as a health professional. Without treatment successes, it is impossible to have real inner confidence in your ability to affect change in your patients' health status. Any confidence that you project in the early years is likely to be exactly that … simply a projection, and little more. As you improve your clinical skills, it would make sense that your inner confidence would increase, and then the confidence that you project is more 'real'. If you are confident of a positive outcome for your patient, whether due to your treatment or due to the natural course of events, you pass that belief along, not only at a conscious level, but undoubtedly at an unconscious level as well.

Little research appears to have been done in this area. While it might seem obvious that a practitioner has confidence, it is important to verify this with a clinical study. A recent study looked at confidence of chiropractic students with two measurement scales, Patient Communication Confidence Scale (PCCS) and Clinical Skills Confidence Scale (CSCS), to measure student confidence in these two areas in manual medicine (Hecimovich et al. 2014). Researchers state in their conclusions that learning new information and skills and dealing with challenging situations can be impacted negatively by a lack of confidence. This study found that as students gained experience, they also gained confidence, which was reflected in their clinical competency. It was also determined that the PCCS and CSCS were valid and reliable instruments in tracking changes in levels of confidence in specific skills over time and the examination of the degree of congruence between confidence and competence. Hopefully more studies will be done in the area of clinician confidence as it relates to clinical outcomes.

In the early years of your practice, it is natural and appropriate to let your ego drink in the joy of a patient's success. This lets you build your confidence; however, it is not wise to let your successes affect your ego. Your ego will definitely interfere with your ability as a clinician. I mention ego but there is an age-old expression, 'pride goes before the fall.* Ego is something that is very hard to see when it does

---

*The origin of this expression is actually from Proverbs 16:18 'Pride goes before destruction, and a haughty spirit before a fall.'

get in the way, so we always need to be on guard personally to make sure that we are not letting patient successes go to our head because, after all, these are patient successes, not our success.

A 1998 North Carolina low back pain study of 189 practitioners, including physicians and chiropractors who were randomly chosen from practices across the state, illustrated that excessive confidence did not lead to improved clinical outcomes. Practitioners in this prospective cohort study enrolled 1633 patients with acute low back pain. While chiropractors had significantly stronger self-confidence scores than physicians, those who received care from practitioners with stronger self-confidence scores did not differ in the time taken to functional improvement, overall patient satisfaction, or their perception of the completeness of care. The level of practitioner self-confidence, as measured by a 4-item scale in this study, did not predict patient outcomes in the treatment of acute low back pain (Smucker et al. 1998).

Why is this? Well, all that we can do is theorize why increased confidence does not have a net-positive effect. As I consider this phenomenon, I am reminded of the Australian Longitudinal Study of Aging (ALSA) that also produced some counterintuitive results. This 1992 study used a series of interviews with nearly 1500 older people to assess how much contact they had with their different social networks, including children, relatives and friends. The group was monitored annually for 4 years and then on an intermittent basis for a decade. The researchers also considered how economic, social, environmental and lifestyle factors affected the health and well-being of the seniors in the study. After controlling for those variables, the researchers were able to make some interesting observations, not the least of which was that close relationships with children and relatives had little effect on longevity rates for older people.* Now aren't you shocked that close family and relatives had no effect on longevity? I certainly was, and once again, the question is why? There are no quick and easy answers, but I will put forward a hypothesis that might answer both conundrums. I will suggest that in both the scenario of practitioner confidence, and 'close' family ties there may be as many positive aspects as there are negative aspects coming in to play. Family is great, but there are also a lot of expectations placed upon family members that are often not met, leading to disappointment. Likewise, confidence is a great thing, but few of us are aware of the role that our ego plays in the therapeutic environment. As our confidence builds, our ego can become deeply invested in this phenomenon, and therein, as they say, lies the rub. Just as our ego is a major impediment to self-actualization, it is also likely a substantial impediment in the professional area as well. To illustrate this more clearly we need to look at the Dunning-Kruger effect.

---

*One very interesting outcome of this study was that people with extensive networks of good friends and confidantes outlived those with the fewest friends by 22%!

The Dunning–Kruger Effect

I am wiser than this man, for neither of us appears to know anything great and good; but he fancies he knows something, although he knows nothing; whereas I, as I do not know anything, so I do not fancy I do. In this trifling particular, then, I appear to be wiser than he, because I do not fancy I know what I do not know.

Attributed to Socrates, from Plato, *Apology*

One of the painful things about our time is that those who feel certainty are stupid, and those with any imagination and understanding are filled with doubt and indecision.

Bertrand Russell, *The Triumph of Stupidity*

If you examine the quotes above, you will probably understand the basics of the concept of the Dunning–Kruger effect. This effect (named after David Dunning and Justin Kruger of Cornell University) occurs when incompetent people not only perform a task poorly, but they also lack the competence to realize their own incompetence at a task. What follows are four phenomena that have been observed with the Dunning–Kruger effect:

1. Incompetent individuals, compared with their more competent peers, dramatically overestimate their ability and performance
2. Incompetent individuals are less able than their more competent peers to recognize competence when they see it
3. Incompetent individuals are less able than their more competent peers to gain insight into their true level of performance
4. Incompetent individuals can gain insight about their shortcomings, but this comes (paradoxically) by gaining competence.

Taken together, these four factors actually contribute to an inverse relationship between confidence and competence; exactly the opposite of what most of us tend to assume. As it turns out, the Dunning–Kruger effect is nothing new, dating back at least to Plato's time. It is, in effect, the arrogance of ignorance. Hopefully, as most of us travel along the road to knowledge we begin to realize that excessive confidence is simply a trap or misstep along the way. Put another way, 'the more you know, the more you realize you don't know'. This is not philosophical navel-gazing, but actually appears to be supported by evidence. As you begin to understand some basic aspects of physiology or healing there is a tremendous temptation to create a new paradigm or system to understand the body and how to treat a broad array of pathologies. You have undoubtedly seen the excessive confidence phenomenon displayed in certain business persons who are marketing their new 'system' that can cure all manner of human ills. Their system is the latest, greatest thing since sliced bread and for only $5000 or $6000 you can become certified and for only $1000 per year you can maintain that certification as one of their registered practitioners. Well, unless they have clinical trials to support their claims, it would probably just be another case of the Dunning–Kruger effect.

Does this mean that you should not project confidence in your approach? Absolutely not! From the patient's perspective, your confidence is an important cue, suggesting a multitude of factors (e.g. that you have made the correct diagnosis, that you are supplying the correct treatment, that the outcome will be positive etc.) but just be aware that your own ego can very easily become wrapped up in your confidence and is likely, at the very least, to create observer bias. Also, if you are perceived as a practitioner with a lot of self-doubt, this is not likely to improve your patient's view of your competence, which brings us to the next part of this section.

Competence

A 1996 study involving 74 general internists and 814 patients randomly selected from their practices identified 125 elements of care that covered nine domains including physician clinical skill; physician interpersonal skill; support staff office environment; provision of information; patient involvement; non-financial access; finances; and coordination of care. Participants rated each element on its importance to high-quality care on a 4-point scale. Patients' ratings and physicians' ratings were compared for individual elements of care and for elements aggregated into domains. Patients and physicians agreed that the most crucial element of out-patient care is clinical skill (Laine et al. 1996).

A study at Stanford University School of Medicine, mentioned earlier, speaks to the patient's perception of competence of the clinician (Sox et al.1981). This study looked at the issue of the patient feeling that the appropriate number of tests had been performed on them to clearly ascertain what exactly was at the root of their malady. As mentioned, these tests are not only for our benefit as practitioners, but they also affect the psychology of the patient. Fewer patients in the group receiving tests reported short-term disability than patients in the no-test group. Statistical analysis confirmed that the use of diagnostic tests was an independent predictor of recovery. Patients in the test group felt that care was 'better than usual' more often than patients in the no-test group. Therefore, it is extremely important to perform any appropriate tests on our patients, both to increase our certainty, and theirs as well. Performing orthopedic tests (most of which can be performed in less than a minute) will give the patient a clear indication that you know what you are doing and increase their belief in your clinical competence.

The topic of practitioner competence is likely to be no shocker to any of us. If you are going to work in health care (or any other realm for that matter) the very first matter at hand is practitioner competence. Anything else is a non-starter. This book is definitely not suggesting that one should use the placebo effect as a replacement for competence. What is up for discussion is whether you are perceived by your patient as being competent. There is the matter of first impressions and this involves such topics as the white coat effect, personal grooming and the atmosphere of your office (covered in the next section). All in all, the matter of patient's first impressions concerning your competence is closely linked to professionalism. As you build the relationship with your patient, there is just no substitute for competence. You have to know your stuff, and you have to know how to apply it. It is really that simple . . . or not so simple if you lack competence.

If you are wondering how to assess your own competence, you might find Rick Brenner's website at Chaco Canyon Consulting (http://www.chacocanyon.com) has useful insights into this matter. Rick's consultancy service helps businesses overcome institutional issues which hinder their ability to solve problems and improve organizational performance. Here are Rick's four generic indicators of competence for application in the workplace:

1. **Awareness of your limitations**. The truly competent understand that their competence is limited – that there are things they cannot do or do not know. This knowledge drives a continued desire to learn.
2. **Desire to learn.** Curiosity, practice, questioning, and continued study are signs of a drive to enhance competence. It is this drive that established the existing level of competence. Where this drive is weak, competence of the individual is questionable.
3. **Constructive response to failure**. Responding to failure in constructive ways is another important way to build competence. This involves setting your ego aside and is essential to building competence.
4. **Ability to assess risk realistically**. Realistic risk assessment requires a reservoir of experience – competence – in the relevant domains. Incompetence leads to mis-assessment of risk. The fearful and incompetent tend to overestimate risks; the brash and incompetent tend to underestimate them. Competence tempers both.

Truly succeeding at the task of assessing and improving one's competence involves setting one's ego aside, honestly analyzing one's performance and then being willing to make changes.

Attire

One of the most obvious, visible and potent symbols in the medical profession is the physician's classic white coat. This one simple piece of attire carries a whole host of meanings beyond cleanliness and hygiene. The following list could probably be a few pages long, but some of the obvious unspoken messages or meanings attached to this one symbol include:

- Specific medical education
- Authority
- Licence to practice medicine
- Confidentiality

- Ability to ask deeply personal questions
- Familiarity with illness, suffering and even death
- Reliability
- Scientific orientation
- Commitment to caring
- Respectability
- Elevated social status
- All other attributes of professionalism.

A recent Canadian study that surveyed 337 family members of patients in three intensive care units offers some insights into this phenomenon (Beach et al. 2013). When asked to select their preferred physician from a panel of photographs, survey respondents 'strongly favored' doctors who wore 'traditional attire' with a white coat, according to the researchers. 'Physicians in traditional dress were seen as most knowledgeable and most honest.' When participants were asked to select the best physician overall, 52% selected doctors wearing traditional attire with a white coat, followed by scrubs (24%), suit (13%) and casual attire (11%).

Interestingly a separate questionnaire that those exact same family members answered provides a contrasting picture of those numbers. That questionnaire found that only 32% of participants believe wearing a white coat is important for physicians. In an accompanying editorial to this piece, another set of authors wrote that the disparity between the numbers likely suggests that patients and their family members have a subconscious preference, not necessarily for white coats but for attire that identifies a physician as a health professional.

It would seem reasonable then to assume that patients associate our appearance with our competence and professionalism. So, since conventional wisdom aligns with research when it comes to attire, it would be highly recommended that you choose wisely. Most of us in the manual therapy professions need to be able to work and manipulate patients' limbs and torsos, so the white coat might not be your first choice, but keep in mind that the more casual you look, the more you may undermine your professional image with your patient.

Enthusiasm of practitioner

Enthusiasm – origin Greek enthousiasmos, from enthousiazein – to be inspired; irregular from entheos – inspired, from en- + theos – god

Merriam Webster Online: Dictionary

Enthusiasm is truly infectious. Most of us are innately drawn to enthusiastic people. Enthusiastic people are often perceived as being more successful and tend to inspire everyone with whom they come into contact. The definition suggests divine origins or inspiration. While this is simply anecdotal, it has been my observation that some of the most enthusiastic people that I know are the most successful practitioners, and their patients typically speak very highly of them. The clinician–patient relationship is a very complex matter, but the patient certainly comes to us looking for something. Some of what they are looking for is quantifiable, while some is not. My own sense is that there is a clear energy exchange that is taking place, and part of what they are expecting to receive is a bit of your energy. If you are enthusiastic, then your energy naturally spills over on to them.

Though little research has been done in this specific area, one important study of dental patients receiving injections (Gryll & Katahn 1978) found that enthusiastic messages of drug effects produced statistically and clinically significant reductions in fear of injection and state of anxiety and markedly lower ratings of pain experienced during injection of local anesthetic. To quote the researchers, *'Although there was a strong tendency for positive placebo effects to occur when the dental staff was perceived as friendly and supportive, only the attitude factors obtained statistical significance.'* Clearly, the staff's enthusiasm was what made the difference in this study.

As mentioned earlier, a 2010 review of evidence, entitled, 'Effectiveness of manual therapies: the UK evidence report', looked at 49 recent relevant systematic reviews, 16 evidence-based clinical guidelines, plus an additional 46 RCT that had not yet been included in systematic reviews and guidelines. The authors spoke of practitioner enthusiasm affecting outcomes in a positive manner in these studies. In their conclusions, the authors state, *'The contextual or, as it is often called, nonspecific effect of the therapeutic encounter can be quite different depending on the type of provider, the explanation or diagnosis given, the provider's enthusiasm, and the patient's expectations'* (Bronfort et al. 2010).

Another example of the importance of enthusiasm with the placebo effect is the power of new treatments of medications. As was discussed in previous sections, whenever a new treatment, therapy or drug arrives on the scene there is a 1- or 2-year honeymoon when the clinical effects are very powerful. After that honeymoon phase, many of these drugs and therapies were found to be no better than a placebo. This speaks to the power of enthusiasm around any given procedure.

What does this mean to you as a clinician? We all have a natural set point for most aspects of our temperament, but that is not to say that you are locked into this manner of presenting yourself. As mentioned, your professional image is an image that you can craft and create. Ways in which you can increase your enthusiasm while interacting with your patients might include:

- **Practice lifetime learning** – lifetime learning is truly the single most important thing that you can do for your career and for your level of enthusiasm. The fact that you are reading this book indicates your desire for improvement, and I commend you for making this effort. I truly believe that learning is the virtual fountain of youth. If you are learning, then you automatically become more enthused about the topic at hand because of the new information that you are taking in. Learning prevents burnout, keeps your mind open to new possibilities and ideally allows you to reassess your current approaches and ideas.

- **Always wear a smile** – this suggestion applies whether you are on the phone or interacting personally with a patient. You would be amazed how people can pick up on someone's mood even in a recorded telephone message.
- **Actively practice gratitude** – gratitude could be a section on its own. Most of us can change our lives by practicing daily gratitudes. This practice yields personal benefit but also spills over into your demeanour improving the clinician–patient relationship.
- **Encourage random acts of kindness** within your office – this involves both inter-office exchanges and interactions with patients as well.
- **Remember the basics** – be aware of your body language. Sit up straight, smile and make eye contact.
- **Verbally demonstrate enthusiasm** – use phrases such as 'I'm so pleased to see you', or 'I would be more than happy to look that up for you'. Like all skills, enthusiasm is an aspect of your professional demeanour that you can choose to cultivate should you wish to improve your interactions with your patients.

CLINICAL/HEALING ENVIRONMENT

The idea of ideal clinical environment changed a lot in the 20th century. At one time hospitals and doctors' offices were austere, clinical environments with few attempts to make the environment warm or relaxing. Now there is recognition of the importance of human elements, and this area has received quite bit of research. Since billions of dollars have been spent building hospitals and we are living in the age of EBM, this would make a lot of sense. Changes in the clinical environment in health care settings have shown that environment can positively influence the health indicators and healing times, as well as improve staff morale and efficiency (Zborowsky & Kreitzer 2008, Schweitzer et al. 2004). Some of these changes include:

- Increased patients' connection to nature (gardens, windows with a view, plants). Viewing nature has been shown to help calm patients, but can also foster improvement in clinical outcomes such as reducing pain medication intake and shortening hospital stays.
- The use of natural lighting, floor-to-ceiling windows and skylights to help keep the patient in sync with respect to chronobiologic principles.
- Diversions that have a calming effect include artwork, depicting scenes of nature, fireplaces, videos of nature, and aquariums.
- Noise reduction.
- Wide hallways that reduce fight or flight response.
- Relaxing music and sounds.
- Glare reduction.
- Improved air quality (which almost always involves fresh air).
- Lounges and waiting rooms with a purpose.

In hospital environments, it has been well established that single rooms are preferable to doubles or wards. Benefits include better communication with staff, minimization of transfers (due to roommate conflicts), fewer medication errors, decreased infection rates, and comfortable inclusion of the family. Orthopedic and psychiatric patients treated in single rooms were more satisfied with their care than those treated in multiple-bed wards (Schweitzer et al. 2004).

Studies of hospital in-patients have linked the lack of windows with high rates of anxiety, depression and delirium. A view of nature has been correlated with shorter postoperative hospital stays, higher satisfaction with nursing care and decreased use of potent analgesics in cholecystectomy patients compared to patients with obstructed views (Schweitzer et al. 2004).

Art

Studies indicate that patients exposed to art with nature images have less anxiety and require fewer strong pain medication doses. Interestingly, abstract art may contribute to less favorable recovery outcomes than viewing no pictures at all and is consistently disliked by patients (Schweitzer 2004).

Music and ambient sounds

It has been shown that music used at times of high stress (e.g. out-patient surgery and recovery) reduces anxiety, resulting in an increase in-patient comfort and endorphin levels, lowering heart rate and anxiety, and reducing the need for anesthesia. In other studies, music in the healing environment led to decreased use of analgesics and hastened recovery from surgery. The use of music in conjunction with surgical procedures was associated with a significant reduction in the amount of perceived pain and decrease in the level of stress hormones in the blood. When music is used with newborn babies, weight gain, reduced stress and shorter hospital stays are seen (Schweitzer et al. 2004).

Sometimes music or sound of some description is required to fill the silence of the room, or sometimes it is used to block sounds from coming outside of the room. If you have worked in a busy office then you might find that it is distractingly noisy, or the noise might affect the patient's ability to relax. In these cases, music can be used as a tool to muffle sounds coming from outside of the treatment area. An alternative to music is nature sounds. These sounds could come from a water fountain in the room, a sound generating machine, or a soundtrack that plays nature sounds.

Color

Certain colors are more relaxing than others. This applies to pharmaceutical drugs, but also to color choices that you make in your treatment rooms and waiting room. Studies have shown that pink pills are more effective at maintaining concentration than blue ones. Yellow placebo pills are the most effective at treating depression, while red pills are the best color for keeping patients more alert and awake. Green pills apparently help ease anxiety while white pills soothe stomach issues. The color of placebo pills is a definite factor in their effectiveness, with 'hot-colored' pills working better as stimulants and 'cool-colored' pills working better as depressants. When administered without information about whether they are stimulants or depressives, blue placebo pills tend to produce depressant effects, whereas red placebos induce stimulant effects (Blackwell et al. 1972). Patients report falling asleep significantly more quickly and sleeping longer after taking a blue capsule versus taking an orange capsule (Lucchelli et al. 1978). Red placebos are more effective pain relievers than white, blue or green placebos (Huskisson 1974, de Craen et al. 1996).

As mentioned earlier, there are many cultural variations with the placebo effect, so culture and environment play a big role. Cultural background has a strong influence on color preference. Studies have shown that people from the same region regardless of race will have the same color preferences (Whitfield 1990).

There is evidence that color preference may also depend on ambient temperature; for example, people who are cold prefer warm colors like red and yellow, while people who are hot prefer cool colors like blue and green. Some studies concluded that women prefer warm colors while men cool colors (Whitfield & Wiltshire 1990).

Color can actually affect our sense of taste. In one study, they found that 14 percent of people thought that pink tablets tasted sweeter than red tablets, whereas a yellow tablet is perceived as salty irrespective of its ingredients. White or blue tablets were perceived as tasting bitter by 11% of participants while 10% said orange-colored tablets tasted sour (Whitfield & Wiltshire 1990).

What colors you choose will also depend upon what type of treatment you actually perform. For example if you are an athletic therapist, your patients are typically active and are not there to relax. Massage therapists on the other hand typically have patients looking for relaxation. The former profession will likely want uplifting colors while the latter will be looking for the opposite.

In the end, much of this stuff is a matter of personal taste. Years ago, the house next to mine went up for sale several times during the years that I lived in my home. (I am positive that this had nothing to do with having me as their neighbor!) The first couple decorated with strong lively colors. The next owners of the house hated the colors, so went with earth tones throughout. The next couple that bought it thought that those colors were boring and bland so repainted with brighter colors. What was the best color for that house? Clearly, it depended upon who was living there.

In the end, it appears that response to color is multi-factorial and can include such factors as your patient`s gender, age, culture, mood and whether they are feeling overheated or chilled at the time. The science is far too contradictory for you to try to make an evidence-based decision on this matter, so in fact it is probably best to follow your own instincts if you have a strong decorating sense. If you do not, then consult with someone who does or hire a professional to guide you in this area. The only caveat to point out here is that professionalism should always be kept in mind when choosing room colors. If you get too far out on a limb with colors, it will negatively affect the perceived professionalism of the office environment.

Design

Feng Shui is used to promote the creation of an optimally productive and harmonious environment that supports the people in that environment. While this is not hard science, Feng Shui principles have gained great acceptance when designing healing spaces (Schweitzer et al. 2004). Like acupuncture, and other aspects of traditional Chinese medicine, Feng Shui has withstood the test of time, so you would be wise to consider incorporating some of its design principles into your workspace. At the most basic level, Feng Shui logic flows out of three principles:

1. Everything is alive
2. Everything is connected
3. Everything is changing.

This sounds good in principle, but what can you do to implement this philosophy into your treatment areas? It might start by purchasing a book on the topic, if you have strong design sensibility. If you feel that you lack this quality then perhaps you might want to hire a consultant. That being said, here some basic Feng Shui design ideas.

- Provide direct views to entrances, so that patients do not have their backs to doorways.
- Avoid placing patients in the direct line of a door in order to protect privacy and avoid the feeling of always being watched. Being in the direct line of a doorway is said to put an individual directly in the rush of chi, with resulting negative effects on health and productivity.
- Utilize warm lighting, as opposed to glaring florescent lighting; overly bright light is believed to irritate people and result in headaches. Sconces (lights mounted on the walls of the treatment area) on dimmers work perfectly. Even at full brightness, they are not in the patient's visual field.

Conclusion

There are a multitude of design and decorating factors that should be taken into consideration when altering a clinic or a treatment space. Your choices will depend upon your practice demographic, whether old or young, ethnic or multicultural, male or female, and it will also depend upon the type of treatments that you offer. No matter what demographic you treat, it is wise to design in such a manner that ambient noise is minimized.

A good exercise for any of us would be to rethink our entire workspace from a different perspective, and not take anything for granted. Music, ambient noise, art, furniture, windows, plants, lighting and patient seating all need to be viewed with an eye to professionalism and patient experience in mind.

Suggestions from workshops on the topic of design

Workshops on this topic have highlighted key elements of a professional treatment space in addition to the previously mentioned topics. From what we have learned in this book, anything that enhances your professional image, which in itself will trigger placebo responses, enhances treatment outcomes. Some of these suggestions include:

- Diplomas and certificates prominently displayed.
- Bookcase(s) with your reference material.
- Patient education brochures and patient reference material.
- Anatomical models giving a clear 3-dimensional perspective on various body structures.

- Professional attire for both practitioners and staff.
- Medical equipment (e.g. laser, ultrasound) prominently displayed.
- Medical and anatomical charts displayed on walls.
- Subscriptions to professional and health magazines in waiting area.
- Attention to detail by you and clinic staff in all manners of clinic operation and appearance.
- Focus on cleanliness and hygiene.
- Awareness and attenuation of ambient noise.
- Monthly newsletter keeping patients up-to-date with clinic and health information.
- **Home clinics** – if one has a home-based office then there needs to be a clear separation from home and clinic. A separate entrance is strongly recommended so that patients are not entering your home (for the patient's sake). In addition, employing soundproofing in clinic walls is recommended so that house noises do not penetrate the treatment space.

Box 2.4

PRACTITIONER'S USE OF HUMOR

A good laugh and a long sleep are the best cures in the doctor's book.

Irish proverb

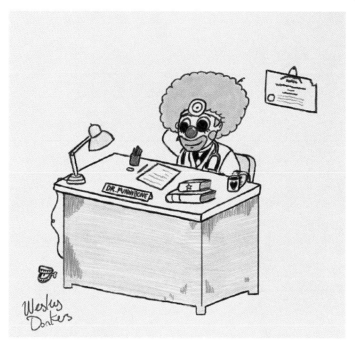

Fig. 2.16

The benefits of humor in relation to health received a lot of publicity with the 1979 publication of Norman Cousins' book *Anatomy of an Illness*. In it, he described how laughter and vitamin C helped his recovery from ankylosing spondylitis. According to Cousins, 10 minutes of laughter resulted in 2 hours of pain-free sleep and a reduction in his erythrocyte sedimentation rate. Around that same time Patch Adams was using humor as an integral part of his approach as a doctor. He founded the Gesundheit! Institute in 1971, but it wasn't till 1998 when the film about his life came out that he became well known. You may know of him and his use of humor, but in reality Patch Adams and his approach is actually so much more. To say that Patch Adams uses humor in his approach is like saying that a car uses spark plugs. Humor is a part of his approach, though, and to this day he can be seen wearing clown pants and is ready to play the clown at the drop of a hat. However, as important as humor is, Patch will say 'Friendship, not laughter is the best medicine', acknowledging the holistic nature of health. Patch has communicated a recurring message in several interviews: there are six qualities that he requires before anyone can work with him in his hospital. These qualities are that the person be *happy, funny, loving, cooperative, creative,* and *thoughtful.* His personal thoughts on humor are that it:

1. Helps prevent burnout
2. Is a painkiller
3. Sets an environment for cooperation, and that
4. It serves to level the issue of hierarchy in the therapeutic relationship, which Adams sees as key.

Therefore, his view is less that it acts a placebo per se, but rather that it performs an extremely important role in the practitioner–patient relationship. The quality of this relationship, as we have seen, directly affects medical outcomes. The area in which he sees a direct effect on the patient is in pain reduction, and he has seen this in the very worst of situations having worked in war zone hospitals with children and spent time with people during the last hours of their life more times that he can remember. If you find the qualities of Patch Adams interesting, you might want to take some time to learn about this amazing man. If so, it is worth noting that the movie about him only looks at his life in a one-dimensional manner, but he has written a few books (see Adams with Mylander1998, Adams 1998 in particular) and you can view interviews of him online. There are plenty of YouTube videos that give insight into his radically holistic approach, dedication, passion and philosophies. Patch Adams is a true medical revolutionary.

In 2003, Howard Bennett conducted an extensive review of the literature on this topic entitled 'Humor in medicine'. According to him, there is support in the literature for the role of humor and laughter in the areas of improved health outcomes, and improved immune function, patient–physician communication, psychological aspects of patient care, medical education, and as a means of reducing stress in medical professionals (Bennett 2003).

A 2011 study looked at 43 children with respiratory pathologies. There were 21 children in the experimental group and 22 in the control group. During their hospitalization, the children of the experimental group interacted with two clowns who were experienced in the field of pediatric intervention. All participants were evaluated with respect to clinical progress and to a series of physiological and pain measures both before and after the clown interaction. When compared with the control group the experimental group showed earlier disappearance of the pathological symptoms, a statistically significant lowering of diastolic blood pressure, respiratory frequency and temperature as compared with the control group. The other two parameters of systolic pressure and heart frequency yielded results in the same direction, without reaching statistical significance. The author conclusions were:

> *Taken together, our data indicate that the presence of clowns in the ward has a possible health-inducing effect. Thus, humor can be seen as an easy-to-use,*

inexpensive and natural therapeutic modality to be used within different therapeutic settings.

(Bertini et al. 2011)

William B. Strean (2009) notes:

> *They are easy to prescribe and there are no substantial concerns with respect to dose, side-effects, or allergies. It seems, however, that the medical community has been reluctant to embrace and support laughter for health.*

Strean noted the shortcomings of studies and the need for more studies on humor, but his conclusion is, '*Let us begin to consider that, along with eating your vegetables and getting enough sleep, laughter is a sound prescription as a wonderful way to enhance health.*'

One point that several papers touch on is the ability for humor to backfire, if it offends or is simply inappropriate. That being said, Patch Adams has had people volunteer to do clown work with him and he steadfastly maintains that in 40 years he has never trained one clown for this task. The only situation in which his clowns are trained is before they enter war zones, because the horrendous circumstances of seeing children experiencing immense suffering, pain and death requires some psychological preparation.

Howard Bennett discusses in his previously mentioned paper ('Humor in medicine') that the area where humor that has shown the most promise is in the use of humor to moderate a patient's response to pain. Several experimental studies in which a patient's pain tolerance was evaluated during or after exposure to comedy videotapes showed an increased ability to tolerate pain. Other studies he reviewed showed that the need for pain medication was reduced after viewing comedies. As one might guess, patients that had a say in what material they were going to watch saw greater improvement. Bennett also notes that humor has been especially important in the field of pediatric medicine.

Bennett's conclusions are much the same as Patch Adam's: that humor's first clear benefit appears to be in the area of the practitioner–patient relationship, in that it has the potential to relieve stress inpatients and medical professionals. At the very least, humor gives patients the opportunity to forget about their anxiety and pain during the treatment, but some studies suggest longer lasting health effects. Humor can put both parties at ease and reduce the power differential, making the doctor or practitioner more human for the patient.

Health and happiness

A recent study by Diener and Chan adds another perspective to this discussion (Diener & Chan 2011). Their review of more than 160 studies of both human and animal subjects found 'clear and compelling evidence' that happy people tend to live up to 10 years longer and experience better health than their unhappy peers. Their 43-page paper looks at seven different measures of happiness which they term subjective well-being and correlates them to health and longevity of the study participants. Their take-home message is worded in a refreshingly unequivocal manner. The reader might want to note the strong language of the authors' conclusions. Their statement is a refreshing break from the typical *'more studies need to be done'* that is often seen in published studies. It is rare indeed to see such a strongly worded conclusion as we see below (Diener 2011):

> *There now are sufficient studies on all-cause mortality and certain diseases to draw relatively strong conclusions. Our overall conclusion is that the evidence for the influence of subjective well-being (SWB) on health and all-cause mortality is clear and compelling, although there is much more uncertainty about how various types of SWB influence specific diseases, and about the role of the possible mediating processes. The effect sizes for SWB and health are not trivial; they are large when considered in a society-wide perspective. If high SWB adds 4 to 10 years to life compared to low SWB, this is an outcome worthy of national attention.*

This extensive study underscores the importance of happiness, which in itself has a very strong take-home message quite apart from the rest of the content of this section. While admittedly happiness is not the same as humor, it would be very hard to argue that one is not happy while one is laughing. Clearly, we have two major emotional release valves – laughing and crying, which lie at opposite ends of the emotional spectrum. Laughing and crying perform the important role of allowing the patient (and every human) to ground themselves emotionally as they release a surge of emotion that could probably be mentally processed, but not in the time required. It is not unlike a lightning bolt during a thunderstorm. We are not the grounding rod in this exchange, but rather we facilitate and participate in the most intimate of human ways by sharing in either of these emotional exchanges.

As with most aspects of the placebo effect, there are cultural variances. One of my patients came from a stern eastern European background. She contends that if a professional tried to use humor with their parents, they would have far less credibility. So like all comedians, 'you need to know your audience' when using humor. Also, all cultural aspects aside, one needs to be judicious in one's use of humor as a medical practitioner because you could be perceived as a joker and not be taken seriously by your patient.

In conclusion, as a practitioner you might want to consider employing humor for the following three reasons:

1. For the benefit of the patient
2. For the benefit of your relationship with the patient, and
3. For your own personal benefit.

Literature and studies indicating the proper use of appropriate humor will provide benefit in all of these areas.

HELPING PATIENTS MAXIMIZE THEIR OWN HEALING RESPONSE

In this section, we will look at any factor that will help with the body's healing response, outside of those that involve the therapeutic encounter. This section is not meant to be an extensive reference on any one of these topics, but rather to be a checklist and a place to start should you have a motivated patient who is interested in maximizing their own healing response. As you will see, there is a whole host of topics that a practitioner should be aware of because:

1. We work in the healing profession, so should be aware of methods to maximize healing for our patients
2. It is also good to be cognizant of these matters because sometimes patients might ask about some of the topics listed below
3. At many times during a treatment, a flag will be raised where the topic can be discussed
4. When you encounter stalled healing, you and your patient will want to consider other strategies for kick-starting their healing response.

In the manual therapy professions we have a lot of contact time with our patients and much peripheral information gets discussed during a treatment, which can veer away from the specific condition that we are treating. We learn a tremendous amount of information about our patients and quickly begin to acquire a broader holistic perspective of the person. Even though we aren't psychologists we cannot help but notice psycho-emotional barriers to our patients' health; and even though we aren't social workers we may notice psychosocial factors that impact on a patient's ability to acquire social support. And while we are not nutritionists, hopefully our training in nutrition, physiology, immunology and pathology should give us a perspective on whether their diet is aiding or impeding their immune system function and whether they are eating foods that tend to exacerbate or minimize inflammation. Some of the pertinent information that we might want to take note of that can be impediments to healing are listed as a checklist for you below:

Important factors affecting the healing response

- Social connectedness
- General anxiety levels
- Ability to manage stress
- Basic nutritional habits
- The inflammatory state of their body
- General attitude, whether positive or negative
- Basic psychological state, i.e. perhaps a gentle suggestion of referral to a professional or support group if you see untreated depression, anger, guilt, or grief

- Level of happiness
- Low self-esteem or poor body image
- Inability to forgive either themselves or others relative to the pathology they are experiencing
- Lack of exercise
- Poor sleeping patterns.

All these factors can affect the treatment that you have just performed, by either augmenting it or sabotaging the patient's return to health. Needless to say, we all have to operate within our scope of practice but we should be cognizant of when to refer to another professional if the matter falls outside of our scope. Secondly, there is always constructive verbal support that we can provide to our patients whenever any of these issues surface during the treatment. Finally, we should be aware of factors such as these that contribute to health, and perhaps keep a file of resources in our community. This way, we can provide resources to patients who are interested and open to the concept of healthy eating, personal growth, and psycho-emotional well-being connected to their health. With this in mind, let us look at factors that can affect a person's health, and therefore their body's ability to battle pathologies, or to bounce back from an injury, illness or infection.

Social support systems

Humans evolved as social beings and still continue to greatly value social connect-edness and benefit in almost every way imaginable from their group approach to everything. Right from the early days in the trees and on the plains of what is now Africa, we have done better in groups than on our own. Almost all of our health benefits come from our social connections and from our social approach to life, whether one considers things such as access to healthcare, the wealth that we enjoy, the comforts of a safe heated home, friends and family with whom we can enjoy life. On the other end of the spectrum are people that are forced to (or occasionally choose to) live on the outskirts of society or on the streets of our metropolitan areas. Their health outcomes are not even a fraction of what one could expect from living in a fully socially-connected manner.

As you look at your practice, you will likely see a few patients in particular whose social connections are scant for various reasons. Sometimes it is mental illness, sometimes it is disability, sometimes income (though this really shouldn't be a large barrier), sometimes it is habit, sometimes it is personality and confidence issues such as shyness or social awkwardness. What is interesting to consider is that doctors might occasionally find themselves in a quandary as to which drug to prescribe for their patients as they sort through the literature and see 3% or 5% improvements of a given drug over another, when in fact if they played some sort of role in helping their patient become more connected, the anticipated health/ longevity outcome would likely be in the double digits. The problem with that idea is that our medical model isn't designed to help people in that way, even though we know it will improve health outcomes. Fortunately, we do have social programs, particularly for the elderly, but still doctors are the sentinels for the many people who are suffering ill health, partly due to social disconnectedness.

The good news is that there has been considerable study in this area over the years, most of it strongly in support of staying socially connected. This ought to come as no great surprise, but still, it is always good to have clinical studies backup conventional wisdom. There have been at least six large longitudinal studies on aging that follow the participants for as long as possible. Studies have been performed in several countries with different cultural traditions. Several have had over 1000 participants in each study and have looked at issues of social interactions and connectedness. One, titled 'Aging in Leganes' is a 1993 cohort study of 2000 residents stratified in age from 65 to 90 with 15 years of follow-up (see Zunzunegui et al. 2009 for an analysis of this Spanish study). Another, The Australian Longitudinal Study of Ageing (ALSA; see References and Further Reading for the website), is an ongoing study of 2087 participants aged 70 years or more. It has had multiple waves of data collection and analysis, beginning in 1992 and following this group forward with several study waves. The 11th wave was in 2010.

So, just what do the studies say? Well, like many other things in life, it is quality not quantity that counts; still, having a larger social circle can confer longevity benefits. ALSA continues to glean information for the Australian government as it reviews its social and health programs for the elderly.

A 2005 ALSA wave (Giles et al. 2005) of this study had 1477 participants aged 70 years and over. It examined different types of social networks including children, relatives, friends and confidants. Participants were living in both the community and residential care facilities. The findings demonstrated that after controlling for a range of demographic, health, and lifestyle variables, greater networks with friends were substantially protective against mortality in the 10-year follow-up period, as summarized here:

- Close relationships with children and relatives had little effect on longevity rates for older people during the 10-year study.
- People with extensive networks of good friends and confidantes outlived those with the fewest friends by 22%! No matter how you look at this statistic, this is a very substantial effect.
- The positive effects of friendships on longevity continued throughout the decade, regardless of other profound life changes such as the death of a spouse or other close family members.

An interesting conclusion of this study was that the effects of social networks with children and relatives were found to be neutral with respect to longevity; neither a positive nor a negative with respect to survival over the following decade. You can draw what you want from this, but it seems clear from this study is that it is beneficial to have friends outside of your family.

Another recent study (Darviri et al. 2009) looked at the habits of centurions (people who lived to 100 or more) and found some interesting social tendencies.

Quoting this study, '*We found that our participants were characterized by selectiveness in their socializing with other people and tendency to avoid conflicts. Also, we found that they predominantly used the 'flight' response whenever confronted with stressors.*' The researchers concluded that the three major psychosocial factors associated with exceptional longevity were:

1. Social selectivity
2. Conflict avoidance, and
3. Adaptiveness.

Teresa Seeman PhD, co-chair of Biostatistics at UCLA School of Public Health, has a particular interest in the role of social and psychological factors on health risks in aging. She has led and participated in a number of studies, which tease out information from previous gerontology studies. Some of the conclusions are very interesting. For example, one of her studies concluded that, 'available data suggest that, although social integration is generally associated with better health outcomes, the quality of existing ties also appears to influence the extent of such health benefits.' Therefore, healthy social integration appears linked not only to longevity, but also better health outcomes. She emphasizes the fact that it is the 'quality' of the ties that appears to be important. However, on the bottom end of the scale, numerous studies support the fact that not just social isolation but also non-supportive social interactions typically lead to poorer health outcomes and shorter lifespan (Seeman 1996, Cerhan & Wallace 1997, Rodriguez-Laso et al. 2007). Her research concluded that 'both social isolation and non-supportive social interactions can result in lower immune function and higher neuro-endocrine and cardiovascular activity, while socially supportive interactions have the opposite effects' (Seeman 1996).

One aspect of social isolation that may not be typically considered is the situation where a person has a social circle but 'feels' useless. People in this situation might have lots of contact with other people but would be defined as poorly socially integrated. A 2009 study by Tara Gruenewald PhD, Assistant Professor of Gerontology at UCLA, looked at feelings of uselessness in the elderly. She found that, 'Older adults with persistently low feelings of usefulness or who experienced a decline to low feelings of usefulness during the first 3 years of the study experienced a greater hazard of mortality during a subsequent 9-year follow-up as compared to older adults with persistently high feelings of usefulness' (Gruenewald et al. 2009). Once again, not a surprising finding, but it is an important reminder of the absolute importance of the concepts being discussed here. These are, in fact, life and death issues.

Another analysis of the Aging in Leganes study, performed at the University of Montreal, found that 'having a poor relationship with at least one child increased mortality by 30%. Elderly persons who felt their role in their children's lives was important had a lower mortality risk than those who felt they played a small role. Feeling loved and listened to by one's children did not have an effect on survival. Maintaining an important role in the extended family was also significantly associated with survival' (Zunzunegui et al. 2009) Another analysis of the Leganes study by Angel Rodriguez-Laso found that having 'a confidant was associated with a 25% reduction in the mortality risk' (Rodriguez-Laso et al. 2007). Several key points raised here are:

1. Perceived role as a parent is very important
2. Perceived role with extended family (grandparent, uncle, etc.) is very important
3. Having a poor relationship with a child was extremely detrimental
4. Having a confidant is also very important.

This study appears to conflict with the Australian study and perhaps cultural differences account for that fact, but what seems to be common in all studies is the need to have some control over your primary role, and be perceived useful in that role. Isolation is not healthy and having a confidant, whether it be a family member or not, is very important. Given the importance of social integration, the obvious question is what role can we play in helping our patients assess their degree of engagement and in becoming more socially engaged if necessary? What is interesting is that as I typed various search terms to find online resources in the area of developing a strong social network, 98% of the results were about 'social media'. I didn't know whether to laugh or cry as these results kept appearing after changing the search terms multiple times. Clearly, it is very much a sign of the times that we live in. Given our busy schedules as practitioners, and for a multitude of professional reasons, it is unlikely that we will have the time to do handholding in this area of the patient's life. What we can do is to create a checklist of suggestions for patients interested in improving their social network. There have been a few patients, during my many years of practice, which have hinted very strongly about their need for a stronger social network. Some patients have asked me if I know of any organizations or clubs that I can suggest for them. For suggestions in this area I recommend that you or they consult the four websites below. There is also a list of suggestions in the Appendix which might be useful:

- Humana.com has a page addressing this issue entitled, *'How healthy is your social life?'* (https://www.humana.com/learning-center/health-and-well-being/mental-health/social-life). It offers several tips on how to become more socially engaged.
- Lifeworks is another site with several suggestions on building a personal support network (https://portal.lifeworks.com/portal/Viewers/HPSArticle.aspx?HPSMaterialID=14691).
- Mayo Clinic has a page with suggestions on building a personal network of connections (http://www.mayoclinic.org/social-support/art-20044445).
- University of Buffalo School of Social Work has an excellent resource area on its website, also included in the Appendix (self-care page: http://www.socialwork.buffalo.edu/students/self-care/support-system.asp).

Exercise

Considering my audience, there should not be a need to emphasize the importance of exercise or to provide the backup research, but let's quickly review it anyway. Apart from remedial exercises and homecare, which needless to say are extremely important and you are presumably already prescribing, here is a list of some of the proven benefits of exercise:

- **Longevity**. People who are physically active live longer. According to one Swedish 20-year follow-up study, regular exercise reduces the risk of dying prematurely (Rosengren & Wilhelmsen 1997). A meta-analysis of research published between 1970 and 2007 showed that walking reduced the risk of cardiovascular events by 31% and it cut the risk of dying during the study period by 32%. These benefits were equally robust in men and women. Protection was evident even at distances of just 5.5 miles per week and at a casual pace of about 2 miles per hour. The people who walked longer distances or walked at a faster pace, or both, enjoyed the greatest protection (Hamer & Chida 2008).
- **Depression.** Multiple studies have shown that exercise promotes mental health and reduces symptoms of depression (Blumenthal et al. 1999, Blumenthal et al. 2007).
- **Cardiovascular health.** Lack of physical activity is one of the major risk factors for cardiovascular diseases. Regular exercising strengthens heart muscle and reduces cardiovascular mortality risk (Janssen & Jolliffe 2006).
- **Cholesterol lowering effect**. Exercise itself does not burn off cholesterol; however, exercise improves blood cholesterol levels by decreasing LDL (bad) cholesterol, triglycerides and total cholesterol, and increasing HDL (good) cholesterol (Kelley et al. 2004).
- **Prevention and control of diabetes**. The link between exercise and type II diabetes is undeniable. A Finnish Diabetes Prevention Study showed that moderate physical activity combined with weight loss and balanced diet can confer a 50–60% reduction in risk of developing diabetes (Lindström et al. 2003).
- **Blood pressure**. All forms of exercise seem to be effective in reducing blood pressure. Aerobic exercise appears to have a slightly greater effect on blood pressure in hypertensive individuals than in individuals without hypertension (Pinto et al. 2006).
- **Stroke**. Research data indicates that moderate and high levels of physical activity may reduce the risk of total, ischemic, and hemorrhagic strokes (Lee et al. 2003).
- **Weight control**. Diet is the most important factor in weight control, but regular exercise also helps to reach and maintain a healthy weight. It is less about the calories burned through exercise than the residual increase in one's metabolic rate after exercise. Use of intervals during exercise

is probably the most efficient method for keeping one's metabolic rate elevated for the longest post-exercise period.

- **Muscle strength and fat reduction**. Health studies repeatedly show that strength training increases muscle strength and mass and decreases fat tissue (Sarsan et al. 2006).
- **Bone strength**. An active lifestyle benefits bone density. Regular weight-bearing exercise promotes bone formation, delays bone loss and may protect against osteoporosis –a form of bone loss associated with aging (Kemmler et al. 2004).
- **Sleep**. Exercise helps promote healthy sleep, but should be done in the morning or afternoon so that it does not interrupt the sleep cycle.
- **Improved cognition and memory**. Researchers found that the areas of the brain that are stimulated through exercise are responsible for memory, learning, decision-making process and problem solving (Wu et al. 2007).
- **Improved sexual function and better sex life.** Regular exercise maintains or improves sex life. Physical improvements in muscle strength and tone, endurance, body composition and cardiovascular function can all enhance sexual functioning in both men and women. Researchers revealed that men who exercise regularly are less likely to have erectile dysfunction and impotence than are men who don't exercise (Bacon et al. 2003).

In addition, you might want to look at the following two quotes and either post them on the clinic wall or bring them up occasionally during treatments to help remind your patients to adopt a regular habit of exercise:

- *'Exercise is the closest thing we have to an anti-aging pill'* says Dr Leaf of the Harvard Medical School. Eighty percent of the health problems once associated with aging are now thought to be preventable or postponable if a person keeps fit.
- 'There is no drug in current or prospective use that holds as much promise for sustained health as a lifetime of physical exercise', *Journal of American Medical Association.*

The health benefits of exercise have been proven in study after study, and no matter what age your patient is, there will be some degree of exercise that you can suggest for them. If their health state is such that you cannot prescribe cardiovascular exercise, then you can undoubtedly suggest strengthening, stretching and movement exercises. At the very least, suggest that all of your patients adopt the following mantra . . . 'movement'.

Sleep

Not getting enough sleep can have profound consequences on our health and well-being both on a short-term and a long-term basis. Short-term consequences include fatigue, bad mood, poor memory and lack of focus. Long-term health consequences include chronic medical conditions, such as diabetes, high blood pressure and heart disease, which may lead to a shortened life expectancy. Additional research studies show that habitually sleeping more than 9 hours is also associated with poor health.

Sleep deprivation studies have revealed a variety of potentially harmful effects such as:

- Increased blood pressure
- Impaired control of blood glucose
- Increased inflammation.

Cross-sectional epidemiological studies indicate that both reduced and increased sleep duration, as reported on questionnaires, are linked with hypertension, diabetes and obesity. However, cross-sectional studies cannot explain how too little or too much sleep leads to disease because people may have a disease that affects sleep, rather than a sleep habit that causes a disease to occur or worsen.

Finally, the third and most convincing type of evidence that poor long-term sleep habits are associated with the development of numerous diseases comes from tracking the sleep habits and disease patterns over long periods of time in individuals who are initially healthy through longitudinal epidemiological studies. Results of these studies are now beginning to suggest that adjusting one's sleep can reduce the risk of eventually developing a disease or lessen the severity of an ongoing disease. The following diseases are linked to lack of or poor sleep:

- **Obesity**. Insufficient sleep has been linked to a high probability for weight gain. Poor sleep leads to an increase in the production of cortisol and the secretion of insulin following a meal. Insulin is a hormone that regulates glucose processing and promotes fat storage; higher levels of insulin are associated with weight gain, a risk factor for diabetes. Insufficient sleep is also associated with lower levels of leptin, a hormone that alerts the brain that it has enough food, as well as higher levels of ghrelin, a biochemical that stimulates appetite.
- **Diabetes**. Researchers have found that insufficient sleep may lead to type 2 diabetes by influencing the way the body processes glucose, the high-energy carbohydrate that cells use for fuel. Numerous epidemiological studies also have revealed that adults who usually slept less than 5 hours per night have a greatly increased risk of having or developing diabetes. In addition, researchers have correlated obstructive sleep apnea – a disorder in which breathing difficulties during sleep lead to frequent arousals – with the development of impaired glucose control similar to that which occurs in diabetes.
- **Heart disease and hypertension**. Even minor periods of inadequate sleep can cause an elevation in blood pressure. Studies have found

that a single night of inadequate sleep in people who have existing hypertension can cause elevated blood pressure throughout the following day. This effect may begin to explain the correlation between poor sleep and cardiovascular disease and stroke. There is also growing evidence of a connection between obstructive sleep apnea and heart disease. Over time, people experiencing sleep apnea are at increased risk of chronic elevation of hypertension, which is a major risk factor for cardiovascular disease. Fortunately, when sleep apnea is treated, blood pressure may go down.

- **Mood disorders**. Chronic sleep issues have been correlated with depression, anxiety and mental distress. In one study, subjects who slept 4.5 hours per night reported feeling more stressed, sad, angry and mentally exhausted. In another study, subjects who slept 4 hours per night showed declining levels of optimism and sociability as a function of days of inadequate sleep. All of these self-reported symptoms improved dramatically when subjects returned to a normal sleep schedule.

- **Immune function**. It is natural for people to go to bed when they are sick. Substances produced by the immune system to help fight infection also cause fatigue. One theory proposes that the immune system evolved 'sleepiness-inducing factors' because inactivity and sleep provided an advantage: those who slept more when faced with an infection were better able to fight that infection than those who slept less. In fact, research in animals suggests that those animals who obtain more deep sleep following experimental challenge by microbial infection have a better chance of survival.

- **Life expectancy**. Considering the many potential adverse health effects of insufficient sleep, it is not surprising that poor sleep is associated with lower life expectancy. Data from three large cross-sectional epidemiological studies reveal that sleeping 5 hours or less per night increased mortality risk from all causes by roughly 15%.

Note that despite its mild sedative qualities, alcohol often contributes to poor sleep. Studies have shown that alcohol use is more prevalent among people who sleep poorly. The reason for this is twofold. First, alcohol acts as a mild sedative and is commonly used as a sleep aid among people who have sleep problems such as insomnia. Second, the sedative quality of alcohol is only temporary. As alcohol is processed by the body over a few hours it begins to stimulate the parts of the brain that cause arousal, in many cases causing awakenings and sleep problems later in the night. If you have patients with sleep issues you might want to advise them against alcohol consumption near bedtime.

It is estimated that while 50–70 million Americans suffer from some type of sleep disorder, most people do not mention their sleeping problems to their doctors, and most doctors do not necessarily ask about them. This is definitely a basic question to have on your intake/case history form. Factors that contribute to healthy sleep are something that patients with sleep issues should look at. This can include diet, exercise schedule, lifestyle and bedroom layout. A quick checklist provided by Harvard University's Division of Sleep Medicine suggests the following: (for more detail on tips to improve quality of sleep, go to http://healthysleep.med.harvard.edu/healthy/getting/overcoming/tips).

1. Avoid caffeine, alcohol, nicotine, and other chemicals that interfere with sleep.
2. Turn your bedroom into a sleep-inducing environment. Consider light levels, noise levels, temperature and ventilation. More drastic measures could include ear plugs, eye mask, black-out curtains and white-noise generator.
3. Establish a soothing pre-sleep routine.
4. Go to sleep when you're truly tired. If you aren't sleeping get up and read.
5. Don't be a night-time clock-watcher.
6. Use light to your advantage. Natural light keeps your internal clock on a healthy sleep–wake cycle, so let in the light first thing in the morning and get out of the office for a sun break during the day.
7. Keep your internal clock set with a consistent sleep schedule.
8. Nap early – or not at all.
9. Lighten up on evening meals.
10. Balance fluid intake. Drink enough fluid at night to keep from waking up thirsty, but not so much and so close to bedtime that you will be awakened by the need for a trip to the bathroom.
11. Exercise early on in the day; not near bed time.

If you suspect a more serious sleep issue, have your patient speak to their doctor about referral to a sleep clinic. A sleep clinic will extensively analyze an individual's quality of sleep. In these studies, approximately 30 wires are attached to the patient to monitor body-wide movements and brain activity during sleep. The results are analyzed by a physician who specializes in sleep disorders and then the patient is consulted directly so that appropriate remedies can be taken. For all sleep-related issues Harvard University's Healthy Sleep website is a valuable resource to recommend to your patients (http://healthysleep.med.harvard.edu/). All information and statistics in this section (on sleep) are drawn from their database, which is a great resource for both practitioner and patient.

Nutrition

Our education as health professionals has taught us the importance of nutrition, but unless we receive the appropriate level of certification, advising on nutritional matters is moving beyond our scope of practice. Still, there are basic concepts that we can communicate to our patients at the appropriate time when the topic comes up during a treatment session. At an energy level, carbohydrates and fats are broken down into glucose which then enters Krebs cycle for the manufacturing of ATP (are your schooldays coming back to you now?). However, the breakdown and digestion of proteins, carbohydrates and fats is a very complex procedure, and so much more than just energy production is taking place. Also, nutrition involves more than macronutrients, it also involves micronutrients like vitamins and minerals. All of the food that we consume provides the raw materials for energy, for the growth and repair of the body, and to continuously rebuild the immune system. Needless to say we need a healthy immune system to allow the body to fight off infection.

Complicating the topic of nutrition are food allergies, food intolerances and food sensitivities. Food allergies run the full gambit from mild annoyance, digestive upset or skin rash to severe anaphylactic reactions and death. This is clearly an area where we are unqualified even to advise our patients. Allergies, sensitivities, and intolerances are typically quite person-specific, and appropriate testing should be done by a qualified health professional. Most people reading this probably know someone who saw immediate health improvements after removing one or two foods from their diet. This is an important health matter, but it is well beyond us to advise or even guide our patients, unless we obtain the proper credentials. All cases of potential food sensitivity, intolerance or allergies should be referred to a health professional qualified in that area.

That being said, basic healthy eating concepts that hopefully most health professionals would agree upon include:

1. **Eat plenty of green leafy vegetables**. Not only are green leafy vegetables low on the glycemic index and among the least calorie-dense (so they will fill you up without adding a high calorie burden), but they are also packed with vitamins and minerals.
2. **Eat fresh vegetables of different colors**.*
3. **Reduce consumption of simple carbohydrates,** especially sugars. Complex carbohydrates in our diet allow the slow release of glucose. Simple carbohydrates cause sugar spikes and predispose us to the risks of type II diabetes. Refined sugars are also linked to premature aging, cardiovascular disease and Alzheimer's disease. Restriction of dietary sugars has been shown to have positive effects on wound healing, insulin resistance and cardiovascular disease (Luevano-Contreras & Chapman-Novakofski 2010).

---

*When it comes to vegetables, I personally prefer to buy organic and/or grow my own in order to reduce the pesticide load on my body, but this is a personal decision based on my reading on this subject. Research shows that there are some vitamins that are specific to food color (e.g. yellow, red, blue/purple, tan/brown/white and, of course, green). Fresh vegetables have similar benefits to those listed under green leafy vegetables above, and remember this – no one ever showed up at a weight disorder clinic with a broccoli or spinach eating disorder. The calorie density of vegetables is quite low so they are an excellent food for people trying to lose weight as long as they are not covered in fats (e.g. butter, oil or gravy), sugars and salt.

4. **Choose whole foods** (e.g. whole grains) over refined foods and grains. Refined foods lack fiber (Canadian Diabetes Association 2014). Fiber has been shown to:
   - Aid digestion by softening and expanding stool volume, speeding up fecal transit and elimination
   - Combat constipation
   - Help regulate blood sugar swings and by lowering serum cholesterol
   - Possibly protect against cancer – in the bowel, bacteria converts fiber into short chain fatty acids, which provide energy for the body and may help protect against cancer.

   In addition to the benefits of fiber found in whole foods, these foods also contain more bio-available vitamins than refined foods. While refined foods often have vitamins added during processing, there is an ongoing debate about the bio-availability of many synthetic vitamins. Finally, whole foods do not cause the sugar spikes seen with refined foods because with these foods glucose is released more gradually into the blood stream.

5. **Avoid processed foods**, whether on the grocery store shelf or in a restaurant. Processed foods contain high levels of sodium and contain preservatives not found in whole fresh foods.

6. **Reduce fat consumption.** Fat is the most energy concentrated food on the planet. We do need a certain amount of fat in our diet, but our needs are very easily met without actively seeking them out or adding them to our diets. There is currently an obesity epidemic in North America, and while dietary fat is not the only reason for this, we still need to be cognizant of the fact that when we eat fat or oils, we are eating concentrated calories. Liberal consumption of fats and oils is especially not a good idea if one is dealing with weight issues. An interesting aside on this matter is the fact that in the 1980s, public health messages suggested reducing our dietary fat intake from the 40%+ mark to 30%. While North Americans' diet is now approximately 33% fats, portion sizes and calorie intake have increased to the point that we are still eating as many calories from fat, even though fats represent a smaller percentage of our calorie intake.

7. **Reduce portion size.** The National Heart, Lung and Blood Institute of America reports that due to increased portion sizes at fast food restaurants, we would consume 1595 more calories per day than if we had the same foods at typical portions served 20 years ago (National Institutes of Health 2013). When foods such as beer and chocolate bars were introduced they generally appeared in just one size, which was actually smaller than or equal to the smallest size currently available. This observation also holds for French fries, hamburgers and carbonated beverages, for which current sizes are two to five times larger than the originals (Young & Nestle 2002).

8.   **Be aware of calorie consumption.** North American calorie consumption
     might finally be levelling out, but the trends over the last 40 years are
     quite troubling. Needless to say, if weight issues are a concern for you or
     your patient (or me), then calorie consumption must be reduced:
     - One study found that US women increased their daily calorie
       consumption 22% between 1971 and 2000, from 1542 calories per
       day to 1877 calories. During the same period the calorie intake for
       men increased 7% from 2450 calories per day to 2618 calories. The
       increase in calories was mainly due to an increase in carbohydrate
       consumption. This has not been an increase in healthy complex
       carbohydrates but rather an increase in sugars. The study also found
       that while the *percent* of calories Americans take in from fat had
       decreased (with most of the drop in saturated fat intake), the actual
       number of fat grams consumed per day has changed little since 1971,
       due to the increase in overall calories consumed daily (Centers for
       Disease Control 2004).
     - In 1981, calorie consumption in the US averaged 3200 per day. In
       2012, that number was 3900 per day (Credit Suisse 2013).
     - The European Association for the Study of Obesity conducted a study
       that looked at relative contributions of food and exercise habits to the
       development of the obesity epidemic. It concluded that the rise in
       obesity in the US since the 1970s was largely due to increased energy
       intake. The study concludes, *'Increased energy intake appears to be
       more than sufficient to explain weight gain in the US population. A
       reversal of the increase in energy intake of ≈2000 kJ/d (500 kcal/d) for
       adults and of 1500 kJ/d (350 kcal/d) for children would be needed for a
       reversal to the mean body weights of the 1970s'* (Swinburn et al. 2009).
9.   **Cook at home more often**. This is really the only way to control sugar,
     salt and fat in your diet and to return to eating whole, unprocessed foods.
     It is extremely hard to control fat and salt when dining out.
10. **Drink more water**. Most of us don't drink enough water. Water fills you
     up, eases the load on your kidneys, and is calorie-free.
11. **Remember SOS!** * Salt, oil and sugar. This amusing acronym is quite
     helpful when pursuing healthier eating habits. Not only are these
     food additives important to avoid when buying products from the
     supermarket or when dining out, but it is also advisable to limit their
     addition to foods prepared at home.

---

*The SOS mantra is espoused by Dr Esselstyn Caldwell MD in his strategy for reversing heart disease, and is also recommended by many other professionals, such as Jeff Novick MS, RD, John McDougall MD, Michael Klaper MD, T. Colin Campbell PhD and Dr Neal Barnard of the Physicians Committee for Responsible Medicine. The caveat that I will provide is that these people are all promoting a vegan diet, but their shared evidence-based reason for doing so is due to the proven cardiovascular, diabetic, and cancer outcomes from eating this type of diet.

Much more could be said about nutrition, of course, but the goal here is to try to keep this discussion as general and as mainstream as possible. There are of course anti-cancer diets, anti-aging diets and thousands of weight-loss diets, which may have lots of validity, but for the purposes of this discussion I have kept with safe, middle-of-the-road suggestions that you may or may not want to pass on to your patients. Below, we will look at some other aspects of nutrition as well as body-wide inflammation.

Inflammation

Presumably most of the readership is well acquainted with methods of treating localized inflammation with hydrotherapy and other methods. Body-wide inflammation, on the other hand, is a topic in which I received no formal schooling, but became interested in after listening to a speech by Neal Barnard MD, head of the Physicians Committee for Responsible Medicine. His published studies, along with the clinical studies performed by Drs Dean Ornish, president and founder of the non-profit Preventive Medicine Research Institute, and Caldwell B. Esselstyn Jr, of the Cleveland Clinic, convinced me to remove all animal protein and animal fat from my diet toward the goal of reversing my heart disease, which is in essence an inflammatory arterial disease. Few patients at this point in human history might be willing to make this sort of radical change, but anyone in enough pain or wishing to take more control of their health is definitely open to suggestions of lifestyle and dietary changes. What follows below are evidence-based suggestions for reducing body-wide inflammation.

One pattern occasionally seen with patients is the development of an idiopathic tendonitis or tenosynovitis or frozen shoulder, without the patient being aware of any activity that may have caused the onset. Sometimes the condition responds positively to treatment initially but then returns in a chronic manner. Sometimes the condition responds to treatment successfully but then you see another idiopathic musculoskeletal issue appear that is inflammatory in nature. At these times it is wise to consider if dietary and other factors might be contributing to the patient's predisposition to inflammation. Their doctor can order a blood test, which will look for three markers:

1. **C-reactive protein (CRP)** – sometimes called an acute phase protein. This means that the level of CRP increases when you have certain diseases that cause inflammation. CRP can be measured in a blood sample.
2. **Erythrocyte sedimentation rate (ESR)** – the ESR measures the rate at which the red blood cells separate from the plasma and fall to the bottom of a test tube. The rate is measured in millimetres per hour (mm/hr). If certain proteins cover red cells, these will stick to each other and cause the red cells to fall more quickly. Therefore, a high ESR indicates that you have some inflammation somewhere in the body. Levels of ESR are generally higher in females, and these levels generally increase with increasing age.

3. **Plasma viscosity (PV)** – the ESR test monitors conditions, which can also be monitored by the PV test. However, it is more difficult to perform and is not as widely used as ESR testing.

While both CRP and ESR both monitor body-wide inflammation, CRP levels will drop more rapidly after making dietary changes, so is largely considered by the complementary health community to be the marker to check after making dietary changes to see if they have had a positive inflammatory effect. Let's take a look at the effect of some foods, lifestyle and health issues on inflammation and CRP levels.

The bad

- Sugar – even moderate consumption of sugar-sweetened beverages raises CRP levels (Livesey & Taylor 2008)
- Smoking raises CRP levels
- High body mass index raises CRP levels
- Low exercise levels will also raise CRP levels
- These factors listed above also have a cumulative effect exacerbating an inflammatory condition (Chun et al. 2008).

The good

- **Whole grains** contain more nutrients, antioxidants, phytochemicals, fiber and other protective components than refined grains. **Fiber rich foods** also help stabilize blood sugars, which may also contribute to lower CRP levels.
- **Magnesium** – most Americans consume magnesium at levels below the RDA. Individuals with intakes below the RDA are more likely to have elevated CRP, which may contribute to cardiovascular disease risk (King et al. 2005).
- **Intake of dietary flavonoids** is inversely associated with serum CRP concentrations. Intake of flavonoid-rich foods may thus reduce inflammation-mediated chronic diseases (Chun et al. 2008):
  - Foods with high flavonoid count include: parsley, onions, blueberries and other berries, black tea, green tea and oolong tea, bananas, all citrus fruits, Ginkgo biloba, red wine, sea-buckthorns and dark chocolate (with a cocoa content of 70% or greater).
- Oddly enough, there appears to be an inverse relationship between **alcohol consumption** and serum CRP levels (Stewart et al. 2002). Studies show that abstainers tend to generally have higher CRP levels. Mild drinkers have slightly lower levels, and moderate drinkers have even lower levels than the mild drinkers. Does this mean you start drinking more? Probably not, but it may help to reduce your guilt if you have a drink. Also, remember from the section on sleep that alcohol near bedtime has a short-term sedative effect but ultimately disrupts the normal sleep cycle,

leading to poor quality of sleep. As well, it is important to remember that there is a positive association between alcohol and many cancers. This is one more reason to limit alcohol consumption.

- **Omega-3 fatty acids** are well recognized for their ability to reduce inflammation. They have also become popular because they may reduce the risk of heart disease. Research shows that omega-3 fatty acids reduce inflammation and may help lower risk of chronic diseases such as heart disease, cancer, and arthritis. Omega-3 fatty acids help reduce inflammation, whereas most omega-6 fatty acids tend to promote inflammation. According to the University of Maryland Medical Center, studies support omega-3 supplementation to be efficacious in the treatment and prevention of the following list of diseases and conditions:
  - High cholesterol
  - High blood pressure
  - Heart disease
  - Diabetes
  - Rheumatoid arthritis
  - SLE
  - Osteoporosis
  - Depression
  - Bipolar disorder
  - Schizophrenia
  - ADHD
  - Cognitive decline
  - Skin disorders
  - Inflammatory bowel disease (IBD)
  - Asthma
  - Macular degeneration
  - Menstrual pain
  - Colon cancer
  - Breast cancer
  - Prostate cancer.

Nutritionally-oriented physicians believe that the typical American diet tends to contain an inappropriate ratio of omega-6 fatty acids to omega-3 fatty acids (University of Maryland Medical Center 2013). They recommend that the average American consumes more omega-3 oils and less omega-6 oils. Omega 3 oils can be found in the following foods, listed from highest to lowest concentration: flax seeds, walnuts, sardines, wild salmon, soybeans, tofu, shrimp, Brussels sprouts, cauliflower and winter squash.

As with all things nutritional, it is best to get your nutrients from whole foods, not supplements. Also, scientific evidence no longer supports fish oil supplementation. Omega-3 oil is very easily damaged by heat and oxygen; it does not store well. This is why it should be consumed in its whole food form. The other concerns about Omega-3 supplements include interactions with medications and an anti-clotting effect on the blood. For these reasons, Omega-3 supplements should really only be taken on the advice of a family physician.

The last approach for treating inflammation, known as 'earthing' (aka grounding oneself), might sound a bit odd, but the science supporting the modality is steadily growing. This topic and the research behind it will be discussed later on in this section. Earthing appears to have many benefits including treatment of both acute and chronic inflammation.

In conclusion, if you feel that your patient is dealing with inflammatory issues, it might be useful for their physician to order a blood test for inflammatory markers. While we are not nutritionists, it is important that we at least be cognizant of the basics of information presented here. If you are so inclined, you could read research referenced in this section and then pass pertinent research along to your patient. This is why you will see a reference after each point raised above. Optimally you could refer your patients to a registered holistic nutritionist for help with their diet. A motivated patient will typically be open to a nutritional approach to health. Finally, grounding is a new (old) modality that also appears to help inflammatory issues.

Patient's outlook

One's outlook on life appears to have a substantial impact on health and longevity. For example, a Yale University study extracted from the Ohio Longitudinal Study of Aging and Retirement (OLSAR) of 660 adults aged 50 and older found that people with a positive outlook on the aging process lived more than seven years longer than those who felt doomed to deteriorating mental and physical health (Levy et al. 2002). This advantage remained after age, gender, socioeconomic status, loneliness and functional health were included as covariates.

ELSA (English Longitudinal Study for Aging) is a longitudinal study following over 10 000 people living in England as they age from 50 years onwards. Its aim is to understand the economic, social, psychological and health concerns of an aging society. One of ELSA's goals is to find out whether seniors' psychological well-being is linked to poorer health outcomes and early death. What researchers found was remarkable. People who were recorded in wave 1 as having a greater enjoyment in life were the ones most likely to still be alive in wave 5 of the study, 10 years later. The results show that persons with a less positive outlook were nearly **three times more likely to have died** when compared with persons with a more positive attitude. Researchers also found measures of psychological well-being from wave 2 (taken in 2004/05, before any impairments had developed) could predict which people would go on to develop coronary heart disease, report more ill health, suffer disability and have a reduced walking speed when they were visited again in wave 5 (2010/11). What is worth noting is that these predictions were just as strong when researchers took into account other possible influencing factors such as age, gender, ethnicity, education, baseline health and wealth.

With this in mind, how can one adjust one's attitude? This is well beyond the scope of this book, and undoubtedly worth a book of its own, but one practical technique is to practice daily gratitude exercises. One expert in this area is Dr Robert Emmons. His primary research interests are in the psychology of gratitude and the psychology of personal goals and how each is related to positive psychological processes, including happiness, well-being and personality integration. He is the Editor-in-Chief of *The Journal of Positive Psychology* and the author of *The Psychology of Gratitude* (Oxford University Press) and *THANKS!: How the New Science of Gratitude Can Make You Happier* (Houghton Mifflin). Here is a sampling of some of the research that Emmons referenced to create his thesis concerning the health/longevity benefits of gratitude (from the Emmons Lab website 2014):

- In an experimental comparison, those who kept gratitude journals on a weekly basis exercised more regularly, reported fewer physical symptoms, felt better about their lives as a whole, and were more optimistic about the upcoming week compared with those who recorded hassles or neutral life events (Emmons & McCullough 2003).
- A related benefit was observed in the realm of personal goal attainment: participants who kept gratitude lists were more likely to have made progress toward important personal goals (academic, interpersonal and health-based) over a 2-month period compared to subjects in the other experimental conditions.
- Participants in the daily gratitude condition were more likely to report having helped someone with a personal problem or having offered emotional support to another, relative to the hassles or social comparison condition. (Acts of altruism have been shown to increase happiness levels.)
- In a sample of adults with neuromuscular disease, a 21-day gratitude intervention resulted in greater amounts of high-energy positive moods, a greater sense of feeling connected to others, more optimistic ratings of one's life, and better sleep duration and sleep quality, relative to a control group.
- Children who practice grateful thinking have more positive attitudes toward school and their families (Froh et al. 2008).

As mentioned, another proven method of altering one's outlook in a positive direction is by performing altruistic acts such as volunteering. A meta-analysis out of University of Exeter Medical School analyzed data from 40 published papers on volunteering and found lower levels of depression, increased life satisfaction and enhanced well-being in the volunteering population (Jenkinson et al. 2013) Additionally it was found in the meta-analysis of five cohort studies that volunteers had a 20% lower risk of death than non-volunteers.

Let me close out this section by saying that research would suggest that people with a more positive outlook on life experience dramatically better health and longevity outcomes. While there are undoubtedly many ways to alter one's outlook on life, one effective method appears to be to perform daily gratitude exercises, and another is the performance of altruistic acts. As we will see in the next section, any strategy that will increase happiness will also improve one's outlook, so these two topics are deeply interrelated.

Happiness

Happiness is closely linked to one's outlook, but there is enough research on this specific subject to warrant treating it as a separate topic. Happiness has undoubtedly been a topic of conversation, contemplation and study for as long as humans have been able to communicate ideas to one another. It has been examined by all of the major religions of the world and by many philosophers as well. The pursuit of happiness is considered an inalienable right in the US, having been included as such into the Declaration of Independence in 1776. Presumably, it is also high on the list of priorities for Canadians because as it turns out we sit 10th in the world for SWB, the scientific term for happiness. This is rightly so, because not only does happiness increase the quality of your life, it also increases the quality of your health. The ancient *Book of Proverbs* says, 'A cheerful heart is a good medicine' (17:22). Recently studies have shown the health benefits of happiness including: increased longevity (Danner et al. 2001) stronger immune systems (Dillon et al. 1985), increased emotional health (Diener 1984), increased vitality and energy (Csikszentmihalyi & Wong 1991), less tendency toward depression (Koivumaa-Honkanen et al. 2001, Diener & Seligman 2002) and greater self-control and coping abilities (Okun et al. 1984, Aspinwall 1998). Happiness doesn't just affect health. Studies also show that happiness also has strong correlations with personal creativity, productivity, the quality of one's work and income. In addition, happier people are less likely to become divorced, have better marriages, are more likely to have more friends and are more likely to enjoy stronger social support (Okun et al. 1984, Berry & Hansen 1996, Marks & Fleming 1999, Harker & Keltner 2001). So, it would seem that the pursuit (or choice) of happiness is indeed worthwhile.

It is very interesting to note that subjective well-being (SWB) studies have debunked some of the myths of our consumer-oriented society. To begin with, happiness is not linked to higher income. Studies show that once your basic needs are met, additional income does little to raise your sense of satisfaction with life. Very interesting to note is that 37% of the people on Forbes' list of wealthiest Americans are less happy than the average American. Surprisingly, neither good education nor higher IQ appear to be linked to life happiness. How about something else that our culture seems to worship…namely, youth? Once again the answer is no. In fact, older people are more consistently satisfied with their lives than the young (Centers for Disease Control and Prevention 2014).

On the other side of the coin, religious faith seems to genuinely lift the spirit. A strong social network is also strongly linked to life happiness (a 2002 study conducted at the University of Illinois by Diener and Seligman found that the most salient characteristics shared by the 10% of students with the highest levels of happiness and the fewest signs of depression were their strong ties to friends and family and commitment to spending time with them). It is interesting to note that the cerebral virtues, such as curiosity and love of learning, are less strongly tied to happiness than interpersonal virtues like kindness, gratitude and capacity for love. Looking at all the factors that affect happiness, researchers have found three major areas that affect our personal happiness.

The concept of happiness set point

We all have a comfortable weight, a comfortable level of activity and also seem to have a pre-set level of happiness. These set points can be altered to some degree; however, they are basic expressions of who we are. An interesting study of lottery winners in 1978 elucidates the concept of set point. This study found that winners did not wind up significantly happier than a control group. Even people who lose the use of their limbs tend to bounce back close to their previous set point. Psychologists call this adjustment to new circumstances 'adaptation'. In his extensive work on adaptation, Edward Diener, Professor of Psychology at the University of Illinois, has found two life events that seem to knock people lastingly below their happiness set point: **loss of a spouse** and **loss of a job.** Either of these experiences can knock you off your set point for many years, despite a new job or relationship. The concept of set point came from Minnesota researcher David Lykken, who gathered information on 4000 sets of identical and fraternal twins. He came to the conclusion that about 50% of one's satisfaction with life, or happiness comes from genetic programming.

While set point is considered to be genetically predetermined, there are three methods of altering it. One way is pharmacologically with drugs such as Prozac and Zoloft. Another method that has been shown to change the level of our set point is meditation. Studies of monks and office employees alike show that meditation can raise one's set point. One final method of raising our set point is by employing cognitive therapy. This involves sessions with a trained therapist to break the negative cycle of your internal thought process to see the world as one of opportunity, rather than danger.

Do life conditions improve our happiness?

Lykken found that certain life circumstances, such as income, marital status, religion and education, do affect our happiness, but to a surprisingly small extent. These factors combined contribute only to about 8% of one's overall well-being. Current studies show that all demographic variables combined, including age, sex, income, race, education, etc. are responsible for only 15% of the difference in happiness levels between individuals (Argyle 1999). What this tells you is that if you are trying to pursue happiness with a better education, better job, newer car or bigger house, you are likely to fail.

Volunteering

Lykken's research on life circumstances coincides with the view of the positive psychology (University of Pennsylvania Positive Psychology Center 2007) http://www.ppc.sas.upenn.edu/) movement, which has put a premium on research showing you can raise your level of happiness. This young science, which began in earnest in 1999, studies mental 'wellness' rather than mental illness by looking at the strengths and virtues that enable individuals and communities to thrive. Research in this field shows that the single most powerful way to increase your happiness is not by altering your life conditions or income, but rather by the voluntary activities that you engage in. Your voluntary activities contribute to at least 40% of your happiness, and unlike your set point, they are always alterable. Several experiments designed to increase participant's happiness demonstrated that individuals could be trained to be 25% happier through various training programs from 2 to 10 weeks (Fordyce 1977, 1983, Lichter et al. 1980). What sorts of activities affect personal happiness? Here are five that your patients can try:

1. One type of voluntary activity is performing acts of altruism or kindness. These activities can include visiting the elderly or infirmed, helping a friend's child with homework, or doing any spontaneous act of kindness. Sonja Lyubomirsky at Stamford University has studied happiness extensively and her work indicates that doing five kind acts per week, especially all in a single day, gives a measurable boost to research subjects.
2. Gratitude exercises (as mentioned earlier) also lift one's mood. Psychologist Robert Emmons found that gratitude exercises improve physical health, raise energy levels and, for patients with neuromuscular disease, relieve pain and fatigue. Keeping a journal devoted to things that you are grateful for is one way to put this concept into practice. 'The ones who benefited most tended to elaborate more, and have a wider span of things they're grateful for,' he notes.
3. The link between our connection to others and our level of happiness is undeniable. Both things tend to feed into one another. Taking concrete steps to get more involved socially is of tremendous benefit, especially if you are socially isolated.
4. Learn to forgive. Hanging on to anger and resentment is associated with ill health and unhappiness. Studies show that people scoring higher on forgiveness scales lead happier, healthier lives. We will look at the topic of forgiveness later on in this section.
5. One final recommendation for lasting happiness is to figure out your strengths and find new ways to deploy them. We all have weaknesses, and

many of them are simply expressions of who we are. Focusing on them typically brings you down, but if you focus on your strengths and use them to your benefit, you will see immediate effects on your level of happiness. This is once again a principle of the positive psychology movement.

6. Lyubomirsky's research also suggests three other activities that one can try:
   - Practicing optimism (i.e. visualizing the best possible future for oneself every week for 8 weeks)
   - Engaging in self-regulatory and positive thinking about oneself (i.e. reflecting, writing, and talking about one's happiest and unhappiest life events for 15 minutes per day during 1 week)
   - Savoring the present (by appreciating what you have over the course of 4 weeks).

Apart from the information covered here there are several websites listed (some cited above and see References and Further Reading at the end of Part 3) if you find you have further interest in this topic. Also, for more information, a web search under 'subjective well-being' or 'positive psychology' will produce evidence-based data.

Forgiveness

Forgiveness is often viewed as a religious concept; however, it has important health implications whether one holds religious views or not. While you might think of it as a practice centred on the actions of others, studies now show the personal health benefits gained from practicing forgiveness. Multiple studies show that people scoring high on forgiveness scales experience fewer health complications, less stress and stress-related symptoms, decreased acute pain and chronic pain, decreased blood pressure, increased pain-related function and decreased mortality (Lawler et al. 2003, Lawler-Row 2008, Toussaint et al. 2012). Researchers also found improved interpersonal relations, increased empathy and improved conflict resolution related to forgiveness. One recent study stated, '*While forgiveness of self and forgiveness of others each appear to have a robust indirect relationship with health, mediation-based associations involving forgiveness of self were nearly twice as frequent. It may be that forgiveness of self is relatively more important to health-related outcomes*' (Webb et al. 2013). There are a tremendous number of studies linking forgiveness (of self, of others, and of feeling forgiven) to health. Virtually every study shows increased health benefits as participants score higher on forgiveness scales.

So what is the mechanism of forgiveness? Well, as a human being moving around the planet, almost no day passes in which you are not injured by the actions of another in some way, or that you don't suffer due to natural or human causes. As these injuries or events happen, we end up taking some of these incidents on psychologically instead of letting the event pass through us. If you do take the event on as an injury, the next step often is to blame someone or something.

You then have a double assault; the original injury and the damage caused by hanging on to the injury psycho-emotionally. We all do this, and no one is able to let go of every injury completely, but the cost of this hanging on can become extremely large. Interestingly enough, the word 'forgiveness' actually comes from the Greek word, afiemi, which has a whole host of similar meanings but one useful translation is 'to let go of'. So forgiveness, in essence, is the *letting go* of these events.

One of the most dramatic examples of applied forgiveness, seen at a national level, is the Truth and Reconciliation Commission, set up after a very bloody civil rights war in South Africa that took tens of thousands of lives. Forgiveness is important at virtually any level of interaction whether it is between marital partners, friends, co-workers, within societies due to civil strife, and across cultures after wars or border disputes. This is undoubtedly the reason that so much money has been poured into research into this topic. The clear unequivocal answer from the research is that it is personally beneficial, psycho-emotionally, to let go of an injury, no matter whom or what caused the insult. Inability to forgive is similar to hanging on to anger. The primary injury ends up being a self-inflicted one, even though you might feel that the energy of the trauma is directed at another individual. One other important level of forgiveness that the research hinted at earlier is forgiveness of self. Forgiveness does not always involve a sense that someone or something has wronged you. Each one of us is far from perfect and our own flaws cause us to act in ways that we can personally regret. This brings to mind the ritual of confession that has existed in the Catholic Church, or what is termed The Sacrament of Reconciliation in the Christian Church at large for over two millennia. One can see, based on the research, the substantial health benefits that are acquired from 'letting go of' the weight of misdeeds, whether they were the actions of others, or your own.

According to Dr Fred Luskin, the director of the Stanford University Forgiveness Project, everyone can learn to forgive. Luskin's approach to forgiveness is scientific and non-parochial; he sees it as a learned skill (just like throwing a baseball) that helps you get control over your feelings:

> *Forgiveness is: – a choice – the peace you learn to feel when let go of injury – for you and not the offender – taking back your power – taking responsibility for how you feel – about your healing and not about the people who hurt you – about becoming a hero instead of a victim.*
> *Forgiveness is not: – condoning unkindness – forgetting that something painful happened – excusing poor behaviour – denying or minimizing your hurt – necessarily reconciling with the offender – giving up on having feelings.*

(Luskin 2002)

If you buy into forgiveness as a tool that would be useful for you or your patients, the next question is, 'How does one go about the act of forgiving.' Well you can just say it and wish it, but that doesn't always work. It's usually a bit more complicated than that. Luskin suggests nine steps that one can practice to let go of major emotional wounds:

1. Know exactly how you feel about what happened and be able to articulate what about the situation is not OK. Then, tell a trusted couple of people about your experience.
2. Make a commitment to yourself to do what you have to do to feel better. Forgiveness is for you and not for anyone else.
3. Forgiveness does not necessarily mean reconciliation with the person that hurt you, or condoning of their action; the goal is to find peace. Forgiveness can be defined as the 'peace and understanding that come from reducing the blame on the person or incident which has hurt you, taking the life experience less personally, and changing your grievance story.'
4. Get the right perspective on what is happening. Recognize that your primary distress is coming from the hurt feelings, thoughts and physical upset you are suffering now, not what offended you or hurt you 2 minutes – or 10 years – ago. Forgiveness helps to heal those hurt feelings.
5. At the moment you feel upset, practice a simple stress management technique to soothe your body's flight or fight response.
6. Give up expecting things from other people, or your life. Recognize the 'unenforceable rules' you have for your health or how you or other people must behave. Remind yourself that you can hope for health, love, peace and prosperity and work hard to get them.
7. Put your energy into looking for another way to get your positive goals met than through the experience that has hurt you. Instead of mentally replaying your hurt, seek out new ways to get what you want.
8. Remember that a life well lived is your best revenge. Instead of focusing on your wounded feelings, and thereby giving the person who caused you pain power over you, learn to look for the love, beauty and kindness around you. Forgiveness is about personal power.
9. Amend your grievance story to remind you of the heroic choice to forgive.

If you were interested in learning more about a pragmatic approach to forgiveness, or you would like to have a resource for your professional lending library then Dr Fred Luskin's 2002 book *Forgive for Good – a Proven Prescription for Health and Happiness* would be a useful addition. Also see References and Further Reading at the end of Part 3 for useful websites on research and information on the health aspects of forgiveness.

This topic has come up with my patients, and I have found a very easy way to broach this or other sensitive subjects if you are empathetic and non-judgemental. If you read non-religious information and studies on forgiveness, you will undoubtedly find some aspect of it to be useful in your own life. Then, if the topic should arise in conversation with a patient, you can simply mention that you found one particular resource to be quite useful. You can then ask them if they would like to borrow the resource. This is a simple and non-judgemental way of broaching an otherwise difficult subject.

Meditation

Years ago, I enrolled in an intensive 6-month course that required me to set aside 2 hours per day for the practice and the study of meditation at a local Buddhist temple. Although I was hoping for a major breakthrough, this was not my destiny. What I experienced was a lot of hard work. It was a constant uphill battle trying to train my mind to be still. Many people in our crazy fast-paced world find that the practice of training one's mind on one word or phrase for an extended period of time, and to keep it from wandering, requires a surprising amount of discipline. The good news is that the science and multiple studies tell us that it is worth the effort.

Meditation has been around for thousands of years, but the North American consciousness awoke to the practice during the late 1960s, thanks, in part, to The Beatles (specifically George Harrison). Eventually, science became interested in this phenomenon and meditation developed more respectability. Since that time there have been almost 3000 entries made to PubMed's database investigating the benefits of meditation. There is clearly no shortage of studies on meditation. There might, however, be a shortage of double-blind studies with large numbers of participants, but if we used this as definitive criteria, we would be looking almost exclusively at drug interventions to treat medical conditions. As a result, we need to accept that there are many valid modalities that are impossible to double-blind or even single-blind when we are studying them.

One book with a unique take on this topic is entitled *Meditation as Medicine* co-written by Dr Dharma Singh Khalsa (Khalsa & Stauth 2002). As a doctor, he was interested in medical application of meditation techniques for his patients. The following statistics were extracted from his book:

- Meditation creates a unique condition, in which metabolism is in an even deeper state of rest than during sleep. (During sleep, oxygen consumption drops by 8%, but during meditation, it drops by 10–20%.)
- Meditation is the only activity that reduces blood lactate, a marker of stress and anxiety.
- Calming hormones melatonin and serotonin are increased by meditation and the stress hormone cortisol is decreased.
- Meditation has a positive effect upon three key indicators of aging: hearing ability, blood pressure and close-up vision.
- Long-term meditators experience 80% less heart disease and 50% less cancer than non-meditators.
- Meditators secrete more of the youth-related hormone DHEA as they age than non-meditators. (Meditating 45-year-old males have an average of

23% more DHEA than non-meditators, and meditating females have an average of 47% more. This helps decrease stress, heighten memory and control weight.)

- 75% of insomniacs in one study were able to sleep normally when they meditated.
- In another study, 34% of people with chronic pain significantly reduced their medication needs when they began meditating.

The claims made above are nothing short of incredible. As it turns out, meta-analyses are less generous in their assessment, but they still support the practice of meditation. Dharma Singh Khalsa's unique spin on meditation, which he calls Medical Meditation, involves meditating on a specific region of the body which needs healing, or meditating with a healthful intent. Dr Khalsa believes that this practice taps into the power of our minds to focus on and heal our bodies. This approach is very similar to guided imagery and visualization which we looked at in the section on reducing your patient's anxiety except that the visualization concerns healing rather than on the reduction of anxiety.

Let's look at a few more recent studies:

- A 2013 study in Seoul, Korea investigated the effects of meditation on anxiety, depression, fatigue and quality of life in 102 women who were receiving radiation therapy for breast cancer (Kim et al. 2013).The subjects included 102 female breast cancer patients who had undergone breast-conserving surgery; these female patients were randomized into equally assigned meditation control groups, with each group consisting of 51 patients. The test group received a total of 12 meditation therapy sessions during their 6-week radiation therapy period, and the control group underwent only a conventional radiation therapy. The breast cancer patients who received meditation therapy compared with the non-intervention group saw improvements in reduction of anxiety, fatigue and improvement in global quality of life.
- A 2012 observational cohort study (Chung et al. 2012) conducted in India enrolled two study groups: 67 participants receiving treatment at the International Sahaja Yoga Research and Health Center (meditation group), and 62 participants receiving treatment from the Mahatma Gandhi Mission Hospital (control group). Researchers measured quality of life, anxiety and blood pressure before and after treatment. At the end of the study the measured improvement in quality of life, anxiety reduction and blood pressure control was greater in the meditation group. The beneficial effect of meditation remained significant after adjusting for confounders.
- In 2012 Balaji and colleagues conducted a Medline search for relevant articles in English literature on evaluation of physiological effects of yogic practices and Transcendental Meditation (TM). Researchers found that

there were considerable health benefits, including improved cognition, respiration, reduced cardiovascular risk, body mass index, blood pressure and diabetes (Balaji et al. 2012).

- A 2012 randomized, controlled trial of 201 black men and women with coronary heart disease randomly placed participants either in a TM program or in a health education program. The average follow-up period was 5.4 years. At that time there was a 48% risk reduction in the TM group. There were reductions of 4.9 mmHg in systolic blood pressure also a reduction in anger expression. Notably, adherence was associated with survival. Researchers concluded that TM *'significantly reduced risk for mortality, myocardial infarction, and stroke in coronary heart disease patients. These changes were associated with lower blood pressure and psychosocial stress factors. Therefore, this practice may be clinically useful in the secondary prevention of cardiovascular disease'* (Schneider et al. 2012).

There seems little doubt that meditation provides health benefits and is a practice which could be beneficial to practitioners and patients alike. The practice is extremely simple; one just needs to set about 15 minutes aside each day in a reasonably quiet undisturbed location to practice. Practice is an extremely good word for this because (in my experience at least) it is very challenging initially to keep one's mind from wandering, but like all endeavours it becomes much easier with continued practice and discipline. There are a host of books on this topic. The classic text that helped to popularize meditation is Dr Herbert Benson's 1975 book, *The relaxation response*. All in all, it would seem that whether the mantra used and the intent of the participant is general or specific (i.e. focused on a body region or an illness), it would appear that there are tremendous health benefits available to those who engage in the practice of meditation.

Earthing (aka grounding)

I first encountered the subject of earthing in 2013 while barefoot in Mexico, researching this book. Grounding oneself capitalizes on the earth's endless supply of electrons. Why is this important? Our bodies are typically electron-deficient. The normal process of metabolism creates highly destructive and highly reactive products known as free radicals. A free radical is an atom (usually oxygen) or molecule that is missing an electron, so it is positively charged and therefore unstable. However, because of their reactivity, these free radicals can participate in unwanted side reactions resulting in cell damage.

As it turns out, if you ground yourself, the free electrons quickly travel throughout your body and cancel out any charges by binding to positive ion radicals. The result is the almost instant neutralization of free radicals. Another body process where earthing appears to have direct effects is acute inflammation. As neutrophils arrive at the site of an injury they deliver the reactive oxygen species (ROS) to the site of injury. ROS is another fancy way to say free radicals. Some of those free radicals can leak into the surrounding tissue and damage healthy tissue. That's what gives the noticeable inflammatory response. Grounding yourself will allow electrons to neutralize free radicals that leak into the healthy tissue, dramatically reducing the collateral damage of the inflammatory response. Another benefit of grounding is the dramatic reduction of the negative effects of electromagnetic fields (EMFs).*

Have you ever considered that we are the only mammal on the planet that isn't constantly grounded? Our shoes and our houses typically prevent us from staying grounded. We all intuitively know that being grounded is a good thing. 'Staying grounded' is a part of our lexicon with positive connotations. My impression is that earthing is not just some new-age belief full of questionable science; in fact the emerging science appears quite solid, but like most natural remedies, appropriate funding is lacking. As a modality it lends itself very easily to double-blinding, since neither the research clinician nor the participant would know if the participant was actually grounded. This makes it infinitely easier to study that manual therapy.

A quote from a 2012 review article on earthing, published in the *Journal of Environmental and Public Health*, states:

Emerging evidence shows that contact with the Earth – whether being outside barefoot or indoors connected to grounded conductive systems – may be a simple, natural, and yet profoundly effective environmental strategy against chronic stress, ANS dysfunction, inflammation, pain, poor sleep, disturbed HRV, hypercoagulable blood, and many common health disorders, including cardiovascular disease. The research done to date supports the concept that grounding or earthing the human body may be an essential element in the health equation.

The idea of grounding for health was developed intuitively by Clint Ober, who actually made billions of dollars in the American communication industry. For him, electricity and electrical experimentation were almost second nature. After a medical crisis where he had to have 80% of his liver removed and almost died, he sold his business to pursue personal and more altruistic goals. He took the 'earthing' idea to his doctor to pursue the scientific/medical basis for this therapy. Clinical trials by Stephen Sinatra MD have shown the incredible benefits of this modality. Earthing claims the following benefits (claims with peer-reviewed research are noted):

- Improved sleep (Ghaly & Teplitz 2004). This is notable since the bulk of all body repair is done during this time, and this is the time period when most of us have the highest exposure to EMFs.

---

*For a great introduction into just how genuine a person Clint Ober is, and for a clear illustration of how earthing reduces EMFs, I suggest watching a video called 'Clint Ober demonstrates earthing'. This 3-part video shows how grounding yourself will dramatically reduce EMFs around you (Ober n.d.).

- Reported body-wide pain and stress level reduction (Ghaly & Teplitz 2004).
- Neutralization of free radicals in the body (Oschman 2007). This is also a very significant finding since free radicals are constantly doing damage in our bodies. Electrons can flow anywhere so are clearly the most effective anti-oxidant out there.
- Improves inflammatory conditions (Oschman 2007). This is highly significant because almost every pathology begins with an inflammatory component. Most chronic conditions involve chronic inflammation.
- Treatment of acute trauma –immediately reduces the negative effects of free radicals released by neutrophils at the site of an injury (Oschman 2007).
- Immediate reduction in muscle tension (as measured by EMG) and blood volume pulse (an indicator of psychological arousal i.e. stress), and immediate levelling of brain activity, as measured on an electron encephalograph (EEG) (Chevalier et al. 2006). These are all objective measurements of human stress levels.
- Reduced recovery times of delayed onset muscle soreness (DOMS) which happens after a heavy workout (which is actually an acute inflammation) (Brown et al. 2010).
- Reduced hypertension (elevated blood pressure). This is achieved by reducing the charges in blood cells, which reduces blood viscosity (Chevalier et al. 2013).
- Reduces cortisol levels (the body's stress hormone) (Ghaly & Teplitz 2004).
- Resynchronizes cortisol hormone secretion more in alignment with the natural 24-hour circadian rhythm profile (Ghaly & Teplitz 2004).
- Reduction of the negative effects of EMF. This is notable because most of us now live and work around EMFs (Chevalier 2010).
- Treatment of autoimmune diseases such as rheumatoid arthritis, lupus, multiple sclerosis, IBS. Since there is an inflammatory component to the chronic autoimmune diseases, it is proposed that earthing should have a positive effect on these conditions. Anecdotal information supports this hypothesis, but double-blind studies have yet to be performed.

So, how does one apply earthing principles in their daily life? One way is to walk around barefoot outside as our ancestors did, but in our climatic region this is impossible for 9 months of the year and impractical for most of the remaining time. The easiest way is to buy a product that is designed to ground you from an earthing company.* If your house was built in North America from about 1960

---

*For earthing products: Canadian source http://earthingcanada.ca/American Source http://www.earthing.com/). Their starter kit includes a bed pad (½ sheet) and an earthing mat that you place your feet on to when you are stationary (for example, when at the computer). It also includes cords that allow you to connect the products to a grounded receptacle in your home, testing equipment and a book on earthing. (I have no financial interest in this product. I am simply making this information available.)

onward, the products from their online store should be very easy to use right out of the box. If your home is older, you may not have grounded plugs; however, the starter kit will inform you how to deal with this challenge. For research on earthing see The Earthing Institute (2014), which reports on double-blind studies showing the efficacy of this therapy.

Stress

Finally, we are going to look at that bad-boy we call 'stress'. This phrase is used in a tongue-in-cheek manner, because although stress constantly gets a bad rap, it often also produces results. Have you ever heard the following phrase, 'a diamond is a lump of coal under stress'? It is actually true. The real issue is not really stress, but 'stress management'. For example, having a life with absolutely nothing to do is stressful because humans are born problem solvers. Having too much to do is also obviously very stressful as well, because this hyperstimulation drains our physical and emotional resources. So, all humans need to be able to manage their stress levels. The reasons should be obvious. Reducing stress will reduce blood levels of adrenaline, cortisol and norepinephrine. The long-term activation of the stress-response system and the subsequent overexposure to stress hormones puts the patient at increased risk of numerous health problems, including:

- Anxiety
- Depression
- Digestive problems
- Heart disease
- Sleep problems
- Weight gain
- Memory and concentration impairment.

It is to this end that we are covering stress management strategies. If you see that your patient is not managing stress well, it is good to know the options that they have available to them and to perhaps steer them in the direction of one that suits their personality, lifestyle and budget. The following subtitles cover techniques that you may want to look at as a practitioner to learn more, or they may be flags that will aid you in helping your patient to identify areas where he or she might want to look to reduce some of the stress and anxiety in their life. Reducing stress will allow their body to more effectively heal itself from illness, or recover from injury. If there is interest on your part or theirs, there is no shortage of books available on this topic.

Stress reduction strategies

In this section I have drawn heavily on the stress reductions strategies offered at HelpGuide.org, a not-for-profit site offering information on matters of mental health and healthy lifestyle (Smith & Segal 2014).

Identify the sources of stress

You can't fix what you can't identify. Stress management starts with identifying the sources of stress in one's life. Sounds easy right? Sometimes the root of these stressors lies in our blind spot. One's true sources of stress aren't always obvious, and it's all too easy to overlook your own stress-inducing thoughts, feelings and behaviours. To identify your true sources of stress you have to look closely at your habits, attitude and excuses, and ask yourself a few hard questions, such as:

- Do you explain away stress as temporary *('I just have a million things going on right now')* even though you can't remember the last time you took a breather?
- Do you define stress as an integral part of your work or home life *('Things are always crazy around here')* or as a part of your personality *('I have a lot of nervous energy, that's all')*
- Do you blame your stress on other people or outside events, or view it as entirely normal and unexceptional?

Until you accept responsibility for the role you play in creating or maintaining it, your stress level will remain outside your control.

Start a stress journal

A stress journal can help your patient in identifying regular stressors in their life. It will also reveal the manner in which they cope with these stresses. Each time one feels stressed they should keep track of it in their journal. As they keep a daily log, they should begin to see patterns and common themes. These are the things that they should write down:

- What caused the stress (make a guess if you're unsure)
- How you felt, both physically and emotionally
- How you acted in response
- What you did to make yourself feel better.

The next step is for the participant to think about the ways they currently manage and cope with stress in their life. Their stress journal can help them identify the management strategies that they use. Then ask, are your coping strategies healthy or unhealthy, helpful or unproductive? Unfortunately, many people cope with stress in ways that compound the problem.

Signs that you are not coping with stress

Here are some examples of avoidance behaviours indicating that you may not be coping with stress, but rather, avoiding it:

- Smoking
- Drinking too much
- Overeating
- Undereating
- Zoning out for hours in front of the TV or computer

- Withdrawing from friends, family, and activities
- Using pills or drugs to relax
- Sleeping too much
- Procrastinating
- Filling up every minute of the day to avoid facing problems
- Taking out your stress on others (lashing out, angry outbursts, physical violence).

Learning healthier ways to manage stress

If your methods of coping with stress are not contributing to your greater emotional and physical health then it is time to find healthier ones. There are many healthy ways to manage and cope with stress, but they all require change. You can either change the situation or change your reaction. When deciding which option to choose, it's helpful to think of the four As:

- **A**void
- **A**lter
- **A**dapt or
- **A**ccept.

Since everyone has a unique response to stress, there is no 'one size fits all' solution to managing it. No single method works for everyone or in every situation, so experiment with different techniques and strategies. Focus on what makes you feel calm and in control; put another way:

- **Change the situation**: **A**void the stressor or **A**lter the stressor
- **Change your reaction**: **A**dapt to the stressor or **A**ccept the stressor.

Stress management strategies

1. **Avoid unnecessary stress**. Not all stress can be avoided, and it is not healthy to avoid a situation that needs to be addressed. You may be surprised, however, by the number of stressors in your life that you can eliminate.
   - **Learn how to say 'no'** – know your limits and stick to them. Whether in your personal or professional life, refuse to accept extra responsibilities and duties. Taking on more than you can handle is a sure-fire recipe for stress.
   - **Avoid people who stress you out** – if someone consistently causes stress in your life and you can't turn the relationship around, limit the amount of time you spend with that person or end the relationship if necessary.
   - **Take control of your environment** – if the evening news makes you anxious, turn the TV off. If traffic's got you tense, take a longer but less-traveled route. If going shopping is an unpleasant chore, do your shopping online.

- **Avoid hot-button topics** – if you get upset over religion or politics, cross them off your conversation list. If you repeatedly argue about the same subject with the same people, stop bringing it up or excuse yourself when it's the topic of discussion.
- **Pare down your to-do list** – analyze your schedule, responsibilities and daily tasks. If you have too much on your plate, distinguish between the 'shoulds' and the 'musts'. Drop tasks that are not truly necessary to the bottom of the list or eliminate them entirely.

2. **Alter the situation**. If you can't avoid a stressful situation, try to alter it. Figure out what you can do to change things so the problem doesn't present itself in the future. Often, this involves changing the way you communicate and operate in your daily life.
   - **Express your feelings instead of bottling them up** – if something or someone is bothering you, communicate your concerns in an open and respectful way. If you don't voice your feelings, resentment will build and the situation will likely remain the same.
   - **Be willing to compromise** – when you ask someone to change their behavior, be willing to do the same. If you both are willing to bend at least a little, you'll have a good chance of finding a happy middle ground.
   - **Be more assertive** – don't take a backseat in your own life. Deal with problems head-on, doing your best to anticipate and prevent them. If you have an exam to study for and your chatty roommate just got home, say up front that you only have 5 minutes to talk.
   - **Manage your time better** – poor time management can cause a lot of stress. When you're stretched too thin and running behind, it's hard to stay calm and focused. But if you plan ahead and make sure you do not overextend yourself, you can alter the amount of stress you're under.

3. **Adapt to the stressor**. If you can't change the stressor, change your internal reaction to the stimulus. You can adapt to stressful situations and regain your sense of control by changing your expectations and attitude:
   - **Reframe problems** – try to view stressful situations from a more positive perspective. Rather than fuming about a traffic jam, look at it as an opportunity to pause and regroup, listen to your favorite radio station, or enjoy some alone time.
   - **Look at the big picture** – take perspective of the stressful situation. Ask yourself how important it will be in the long run. Will it matter in a month? A year? Is it really worth getting upset over? If the answer is no, focus your time and energy elsewhere.
   - **Adjust your standards** – a perfectionist mindset is a major source of avoidable stress. Stop setting yourself up for failure by demanding perfection. Set reasonable standards for yourself and others, and

learn to be okay with 'good enough.' Much of this attitude comes from misplaced 'control issues.'

- **Focus on the positive** – when stress is getting you down, take a moment to reflect on all the things you appreciate in your life, including your own positive qualities and gifts. This simple strategy can help you keep things in perspective.
- **Adjust your attitude** – how you think can have a profound effect on your emotional and physical well-being. Each time you think a negative thought about yourself, your body reacts as if it were in the throes of a tension-filled situation. If you see good things about yourself, you are more likely to feel good; the reverse is also true. Eliminate words such as 'always,' 'never,' 'should,' and 'must.' These are telltale marks of self-defeating thoughts.

4. **Accept the things you cannot change**. Some sources of stress are unavoidable. You can't prevent or change stressors such as the death of a loved one, a serious illness or a national recession. In such cases, the best way to cope with stress is to accept things as they are. Acceptance may be difficult, but in the long run, it's easier than railing against a situation you cannot change.
   - **Don't try to control the uncontrollable** – many things in life are beyond our control, particularly the behavior of other people. Rather than stressing out over them, focus on the things you can control such as the way you choose to react to problems.
   - **Look for the upside** – as the saying goes, 'What doesn't kill us makes us stronger.' When facing major challenges, try to look at them as opportunities for personal growth. If your own poor choices contributed to a stressful situation, reflect on them and learn from your mistakes.
   - **Share your feelings** – talk to a trusted friend or make an appointment with a therapist. Expressing what you're going through can be very cathartic, even if there's nothing you can do to alter the stressful situation.
   - **Learn to forgive** – let's face it. We live in an imperfect world where people make mistakes. Some people even do things out of malice. It is our personal interest to let go of the anger and resentment that we develop due to these injuries.

5. **Make time for fun and relaxation**. Beyond a take-charge approach and a positive attitude, you can reduce stress in your life by nurturing yourself. If you regularly make time for fun and relaxation, you'll be in a better place to handle life's stressors when they inevitably come. A list of healthy ways to relax and recharge might include:
   - Going for a walk.
   - Spending time in nature.

- Calling a good friend.
- Sweating out tension with a good workout.
- Writing in your journal.
- Taking a long bath and lighting scented candles.
- Savoring a warm cup of coffee or tea.
- Playing with a pet.
- Working in your garden.
- Getting a massage.
- Curling up with a good book.
- Listening to music.
- Watching a comedy.
- **Fill your cup** – most of all do what you love doing; that activity that fills your spiritual and emotional cup. Nurturing yourself is not a luxury, but a necessity.
- **Set aside relaxation time** – include rest and relaxation in your daily schedule. Don't allow other obligations to encroach. This is your time to take a break from all responsibilities and recharge your batteries.
- **Connect with others** – spend time with positive people who enhance your life. A strong support system will buffer you from the negative effects of stress.
- **Do something you enjoy every day** – make time for leisure activities that bring you joy, whether it be stargazing, playing the piano, or working on your bike.
- **Keep your sense of humor** – this includes the ability to laugh at yourself. The act of laughing helps your body fight stress in a number of ways.

6. **Adopt a healthy lifestyle**. You can increase your resistance to stress by strengthening your physical health:
   - **Exercise regularly** – physical activity plays a key role in reducing and preventing the effects of stress. Make time for at least 30 minutes of exercise, three times per week. Nothing beats aerobic exercise for releasing pent-up stress and tension.
   - **Eat a healthy diet** – well-nourished bodies are better prepared to cope with stress, so be mindful of what you eat. Start your day right with breakfast, and keep your energy up and your mind clear with balanced, nutritious meals throughout the day.
   - **Reduce caffeine and sugar** – the temporary 'highs' caffeine and sugar provide often end in with a crash in mood and energy. By reducing the amount of coffee, soft drinks, chocolate and sugar snacks in your diet, you'll feel more relaxed and you'll sleep better.
   - **Avoid alcohol, cigarettes, and drugs** – self-medicating with alcohol or drugs may provide an easy escape from stress, but the relief is only temporary. Don't avoid or mask the issue at hand; deal with problems head on and with a clear mind.

- **Get enough sleep** – adequate sleep fuels your mind, as well as your body. Feeling tired will increase your stress because it may cause you to think irrationally.

7. **Practice effective time management**. Good time-management skills are very important for stress control. Not only does this apply to our patients, it is important for everyone. In particular, learning to prioritize tasks and avoid over-commitment are important measures to make sure that one is not overscheduled. One way to develop time-management skills is fastidious use of a calendar or planner, and then checking it faithfully before committing to anything. If someone is finding that they just don't have enough time in their day, then keeping a diary for a few days and noticing where you may be losing time is one way of identifying time-wasting tasks. One example of time management is setting aside a specific time(s) each day to check and respond to email and messages, rather than being a continual slave to incoming information. Procrastination is another enemy of time-management, and oft time those things that you aren't getting done, because you have put them off contribute to stress levels and background anxiety levels (I'm speaking from personal experience here!). While we may not be experts in time-management, it can at the very least be a question that we might ask of patients who appear to be highly stressed.

8. **Develop improved organizational skills**. This is another large topic, and we will only have time to touch on it. Admittedly, some people's organizational skills are innately high and some ... not so much. Like most things, it is a spectrum and there are hazards with being too far out on either end of the continuum. One example of applied organizational skills is if your physical surroundings (office, desk, kitchen, closet, or car) are well-organized, you won't be faced with the stress of misplaced objects and clutter. Making a habit of periodically cleaning out and sorting through the messes of paperwork and clutter that accumulate over time definitely reduces one's stress levels. Taking the time to do this requires time-management (see Point 7 and try not to get caught in an infinite loop!).

   This is last topic probably a more sensitive one to broach with a patient than time-management skills as it sounds more judgmental. Presumably if they begin to look at time-management skills, this topic will surface in literature that they encounter. Ultimately, as suggested earlier, the best way that we as health care practitioners can facilitate effectively in the area of stress management, apart from offering stress-reduction treatments, is to answer any questions and to perhaps provide a handout with some of the information provided above in a generic fashion coupled with resources from your local community. This way you are not moving outside of your scope of practice and it does not sound as if you are making a judgment on your patient's behaviour.

Techniques to maximize healing previously covered

Before we close out this section, let me remind you of techniques that will help your patients to maximize their own healing response that were previously discussed in the earlier section, 'Reducing your patients' anxiety levels (p. 135). For information on these techniques, refer back to that section under the following subheadings:

- Guided or auto relaxation techniques
  - Autogenic training
  - Progressive muscle relaxation
  - Guided imagery aka visualization techniques focused on a specific area of healing. In his book, *The placebo response: how you can release the body's inner pharmacy for better health*, Howard Brody (2000a) suggests visualizing what he calls 'the inner pharmacy' to awake the body's resources to respond to illness and injury and to heal the body.
- Movement therapies
  - Qigong
  - Tai chi
  - Yoga.
- Biofeedback.

CONCLUSIONS

We have now reached the end of this exploration of methods for improving therapeutic outcomes, and we have covered a lot of ground. There have actually been many surprises for me as I researched this book, and I hope that some of the information presented has caused you to reconsider some of your beliefs and approaches. One thing that has constantly struck me while researching this book, which is quite separate from the placebo effect or the larger topic of improving therapeutic outcomes, is that factors which reduce pain and disease symptoms and improve health almost invariably increase life expectancy. Quality of life (from a health point of view) and length of life are inextricably intertwined. We have all met someone who says that they are here for a good time, not a long time, and then use that as an excuse for a self-destructive lifestyle. Speaking as someone who has now entered his sixth decade on the planet, I now rarely hear that sentiment from my peers. Why is this? Well one reason is that with that self-destructive approach to life and health, your odds of making it to your 60s and 70s are somewhat diminished. Most of the research that we have viewed here supports the linking of improved health outcomes with increased longevity. This is a selling point that you can use with your patients in motivating them to make healthier lifestyle and nutritional choices.

As was mentioned several times throughout the book, in no way am I trying to create a definitive view of any aspect of the body's ability to heal itself in this part of the book. Instead, there has been an earnest attempt to touch on as many ways to access and augment the body's amazing healing system, in the hope of giving you a new perspective on healing, and to provide you with new tools to improve therapeutic outcomes in your practice. If you find that you have a deep interest in one of these topics, then definitely take the ball and run with it. For me, I had to walk a line with this book. My goal was to view and examine the placebo effect in its broadest manner possible; so this necessarily prevented me from providing the depth of coverage that many topics deserved. As you can see, a great many factors contribute to the topic of accessing your patients' inner healing system, and while an earnest effort was made to touch on as many as possible, undoubtedly some were missed. If you feel so inclined, please feel free to contact me with suggestions for a possible future edition of this book. I welcome any feedback from the readership. While some topics may lack the depth that they might have deserved, I have now exceeded 110 000 words, and at some point one just has to 'wrap things up'. I hope that the information presented in each chapter and each section of individual chapters has encouraged you to learn more about the subject at hand. Any individual section in Part 2 could be a book on its own. Indeed hundreds of books have already been written on many of the topics covered in this book.

Health, like many things in life, is an amazing complex matter and a complicated subject to dissect and analyze. As we can see from this book, the elements that contribute to health and the placebo response is definitely multi-factorial, and each of these individual factors is deeply interconnected to other processes in the body. Trying to find good evidence to back up a thesis is challenging, so in some cases I ended up working in reverse, seeing a trend in the research and then formulateding a theory. It is likely that a percentage of the readership might approach the placebo effect as I did, by initially being interested in this mysterious phenomenon but eventually came to see the effect as something less mysterious than they thought it once was. The hope and intent here is that now that you understand the topic better, you can institute subtle ways to change your practice to maximize the hidden healing powers that exist within all of your patients. Undoubtedly, you now realize that you have actually been using the placebo effect in your practice all along, but now you understand it much better, so are in a far better position to apply the principles in your daily treatment sessions.

I wish that I had some marvellous grand conclusions that I could convey at this time, but a lot of ground has been covered since the opening pages of this book. So much has been covered, that it is very difficult to make grand encompassing statements at this time. What I hope instead is that I have reawakened your sense of wonder, but at the same time, shown you that while this phenomenon is deeply mysterious, there are many elements of it that you can manage. In so doing, you *will* improve clinical outcomes with your patients. The two leading, well-supported theories concerning the placebo effect suggest that patient expectations, and patient conditioning are involved in this phenomenon. Therefore, you should always be cognizant of these two powerful components of this phenomenon in your daily practice. The third placebo theory, which involves 'meaning' or 'context', is an extremely complex, multi-faceted situation, and varies dramatically from patient to patient, so success with this phenomenon requires you to be able to 'read' your patients and make subjective decisions. This is where art meets science. I would guess that this would be nothing new to you, since most manual therapy is a complex blend of art and science.

Another point that I hope most readers could agree on is that, as practitioners, we should be far less interested in what we might 'call' this phenomenon than our actual interest in seeing our patients getting healthier more quickly. The *semantics* around this healing phenomenon will eventually sort itself out, and much of the criticism of the placebo effect strikes me as being ego-driven. The phrase 'placebo effect' or 'placebo response' will eventually give way to another term that more adequately describes this phenomenon. This will happen as research uncovers more of the underlying neural, hormonal and biochemical processes involved. Eventually there will be a push among the scientific community to settle on one term, and this will undoubtedly happen over time. For now, what we all should want is for our patients to get better, not to argue over what we will call this phenomenon.

Everyone's body has an amazing capacity to heal itself. The wisdom of the body really ought to leave each and every one of us in absolute pure awe! However, occasionally the body reaches a point of stalled healing, and that is when patients come to us looking for help. It can sometimes be easy to become frustrated ourselves by the stalled healing that we see in our patients, but I hope that the techniques and ideas presented in this book afford you with new ways to kick-start and maximize healing in your patients. In addition, I hope that this book presents you with solid reasons to never get discouraged as a practitioner or a therapist, and that this positive attitude can be something that you can pass on, not only to the patient's conscious mind, but also to their unconscious mind that actually handles the bulk of the healing processes.

One thing to keep in mind when applying the principles in this book is to always tailor the approach to the patient. This is really nothing new for you as a practitioner. Few of us are successful with a cookie-cutter approach to treating patients, even though many of these treatment protocols were hammered into us during our formal schooling years. Every good practitioner knows that each and every patient that walks through your door is not just unique, but everybody (or every 'body') responds quite differently even to the same treatment modality. What works for patient A, doesn't necessarily work for patient B, or patient C. Applying the principles contained within this book is no different. Some people will be extremely open to the idea of visualization techniques, while others will pretty much think that it is a bunch of nonsense. You can try to make believers of your patients with techniques that they are likely to balk at, but instead, since this book presents so many ways to achieve the goal of health, I would suggest that you simply offer up another method.

It is also good to remember, depending upon where you practice, that there is a broad cultural variability surrounding certain aspects of the placebo effect. This was clearly shown by Daniel Moerman's analysis of cimetidine studies. He examined 31 studies of identical design of the same drug (cimetidine) against a placebo. The trials took place in many different counties. The responses to cimetidine were fairly uniform across all of the studies. The placebo arm, on the other hand, varied from 10% in Denmark to 90% in Germany, and anywhere in between in other countries. Moerman speculated that either the study design was highly flawed, or the cultural perspectives of participants coloured their response to the placebo. There are no hard and fast rules where culture comes in to play. You have to feel out each patient and tailor all aspects of your treatment to the specific patient.

When I first met Stuart Taws, creator and developer of Soft Tissue Release, he indicated that he was working on the 'No-technique-technique.' This might actually have made a fun title for this book. Everyone working in the manual therapy profession necessarily works with their hands, and I am sure that most of us wouldn't want it any other way. However, after many years of practice and postgraduate education, I found that I was becoming somewhat 'technique-weary'; meaning, that I really didn't need to learn more techniques. What I needed were more ways to employ the techniques that I was already using. This fueled my interest in the subject matter of this book. I sincerely hope that you found Part 2 to be rich with new and different ways for you to apply the techniques that you already use, improving the clinical outcomes for your patients, in other words, employing these 'no-technique-techniques'.

I wish you well on your journey as a practitioner, and I thank you for taking the time to read this book. It has been a joyful rewarding process, which I affectionately call *The Mexican Project*, because most of it was written while on various holidays in sunny warm Mexico; an absolutely wonderful place to immerse one's self in any project. At this time I would like to say, 'Adiós mis amigos; hasta luego!'

Part 3

Perspectives on Healing

INTRODUCTION TO PART 3

If you are still reading, then you must just be a glutton for punishment, as I am. Often when looking at any subject, it is good to consider alternative conceptual views so that you can open your mind to new possibilities. In this case, the subject at hand is that of health and healing. In the course of gathering research and theories for Part 2, I encountered several interesting ideas from what might be described as alternative thinkers. The ideas considered in Part 3 are not mainstream, nor do they have strong clinical orientation, hence the decision to place them at the end of the book after the clinical sections. These ideas challenge existing paradigms by proposing alternative explanations to the complex matter of biological systems. I am not saying that these ideas are right or wrong, but rather they represent a viewpoint that is worth considering, or at least interesting to ponder.

I hope that you find some of the following perspectives interesting, but you might also think that they are way too far out there for your liking. If so, then just ignore this final section. They are not integral in any way to the message of this book, and are only offered up as a 'dessert portion' after the big meal of Part 2.

WHERE DO WE GO FROM HERE?

We still do not know one thousandth of one percent of what nature has revealed to us.

Albert Einstein

Do not fear to be eccentric in opinion, for every opinion now accepted was once eccentric.

Bertrand Russell

Where do we go from here? Hopefully research will begin to unravel more of the mechanism of the placebo effect and personal healing, but are likely real limits to our ability to understand this phenomenon. If we ever completely understand the placebo effect, then we will completely understand healing, and we are a long way from there right now. Currently medicine is still locked into the Newtonian mechanistic paradigm and seems unwilling to look at the bigger picture of health. One can always hope that the human spirit alone will unlock doors and create new paradigms, but the major factors affecting development and implementation of new ideas is always heavily affected by money and power. Clearly the power right now, as far as research dollars is concerned, lies with the drug companies. However, as health-care costs climb higher and higher, our governments will look for ways to spend their health dollars more wisely. We have already seen a large number of services cut as our government here in my home province of Ontario attempts to control ballooning health-care costs.

To counter the tendency for governments to only consider the idea of slashing health services to control costs, there needs to be a push from our community of manual practitioners and other holistic practitioners to show decision-makers that it is much cheaper to invest money in prevention than it is to treat a pathology, or a disorder after it appears. The cost of our medical system has become higher and higher, and instead of always tearing the system down with service cutting, we need to show decision-makers how to build up health-care in an efficient manner, and that is almost necessarily by using a holistic approach. This change in thinking would not be a few token measures; it would involve adopting a truly holistic health model from which decisions will flow. One existing example of this is 'health spending accounts' that some employees have through their extended health-care coverage through their place of work. This empowers the patient to spend dollars where they feel they get the most benefit. It is bottom-up thinking rather than top-down thinking. There is no argument that allopathic trauma-based medicine is extremely important and that it saves lives. It certainly saved my life when my appendix ruptured. However, if people eat badly, are exposed to health hazards in their daily life, have poor lifestyle habits and are engaged in behaviours and thought patterns that are ultimately destructive, it is a lot to ask of the medical establishment to 'fix' them.

There are no surprising facts, only models that are surprised by facts; if a model is surprised by the facts, it is no credit to that model.

Eliezer Yudkowsky

Few biomedical scientists seem willing to think outside of the box and those that do are typically ridiculed by their peers and the mainstream establishment. Fortunately, a few scientists are willing to consider other paradigms, fully aware that they are risking their reputation. One such man was Galileo, and it didn't end well for him as he spent his last years under house arrest after being forced to recant his theories. For others like Antoine Lavoisier, it ended much worse; in his case it was the guillotine. History is full of many examples of people who stuck their necks out and questioned the status quo, who became ostracized and vilified during their lifetime, only to have their reputations resurrected after their death. We are now going to look at a few modern-day scientists who might fall into that category. These individuals are trying to promote a new paradigm and a larger way of explaining what is going on in the healing process than Newtonian physics seems able to explain. This is achieved partly by incorporating the knowledge that has been derived from quantum mechanics.

Rupert Sheldrake PhD

Rupert Sheldrake graduated with double first class honours degree in biochemistry, and won the University Botany Prize. He won a Frank Knox fellowship to study philosophy and history at Harvard University. He returned to Cambridge, where he obtained his PhD in biochemistry. His books and papers stem from his theory of morphic resonance (MR) and cover topics such as animal and plant development and behaviour, memory, telepathy, perception, and cognition in general.

Sheldrake describes MR as a feedback mechanism between the field and the corresponding forms of morphic units. To quote Sheldrake:

The greater the degree of similarity, the greater the resonance, leading to habituation or persistence of particular forms. So, the existence of a morphic field makes the existence of a new similar form easier.

He uses MR to explain a number of common but not yet understood phenomena such as flock behaviour of birds in flight, embryonic development, social learning and instincts. Sheldrake proposes that the process of MR leads to stable morphic fields, which are significantly easier to tune into. Sheldrake views fields as existing in fractal forms where smaller fields exist within other larger fields and any number of fields can exist within a larger one. His field theory attempts also to explain one mechanism by which you as a practitioner can affect change. This change can actually happen without you really doing anything substantial other than being present with intent. This theory might explain why practitioners achieve success with highly divergent modalities with everything from very deep work such as Rolfing to Reiki and Therapeutic Touch where the practitioner doesn't even touch the patient. I don't know about you, but it has always left me curious when I see practitioners using totally different approaches on the same pathology and still getting positive results. This spurred me on to pursue the placebo effect as one possible explanation; morphic energy fields might be another. If you find Sheldrake's ideas interesting you can view his TED talk on YouTube. He has a great sense of humor and typically comes across very well in interviews.

James L. Oschman PhD

James L. Oschman has an undergraduate degree in biology and a PhD in biophysics from the University of Pittsburgh. He has worked in major research labs in Cambridge, Case-Western Reserve, University of Copenhagen and Northwestern University in Evanston, Illinois, where he was on the faculty. He is the author of, *Energy medicine: the scientific basis and energy medicine in therapeutics and human performance.* He currently sits on the Scientific Advisory Board for Neuro Resource Group and the Scientific Advisory Board of the National Foundation for Alternative Medicine and is president of Nature's Own Research Association.

Oschman's consuming interest is energy medicine. Now if this phrase gets your hackles up, then don't worry, because it does for me as well! Energy medicine is a field that I have always viewed as being full of some very 'interesting' people, and that alone has typically steered me away from this pursuit. I have long viewed myself as a 'muscle mechanic'; very practical and empirically minded, so I enter the area of energy medicine kicking and screaming. Oschman has a strong background in electrical theory and electronics. His lectures go on about such things as Ampere's Law, and Faraday's Law of Induction so that he can explain his concepts. One way which he attempts to diffuse the 'energy' word is with this introduction: '*So what is energy medicine? First what is energy? Nothing happens in nature without an energy exchange; communication, or acquisition of knowledge of any kind occurs only with an energy transfer. There are no exceptions. This is a rule of nature.*' Okay, I'll buy that! Makes sense to me. Oschman then goes on to say that Newtonian physics explains the mechanistic world, the world of machines, and is invaluable in predicting and explaining most physical interaction in the world. However, there is another level, the subatomic level where quantum physics explains what is going on. Quantum physics doesn't go against Newtonian physics, it just says that there's another subtle level of interaction and that level of interaction concerns all space, the energy that is present everywhere in space, the way that we 'affect' the properties of space, and the possibility is that space has information that we can tap into. He mentions scalar fields, quantum fields and quantum potential as energies that are out there and are potentially affecting us.

Now I don't pretend to understand quantum physics at all myself. Here I depend on experts to interpret these theories and make them digestible for you and me to understand and relate to. One thing that many of these experts seem to be saying is that so much of what goes on in the world of living organisms is unexplained by Newtonian physics, because living things are much more than mechanistic machines. Oschman is also a supporter of the concept of the 'living matrix' a concept that I was introduced to by Dr George Roth of the Matrix Institute whose applied technique called 'matrix repatterning' is doing amazing things with a therapy that is extremely subtle. The cellular matrix is a well-established concept, but Oschman also believes that there is also a matrix surrounding us (often referred to as our aura or biomagnetic field), and that there is also the matrix of space (Sheldrake's morphic field).

What I hope that you get from Oschman's and Sheldrake's perspectives is that the world (and the world of healing) is far stranger than you had ever thought it was and that miracles are entirely possible; maybe even normal. If you truly believe that, then you open the door to possibility. If you project that belief upon your patient, you allow them to open the door to the possibility.

Bruce Lipton PhD

Finally, there is one other 'cowboy' that we looked at in the section entitled 'The nature of belief'. Bruce Lipton has an undergraduate degree in biology at Long Island University, and a PhD in developmental cell biology at University of Virginia. For years, Lipton was a professor at several universities teaching undergrad and graduate level courses to medical students on topics such as histology-cell biology, medical embryology and graduate level physiology. He is the author of two books, *The biology of belief: unleashing the power of consciousness, matter and miracles* (2005) and *Spontaneous evolution: our positive future* (2009).

One of Bruce's mantras is to refer to the cell membrane as a mem-brain. Like the two previous scientists, Bruce's work has also gone against the grain and his ideas are quite interesting. Central to his (and Sheldrake's and Oschman's) theories is the idea that the DNA isn't the master controller of our, or any other species' development. He views DNA as more or less a template or a library where information is stored, but the membrane is the cellular structure with the ability to communicate with the outer world. This is achieved by a multitude of receptor and effector and proteins that constantly interact with the surrounding environment. It is from the membrane that all things in the outside world are sensed and all action is initiated. The environment is the cue for all cells to either advance, retreat (in the case of single-celled organisms); and to grow, atrophy, undergo mitosis or even die (in the case of all organisms whether multicellular or unicellular). Lipton does a great job of explaining the fact that humans are a community of over 30 trillion cells all working in harmony. He has been adamantly against the DNA-centered thinking that was very much a 20th century dogma, because he is so sure that it is the membrane where most decisions are being made.

The results of the Human Genome Project (HGP) clearly indicate that there is a whole lot more going on than just DNA. When the project was begun, it was expected that they would find over 100 000 genes. This was the number of genes it was expected to be needed to produce all of the body's proteins. The HGP was supposed to unlock the keys to provide individual treatment for each and every human illness. Venture capitalists jumped on board. Unfortunately the project only found 21 000 genes, and shares for the privately funded HGP fell from $230 per share to only $7 per share at the end of the project. This tells you that the despite the fact that the press still touts the HGP as a master achievement, its investors clearly did not. If you want to put our 21 000 genes in perspective, you only need to look at the simple roundworm *C. elegans*. It has 20 000 genes. This simple animal with no arms, no legs and no sentient consciousness (that we know of) has almost as many genes as us! The translucent water flea, *Daphnia pulex*, which lives in ponds and lakes throughout North America, Europe and Australia has 31 000 genes! What this all suggests to Lipton is that the controls for so much of what we are, what we do and how we develop is not in the genes but somewhere else. Lipton thinks that it is the cell membrane where many of those decisions are made, and he presents strong arguments to suggest that this is the case.

The growing field of epigenetics recognizes that genes alone do not control our lives. This field exploded after the HGP failed to produce the results expected and it was obvious that there was a whole lot more going on than just our DNA. Epigenetics looks at the many factors outside of the cell and the organism that affects its growth, development and its health; even its offspring. For example, several hundred million people worldwide chew areca nut, a seed from a palm tree, and people who engage in this habit tend to develop high blood pressure, diabetes and metabolic syndrome. The children born to these people are likely to develop metabolic syndrome as well, even if the children themselves have never chewed areca. This idea was actually proposed by Jean-Baptiste Lamarck in the early 19th century and was actually championed by Charles Darwin because it fit with his theory of natural selection. The idea was challenged by many at the time and near the end of the 19th century German biologist, August Weismann, decided to put an end to Lamarck's theory. Weismann snipped the tails off mice, bred the animals and observed the offspring for 'taillessness'. After hundreds of mice were born, all with normal tails, Lamarckism was considered disproved. In the 20th century, there was little support for Lamarckism. It was generally accepted through the 20th century that acquired characteristics could be inherited only through direct mutation of the DNA contained in germ cells (sperm and eggs), but no environmental factors capable of inducing germ-line mutations in humans were identified. Recently scientists have identified several acquired characteristics that can be passed from one generation to the next. The mechanism by which these characteristics are inherited involves transmission of subtle chemical modifications to DNA and DNA-associated proteins to offspring. These modifications, which are acquired during childhood and adulthood, can manifest as detectable traits in offspring. What would have been called fantasy or science fiction 20 years ago is now the highly credible field of epigenetics.

Lipton further believes that through our consciousness we can actually affect how our genes are expressed, and therefore affect our health. He sees genes as what people in the construction industry call a 'bill of materials'. The cell membrane is the contractor. So then, where is the blueprint? Sheldrake sees the morphogenic field as the blueprint. Lipton is very interested in consciousness. He believes that to change our behaviour and heal ourselves, requires that we reprogram our unconscious selves. Lipton states that our conscious minds only control 5–10% at best of what we do.*

He sees the subconscious mind as a super-computer loaded with a database of programmed behaviors, most of which we acquire before we reach the age of six. Like all learning, these beliefs, attitudes and prejudices then become a part of our unconscious or subconscious programming.

Neuroscience has other findings that are helpful to this discussion. A number of meditation experiments have shown that people can actually change their brain structure (regardless of their age) by creating new neural pathways just by conscious thinking. Until around the 1970s, neuroscientists believed that the nervous system was essentially fixed throughout adulthood, both in terms of brain functions, as well as the idea that it was impossible for new neurons to develop after birth. We now know that this is not the case. The concept of neuroplasticity is now extremely well established both in theory and in practice. Brains can, in effect, rewire themselves. This cannot be understated that the brain can be rewired, and that consciousness can alter physiology. These two concepts, Lipton believes, have broad implications in the area of health and healing. So then, if this is true, why doesn't positive thinking alone produce changes in anyone attempting this practice? Lipton believes that it is not enough to change your conscious mind if your unconscious programming is giving the body the opposite message. In other words, if your unconscious program running in the background of your mind believes that achieving a certain goal, or self-healing is not possible, then all of the positive self-talk won't change a thing.

---

*There appears to be no number that neuroscientists can currently agree upon in reference to conscious control versus unconscious control; however, there is strong agreement that majority of mental processes do *not* take place at a conscious level. Dr David Eagleman, a neuroscientist at Baylor's College of Medicine, and director of both the Laboratory of Perception and Action and the Initiative on Neuroscience and Law has a fun term to describe mental processes that do not take place at a conscious level. In his book, *Incognito: the Secret Lives of the Brain*, he uses the phrase, 'under the hood'. This light-hearted term avoids all of the baggage and the multiple definitions that come with words like unconscious or subconscious and preconscious. When interviewed on NPR, Eagleman stated that, *'Just lifting a cup of coffee to your mouth is an enormously complicated act, as we know from trying to make robots do even simple things. And yet all of this happens invisibly for you. When you lift the coffee, you don't know anything about the nerves and the tendons and the muscles and the exquisite symphony of signals that allows it to happen.'* So if lifting a coffee cup involves all sorts of 'under the hood stuff', imagine how much else is going on under the hood from heart rate to respiration, digestion, immunological activity and healing to name just a few. Eagleman feels that the bulk of our mental processes happen under the hood. The typical analogy used to represent this view is that of an iceberg, where conscious mental activity represents the part above the water, with the bulk of the iceberg (mental processes) being below the surface.

Clinical implications

Lipton's concept would be used in much the same manner as expectancy theory in Part 2 of this book. Clinical implications of this can involve everything from rehabilitation to stalled healing. We need to remind ourselves and remind our patients that neuroplasticity when combined with conscious thought has tremendous implications in recovery, and in matters of stalled healing. We need to be able to confidently project these beliefs, and our patients need understand that this is not science fiction, but reality. One of our roles then is to feed the conscious mind with positive messages concerning its power in shaping health. As you treat the body, you need to give messages at least to the conscious mind that the body can heal this area after your intervention. Instilling positive mental programming is probably one of the most important things that we can do for our patients in their time with us. We obviously do that at a conscious level, but what about everything under the hood? This is where referral would be appropriate. There are many approaches out there to help people 'reprogram their minds' but before you make referral suggestions, you should know that this is an area fraught with charlatans. Much of what you will find in the area of subconscious programming is materialism-centred approaches, which are supposedly based on 'personal success' (wink-wink), but which actually are catered to appeal to people's sense of greed; because success is typically suggested to be monetary success. This strikes me as a rather shallow, greed-based approach to true health and happiness. So what can you suggest for your patient who is stuck? Please see the Box 3.1 for a few suggestions for referrals.

Auto-suggestion is another method that anyone can use without taking a course or enrolling in a program. It involves the repetition of certain positive sentence/phrase before sleeping and when you wake up. It is implemented as follows. Create a simple single sentence. You only tackle one idea at a time that you must repeat before going to sleep and when you wake up. You must repeat it for an extend period of time, a minimum of 20 days. The phrase must have a meaning to the participant. In the area of healing it might be something like, 'My body (or shoulder or back etc.) can heal itself.'

Cognitive Behavioral Therapy is a psychotherapeutic approach that addresses dysfunctional emotions, maladaptive behaviors and cognitive processes through a number of goal-oriented, explicit systematic procedures. It is very much a mainstream modality and it is considered to have a high degree of efficacy. This modality is used by psychotherapists as well as social workers.

Clinical Hypnotherapy is the most obvious method of entry into the subconscious. A 2003 meta-analysis by Flammer and Bongartz examined data on the efficacy of hypnotherapy in studies of psychosomatic illness, test anxiety, smoking cessation and pain control during orthodox medical treatment. The authors considered a total of 444 studies, and then narrowed their focus down to 57 controlled trials. These showed that, on average, hypnotherapy achieved at least 64% success compared with 37% improvement among untreated control groups. According to the authors, this was an intentional underestimation. Their stated aim was to discover whether, even under the most skeptical weighing of the evidence, hypnotherapy was still proven effective. They concluded that it was effective (Flammer & Bongartz 2003).

Eye Movement Desensitization and Reprocessing (EMDR) is a psychotherapeutic technique developed to treat PTSD and has been judged efficacious by numerous professional bodies. In EMDR treatment, the patient first recalls traumatic events, then uses free association on their own to sequences of linked material, both traumatic and non-traumatic. During this time the patient is simultaneously attending to inner thoughts while the therapist applies sensory stimulation from a rhythmic, bilateral source. The sensory stimulus is most typically visual (hence 'eye movement'), but can be auditory, tactile or proprioceptive. The goal of EMDR therapy is to process these distressing memories, reducing their lingering influence and allowing patients to develop more adaptive coping mechanisms. A referral to a practitioner would be indicated if you felt the patient's healing was stalled due to traumatic experiences from their past.

Holographic Memory Resolution (HMR) is a relatively new approach to therapy developed by Brent Baum, which allows the patient to access their past experiences swiftly and without emotional associations. The patient does not relive the ordeal but instead they can identify and address specific memories and gain the ability to self-heal. HMR employs techniques that encourage visualization and discovery of memories in a safe and secure environment. This therapy strives to remove the unconscious factors that are responsible for eliciting powerful and often negative emotional and physical responses to disturbing memories. HMR theorists surmise that the restoration of properly functioning cellular structures can serve to increase our immune system's effectiveness and prevent disease.

Psychological Kinesiology* (PSYCH-K) is a self-help tool developed by Robert M. Williams in 1988 which attempts to change beliefs harbored in the subconscious mind. Subconscious beliefs are seen to be the 'invisible' cause of self-sabotaging behaviors. The PSYCH-K program was designed to help people change the way they feel, behave and interact in life. In PSYCH-K, applied kinesiology is used to communicate with the subconscious mind. Specific body postures and movements cause neuron firings in both hemispheres of the brain, creating a state in which change can occur more readily. The creator of the program claims that, using this method, it is possible for subconscious beliefs to be recognized, and a debilitating belief could be replaced with one more desirable.

---

*For more on psychological kinesiology visit http://psych-k.com/

Box 3.1

QUANTUM HEALING

Everything we call real is made of things that cannot be regarded as real. If quantum mechanics hasn't profoundly shocked you, you haven't understood it yet.

Niels Bohr

For my last and final trick, I will tackle quantum mechanics. No, actually I won't. Okay, let's be completely honest, only an idiot or a quantum physicist would tackle this topic (and I'm definitely not a quantum physicist). Experts have trouble describing quantum theory, and even they admit that they don't understand it, they just accept it, because the concepts involved defy rationality. This is a field where I hold absolutely *no* expertise (notice how I emphasized 'no'). As a matter of fact, I really didn't even want to write this section. So why am I touching on it? Well, it's because I keep encountering the suggestion that quantum mechanics is involved in biological processes and the stuff of life by so many people whose ideas I find quite appealing and somewhat logical. In researching basic quantum mechanics principles, I found out that without realizing it, we are all actually using applied quantum mechanics every day. For example, you use quantum mechanics to see. Your retina converts electromagnetic radiation into nerve impulses. The business of light absorption necessarily involves quantum mechanics. Also, almost every one of us is using quantum mechanics on a daily basis every time we use a computer or a cell phone, for example. Semi-conductors, which are used in virtually everything these days, are built on the principles of quantum mechanics. As you will see shortly, quantum mechanics explains the flow of electrons (aka electricity or energy) through those semi-conductors (and even us).

One field of inquiry that welcomes new ideas and seems to be less threatened by a new explanation of the world is physics. The world of quantum physics emerged when classical physics failed to explain certain phenomenon. Light, for example, as we now know, behaves both like particles and waves; but this is a modern understanding of the phenomenon. Interestingly enough this debate goes back to the 17th century. Isaac Newton proposed that light was a particle, as this fit more comfortably with his model. One of Newton's contemporaries, Christiaan Huygens proposed that it was in fact a wave. Newton's idea won out initially, but the controversy was not going to go away. Newtonian physics failed to explain certain phenomena concerning the behaviour of light, so a more complete model was needed. In the 19th century, James Clerk Maxwell discovered that he could combine four simple equations, to describe the self-propagating waves of oscillating EMFs. When the propagation speed of these electromagnetic waves was calculated, the speed of light was mathematically produced. It then became apparent that visible light, ultraviolet light and infrared light were all electromagnetic waves of differing frequency. So now light was a wave. However, this still presented a problem, and it wasn't until the 20th century that this debate was more or less wrestled to the ground with the cumbersome wave/particle duality theory. Einstein was never comfortable with this theory and to this day, the debate continues. What is interesting to note here is that the field of physics continues to be open to new ideas and theories without needing to attack individuals for their alternative explanations of phenomenon that do not fit into the current model or theory. Researchers are genuinely excited, rather than threatened when new information appears. They are like kids with new candy when new data and theories appear. It would be great if this were the case in the biomedical field, but it would seem that too many people and corporations are protecting their own interests or their own egos, and this severely hampers creative open-minded thinking.

Is it a particle, or a wave? Newtonian physics explains the movement of electrons through a vacuum. Vacuum tubes were common in radios and televisions when I was growing up, but in the 1950s and 1960s 'solid state electronics' appeared. It turns out that when electrons flow through a solid, they behave both like a particle (containing a charge) and a wave (as they move through the solid material). As a result, one needs to understand quantum physics to build electronic components, because in the medium of semi-conductors, electrons behave both as waves and as particles. These solid semi-conductors include everything from transistors to integrated circuits, diodes, transistors, microprocessor chips, flash drives, the light-emitting diode (LED), and the liquid-crystal display (LCD). So in case you didn't know it, every time you turn on and use a computer (or a radio, TV, cell phone or any other electronics device), you are actually applying quantum mechanics.

Free electrons are floating throughout our body, another semiconductor and as you might guess, they obey the laws of quantum physics. Something that I didn't realize until researching this book was the importance of grounding oneself. The earth can be viewed as a reservoir of electrons and these electrons help us to fight inflammation (both chronic and acute), all inflammatory diseases including autoimmune diseases, and free radicals. Positively-charged free radicals are stopped in their tracks, becoming electrically neutral, the moment that they bind to a free electron. Once a free radical has become electrically neutral, it ceases to do damage in the body. One of the most basic things that you can do for yourself, and suggest to your patients to prevent free radical damage, is by using earthing, also known as grounding technology (which was discussed in the last section of Part 2 (p. 232).* But I digress.

The first person to write on the implications of quantum mechanics on biological systems was Austrian born physicist and theoretical biologist Erwin Schrödinger (yes, the cat guy, but don't worry, he never killed any cats!). His 1946 book, *What is Life?*, was based on a course of public lectures that he delivered

---

*Research on grounding can be found at: http://www.earthinginstitute.net/index.php/research

in February 1943* Schrödinger's original lecture focused on one basic question: 'How can the events in space and time which take place within the spatial boundary of a living organism be accounted for by physics and chemistry?' In his book, which was written before DNA was discovered, Schrödinger hypothesized that the carrier of hereditary information had to be both small in size and permanent in time, contradicting a 'naïve' physicist's expectation. This contradiction, he said, could not be resolved by classical physics. Ten years later James Watson and Francis Crick discovered the molecular structure of DNA, bringing to life the concept of a small storage medium for genetic material but, unfortunately, inquiry into non-mechanistic aspects of inheritance seems to have ended at that point. It seems ironic that one of the leaders in quantum mechanics was already suggesting back in 1946 that we needed to look beyond classical physics to explain genetic inheritance, and yet no one has really taken up that torch and run with it in the mainstream medical research community.

In Chapter VI of his book Schrödinger states:

> … *living matter, while not eluding the 'laws of physics' as established up to date, is likely to involve 'other laws of physics' hitherto unknown, which however, once they have been revealed, will form just as integral a part of science as the former.*

This is an impressive statement from one of the great minds of the 20th century, that life is in fact far stranger than we could imagine, and this man had a firm grasp on Newtonian and quantum physics.

Today it is understood and accepted that many biological processes involving the conversion of energy into forms that are usable for the cell are quantum mechanical in nature. Such processes involve chemical reactions, light absorption, photosynthesis, formation of excited electronic states, conversion of chemical energy into motion, transfer of excitation energy, transfer of electrons and protons in photosynthesis and cellular respiration, DNA mutation, and Brownian motors (e.g. the ATPase motor that hydrolyzes ATP) in many cellular processes. To make you comfortable with the idea of quantum mechanics, consider that even our own vision has been found to be quantum mechanical in its nature.

Admittedly, our brains are not wired to understand quantum mechanics. It moves well beyond logic and requires some very creative math to describe and predict. Even to make predictions about locations of quantum particles there is always an aspect of uncertainty. This is what is known as the uncertainty principle. This has also been stated as 'probability rules!' Einstein himself was uncomfortable with this notion as it suggested to him that God plays with dice. This caused Einstein to spend the last 20 years of his life trying unsuccessfully to disprove

---

*Schrödinger's book, *What is Life?* is available as a free download at http://whatislife.stanford.edu/LoCo_files/What-is-Life.pdf

this aspect of quantum theory, also known as probability aspect, because of the uncertainty.

If we return to why I am touching on this massive subject, there appears to be nothing in Newtonian physics that can explain the fields that as practitioners we intuitively sense are around us and our patients. Newtonian physics also cannot explain how you just 'know' something about a patient, a loved one or a situation. Oschman considers this a manifestation of quantum non-locality, another aspect of quantum physics. The field of quantum non-locality involves the interconnection of two particles over space and time. Their connection does not appear to be affected by distance, like other conventional fields. Einstein referred to this as the 'spooky action at a distance'.

Another word commonly used to describe quantum non-locality is entanglement. The new-age translation of this is that 'we are all connected' or even 'we are all one'. It may or may not be a view that you hold, but it is something that has become obvious to me over time. If you don't accept the latter, I hope that the idea that we are all connected becomes abundantly clear to you in your lifetime; not just through belief, but rather through experience. This may or may not be an aspect of quantum entanglement, but those of us with holistic perceptions do find the idea appealing. My explanations of entanglement will not satisfy any physicists in the crowd, but for the purposes of this discussion, entanglement refers to the correlation between the results of measurements performed on entangled pairs. These pairs could be subatomic particles, molecules and even large spherical molecules known as 'buckyballs'. These measurable correlations have been observed even when the entangled pair was separated by arbitrarily large distances. In quantum entanglement, part of the transfer of information happens instantaneously. Repeated experiments have verified that this works even when the measurements are performed more quickly than light could travel between the sites of measurement. (Recent experiments (Yin et al. 2013) have shown that quantum entanglement transfer occurs at least 10 000 times faster than the speed of light.)

Recognition of the interconnection of all life at all levels whether at a physical, spiritual, biological, ecological or at a quantum level is, I believe, a wonderfully appealing concept to most of us in the healing arts. Often, one's perception of our separateness is the beginning of dysfunction or illness. If our patient is feeling disconnected it is all the more important that we establish that bond... that trust... that connection. Our connection with the patient is undoubtedly central to the healing that will take place, and is a large part of the healing/placebo effect.

Here ends my mangling of quantum theory. This was not meant to be a treatise on the topic, just a cursory view meant to open up our minds to the idea that there is a whole lot more going on than we currently understand. Our medical models fall far short of explaining much of what goes on with healing. As the quote goes, 'There are no surprising facts, only models that are surprised by facts.' Healing exceptions are not really exceptions. They demonstrate inadequacies of the model used to describe them. We need to think bigger in the matter of healing, and we need researchers and practitioners who are open to newer, larger, and more inclusive interpretations of what is going on in the human body. Our bodies are strange and complex, and everything that goes on is deeply interconnected. We should never be afraid of examining and testing out new hypotheses as we search for a more complete understanding of the body-placebo or no placebo.

Appendix: Developing Strong Social Support

Here is a list of ideas from University of Buffalo School of Social Work for developing strong social support.
Source: http://socialwork.buffalo.edu/social-research.html.

Sustaining your current relationships

Successful relationships require give-and-take. A good rule of thumb is to treat your friends as you want to be treated. In other words, be the friend you want to have. Many factors contribute to healthy, happy relationships. Here are some tips:

Show your appreciation. Cherish your relationships. Tell your friends and family how important they are to you and thank them for all they give you.

Stay in touch. Return phone calls, texts, and emails in a timely manner (when possible) and reciprocate invitations. Doing these things is not only polite but it lets people know they are important to you.

Be available when you're needed. True friends come through when times are tough. Be a good listener and allow your friend to confide freely and without being judged. Let them know you are in their corner. Ask what you can do to help.

Accept their help. Some people find it hard to accept support, preferring to be the one always offering it instead. Some may fear becoming dependent or want to maintain their self-image as the 'strong' and 'together' one. But friends and family often want to feel they have done something for you. Let them! Accepting help can help you. It also keeps the relationship balanced (as it should be) and lets your friends and loved ones know that they have something to offer that you value.

Support successes. When you genuinely care about someone, you will be excited when they succeed. If you find yourself feeling a little jealous too, you can acknowledge that to yourself, but don't let it poison your friendship.

Keep the lines of communication open. Open, honest communication is the lifeblood of healthy, happy relationships. If a friend does or says something that hurts your feelings, try to deal with it directly. Start by assuming that it is a misunderstanding or that the misstep was unintentional, but ask them about it. (Don't stuff bruised feelings.) Your friend will likely appreciate the opportunity to remedy the situation. Whatever the case, accept apologies graciously (as you would hope others would accept yours).

Respect needs and limits. Each person has their own setting for how much social interaction they need and want. Know your own and respect that of others, even if it differs from yours. Sometimes finding this balance can be hard with a new friend and may require adjustments. However, if a friend starts to pull away or initiate less communication, it may be that you have overstepped. Don't assume though. Ask them, address the issue, and apologize (if appropriate). Remember, friendships are two-way streets.

Know when a relationship isn't working for you. If you find that you are drained whenever you see a particular friend, or that he or she is inconsiderate of your time or feelings, or is unreliable, highly critical of you, or generally negative, they may not be the friend for you. Similarly, if they engage in unhealthy behaviors, such as alcohol or substance abuse, particularly if you have had trouble with such issues, they also may not be a good choice for your social support network. Remember, those in your support system should help you reduce stress, not increase it. They should support your goals and efforts to achieve them, not belittle or undermine them.

Some ideas for building your social support system

Volunteer. Identify a cause that is important to you and get involved. Give some of your time to help a community organization, a local church, synagogue or mosque, or the local section of a national organization. Volunteering can give you the gratification of taking action to further your values and will bring you into contact with others who share your interests and ideals.

Take up a sport or join a gym. Regular exercise is good for your physical and psychological health and it may also provide the opportunity to build new friendships.

Start a book club and invite some people to join who you don't already know well. Discussing interesting ideas and sharing thoughts and observations is a wonderful way to make new friends.

Meet your neighbors. Make an effort to get to know some of the acquaintances you see on a regular basis. Chances are some of them are gems.

Join professional organizations. Taking this step is good not only for your future career but it will also extend your social network to encompass others in your field. Sometimes friends in the same profession can understand the stresses you face better than anyone.

Use online resources. Social networking sites can help you stay connected with friends and family. Sending emails and electronic greetings for holidays and birthdays, posting pictures, and forwarding interesting articles are all ways to stay in touch that can sustain relationships over time and distance, even when in-person time is limited.

REFERENCES AND FURTHER READING

Adams P with Mylander M (1998) Gesundheit!: bringing good health to you, the medical system, and society through physician service, complementary therapies, humor. Vermont, Healing Arts Press.

Adams P (1998) Joy and house calls – how we can all heal the world one visit at a time. Bandon, OR, Robert D. Reed Publishers.

Ader R (2000) The role of conditioning in pharmacology. In: Harrington A (2000) The placebo effect: an interdisciplinary exploration. Cambridge, MA, Harvard University, pp 138–165.

Ader R, Cohen N (1975) Behaviourally conditioned immunosuppression. *Psychosom Med* 37: 333–340.

Albring A et al (2012) Placebo effects on the immune response in humans: the role of learning and expectation. *PLoS ONE* 7(11): e49477.

ALSA (1992 - present) The Australian Longitudinal Study of Ageing. Online. Accessed June 2014. Available: http://www. flinders. edu. au/sabs/fcas/alsa/.

Apóstolo JL, Kolcaba K (2009) The effects of guided imagery on comfort, depression, anxiety, and stress of psychiatric inpatients with depressive disorders. *Arch Psychiatr Nurs* 23(6): 403–11.

Argyle M (1999) Causes and correlates of happiness. In: Kahneman D, Diener E, Schwarz N (eds). *Well-being: the foundations of hedonic psychology*. New York, Russell Sage Foundation.

Aspinwall LG (1998) Rethinking the role of positive affect in self-regulation. *Motivation and Emotion* 22: 1–32.

Avis A (1994) Choice cuts: an exploratory study of patients' views about participation in decision-making in a day surgery unit. *Int J Nurs Stud* 31 (3): 281–298.

Bacci I (2005) Effortless pain relief. New York, Free Press, Simon & Schuster.

Bacon CG et al (2003) Sexual function in men older than 50 years of age: results from the health professionals follow-up study. *Ann Intern Med* 5; 139(3): 161–8.

Balaji PA et al (2012) Physiological effects of yogic practices and transcendental meditation in health and disease. *N Am J Med Sci* 4(10): 442–8.

Barak Y (2006) The immune system and happiness. *Autoimmun Rev* 5(8): 523–527.

Bargh J (2009) The 'subatomic' world of unconscious causation. Psychology Today. Online. Accessed June 2014. Available: http://www. psychologytoday. com/blog/cultural-animal/200906/john-bargh-and-some-misunderstandings-about-free-will/comments#comment-64745.

Barrier PA, Jensen NM (2003) Two words to improve physician-patient communication: what else? *Mayo Clinic Proceedings* 78(2): 211–4.

Bass MJ et al (1986a) The physician's actions and the outcome of illness in family practice. *J Fam Pract* 23: 43–47.

Bass MJ et al (1986b) Predictors of outcome in headache patients presenting to family physicians: a one-year prospective study. *Headache*. 26: 285–29.

Bates MS et al (1993) Ethnocultural influences on chronic pain perception. *Pain* 52: 101–112.

Baumeister RF (2009) The 'subatomic' world of unconscious causation. Psychology Today. Online. Accessed June 2014. Available: http://www. psychologytoday. com/blog/cultural-animal/200906/john-bargh-and-some-misunderstandings-about-free-will/comments#comment-64745.

Beach MC et al (2013) White coat hype: branding physicians with professional attire. *JAMA Intern Med* 173(6): 467–468.

Beecher HK (1955) The powerful placebo. *JAMA* 159: 1602–1606.

Beecher HK (1956) Relationship of significance of wound to pain experience. *JAMA* 161: 1609–161.

Benedetti F (2008) Mechanisms of placebo and placebo-related effects across diseases and treatments. *Annu Rev Pharmacol Toxicol* 48: 33–60.

Benedetti F (2012) The placebo response: science versus ethics and the vulnerability of the patient. *World Psych* 11(2): 70–72.

Benedetti F, Amanzio M (2011) The placebo response: how words and rituals change the patient's brain. *Patient Educ Couns* 2011 84(3): 413–9.

Benedetti F, Amanzio M (2013) Mechanisms of the placebo response. *Pulm Pharmacol Ther* Jan 28. pii: S1094–5539(13)00052-7.

Benedetti F et al (2003a) Open versus hidden medical treatments: the patient's knowledge about a therapy affects the therapy outcome. *Prev Treatm* 6(1) Jun 2003 No Pagination Specified Article 1a.

Benedetti F et al (2003b) Conscious expectation and unconscious conditioning in analgesic, motor, and hormonal placebo/nocebo responses. *J Neurosci* 15; 23(10): 4315–23.

Benedetti F et al (2005) Neurobiological mechanisms of the placebo effect. *J Neurosci* 25(45): 10390–10402.

Benedetti F et al (2006a) The biochemical and neuroendocrine bases of the hyperalgesic nocebo effect. *J Neurosci*. 26(46): 12014–12022.

Benedetti F et al (2006b) Loss of expectation-related mechanisms in Alzheimer's disease makes analgesic therapies less effective. *Pain* 121(1–2): 133–44.

Benedetti F et al (2011) How placebos change the patient's brain. *Neuropsychopharmacology* 36(1): 339–354. Online. Accessed June 2014. Available: http://www. nature. com/npp/journal/v36/n1/full/npp201081a. htmlBennett HJ (2003) Humor in medicine. *South Med J* 96(12): 1257–61.

Benson H, with Klipper, MZ (1975) The relaxation response. New York, HarperCollins.

Benson H, McCallie DP (1979) Angina pectoris and the placebo effect. *N Engl J Med* 300: 1424–1429.

Benson H (1997) Timeless healing: the power of biology and belief. New York, Fireside, Simon & Schuster.

Berndt ER, Cockburn IM (2013) Price indexes for clinical trial research: a feasibility study. *The National Bureau for Economic Research*. NBER Working Paper No. 18918.

Berry DS, Hansen JS (1996) Positive affect, negative affect, and social interaction. *J Pers Soc Psychol* 71: 796–809.

Bertini M et al (2011) Clowns benefit children hospitalized for respiratory pathologies. *Evid Based Complement Alternat Med* 2011: 879125.

Bialosky JE et al (2011) Placebo response to manual therapy: something out of nothing? *J Man Manip Ther* 19(1): 11–19.

Bianconi E et al (2013) An estimation of the number of cells in the human body. *Annals of Human Biology* 40(6): 463–471.

Bingel U et al (2011) The effect of treatment expectation on drug efficacy: imaging the analgesic benefit of the opioid remifentanil. *Sci Transl Med* 16; 3(70): 70ra14.

Bishop FL et al (2015) Psychological covariates of longitudinal changes in back-related disability in patients undergoing acupuncture. *Clinical Journal of Pain* 31 (3): 254–264. doi: 10. 1097/AJP. 0000000000000108.

Blackwell B et al (1972) Demonstration to medical students of placebo responses and non-drug factors. *Lancet*. 10; 1(7763): 1279–82.

Blau JN (1985) Clinician and placebo. *Lancet* 1: 344.

Blumenthal JA et al (1999) Effects of exercise training on older patients with major depression. *Arch Intern Med* 159(19): 2349–56.

Blumenthal JA et al (2007) Exercise and pharmacotherapy in the treatment of major depressive disorder. *Psychosom Med* 69(7): 587–96.

Boileau I et al (2007) Conditioned dopamine release in humans: a positron emission tomography. *Journal of Neuroscience* 27(15): 3998–4003.

Boissel JP et al (1986) Time course of long-term placebo therapy effects in angina pectoris. *Eur Heart J Dec*: 7(12): 1030–6.

Booth-Kewley S et al (2014) A prospective study of factors affecting recovery from musculoskeletal injuries. *J Occup Rehabil* 24(2): 287–96.

Bovbjerg DH et al (1990) Anticipatory immune suppression and nausea in women receiving cyclic chemotherapy for ovarian cancer. *J Consult Clin Psychol* 58: 153–157.

Branthwaite A, Cooper P (1981). Analgesic effects of branding in treatment of headaches. *Br Med J (Clin Res Ed)* 282(6276): 1576–8.

Breach C et al (2007) Is patients' preferred involvement in health decisions related to outcomes for patients with HIV? *J Gen Intern Med* 22 (8): 1119–1124.

Brody DS et al (1989) Patient perception of involvement in medical care. Relationship to illness attitudes and outcomes. *J Gen Intern Med* 4(6): 506–511.

Brody H (2000a) The placebo response: how you can release the body's inner pharmacy for better health. New York, HarperCollins.

Brody H (2000b) The placebo response: recent research and implications for family medicine. *J Fam Pract* 49 (7): 649–654.

Brody H (2003). Stories of sickness. New York, Oxford University Press.

Brody H (2012) Placebo effects and implications for the doctor-patient relationship. In: *Samueli Institute. Using placebo responses in clinical practice: is there a there, there? What do we need to know?* January 19–20, 2012, p. 15 Online. Accessed June 2014. Available: http://www. samueliinstitute. org/File%20Library/Unassigned/ RPT_Using-Placebo-In-Clinical-Practice-1-20-12. pdf.

Bronfort G et al (2010) Effectiveness of manual therapies: the UK evidence report. *Chiropr Osteopat* 18: 3.

Brown D et al (2010). Pilot study on the effect of grounding on delayed-onset muscle soreness. *J Altern Complement Med.* 16(3): 265–73.

Brown WA (2013) The placebo effect in clinical practice. New York, New York, Oxford University Press, p. 99,137.

Buckalew LW, Ross S (1981). Relationship of perceptual characteristics to efficacy of placebos. *Psychol Rep.* 49 (3): 955–61.

Campbell J (2003) The myths and masks of God. Audio Collection, Disk 5, track 9. Minneapolis, HighBridge Company.

Campbell J (2012) The hero with a thousand faces (Collected works of Joseph Campbell). San Francisco, New World Library.

Campos de Carvalho E et al (2007) A pilot study of a relaxation technique for management of nausea and vomiting in patients receiving cancer chemotherapy. *Cancer Nursing* (2): 163–7.

Canadian Diabetes Association (2014). Fibre. Online. Accessed September 2014. Available: http://www. diabetes. ca/diabetes-and-you/healthy-living-resources/diet-nutrition/fibre.

Cannon WB (2002. Walter B. Cannon and 'Voodoo death': a perspective from 60 years on. *Am J Public Health* 92(10): 1564–6.

Centers for Disease Control (2004) Trends in intake of energy and macronutrients – United States, 1971–2000. Online. Accessed June 2014. Available: http://www. cdc. gov/mmwr/preview/mmwrhtml/mm5304a3. htm.

Centers for Disease Control and Prevention (2014) http://www. cdc. gov.

Cerhan JR, Wallace RB (1997) Change in social ties and subsequent mortality in rural elders. *Epidemiology* 8(5): 475–81.

Chen JA et al (2011) Association between patient beliefs regarding assigned treatment and clinical response: reanalysis of data from the Hypericum Depression Trial Study Group. *J Clin Psychiatry* 72(12): 1669–76.

Chen WC et al (2009). Efficacy of progressive muscle relaxation training in reducing anxiety in patients with acute schizophrenia. *J Clin Nurs* 18(15): 2187–96.

Cheung W et al (2007) Maternal anxiety and feelings of control during labour: a study of Chinese first-time pregnant women. *Midwifery* 23 (2): 123–130.

Chevalier G et al (2006) The effect of earthing (grounding) on human physiology. *European Biology and Bioelectromagnetics* 2006: 600–621.

Chevalier G (2010) Changes in pulse rate, respiratory rate, blood oxygenation, perfusion index, skin conductance, and their variability induced during and after grounding human subjects for 40 minutes. *J Altern Complement Med* 16(1): 81–87.

Chevalier G et al (2012) Earthing: health implications of reconnecting the human body to the Earth's surface electrons. *J Environ Public Health* Article ID 291541, 8 pages http://dx.doi.org/10.1155/2012/291541

Chevalier G et al (2013) Earthing (grounding) the human body reduces blood viscosity – a major factor in cardiovascular disease. *J Altern Complement Med* 19(2): 102–110.

Chun OK et al (2008) Serum C-reactive protein concentrations are inversely associated with dietary flavonoid intake in U.S. adults. *J Nutr* 138(4): 753–60.

Chung SK et al (2007) Revelation of a personal placebo response: its effects on mood, attitudes and future placebo responding. *Pain* 5; 132(3): 281–8.

Chung SC et al (2012) Effect of Sahaja yoga meditation on quality of life, anxiety, and blood pressure control. *J Altern Complement Med.* 18(6): 589–96.

Cobb LA et al (1959) An evaluation of internal mammary artery ligation by double-blind technique. *N Engl J Med.* 20: 1115 –1118.

Colloca L et al (2004) Overt versus covert treatment for pain, anxiety, and Parkinson's disease. *Lancet Neurol* 3(11): 679–84.

Colloca L et al (2005) The placebo response in conditions other than pain. *Semin Pain Med* 3: 1; 43–47.

Coulehan J et al (2001) 'Let me see if I have this right…': words that help build empathy. *Ann Intern Med* 135 (3): 221–7.

Cousins N (1981) Anatomy of an illness as perceived by the patient. New York, Bantam Books.

Covey SR (2004) The 7 habits of highly effective people: powerful lessons in personal change. New York, Free Press.

Credit Suisse Research Institute (2013) Sugar. Consumption at a crossroads. Online. Accessed June 2014. Available: https: //doc. research-and-analytics. csfb. com/docView?language=ENG&source=ulg&format=PDF& document_id=1022457401&serialid=atRE31ByPklJEXa%2Fp3AyptOvIGdxTK833tLZ1E7AwIQ%3D.

Crum AJ, Langer EJ (2007) Mind-set matters: exercise and the placebo effect. *Psychol Sci* 18(2): 165–171.

Crum AJ et al (2011) Mind over milkshakes: mindsets, not just nutrients, determine ghrelin response. *Health Psychol* 30(4): 424–9.

Csikszentmihalyi M, Wong MM (1991) The situational and personal correlates of happiness: a cross-national comparison. In: Strack F, Argyle M, Schwarz N (eds). *Subjective well-being: an interdisciplinary perspective*, pp 193–212. Elmsford, NY, Pergamon Press.

Danner DD et al (2001) Positive emotions in early life and longevity: Findings from the nun study. *J Pers Soc Psychol* 80: 804–813.

Darragh M et al (2014) Investigating the 'placebo personality' outside the pain paradigm. *J Psychosom Res* 76(5): 414–21.

Darviri C et al (2009) Psychosocial dimensions of exceptional longevity: a qualitative exploration of centenarians' experiences, personality, and life strategies. *Int J Aging Hum Dev* 69(2): 101–18.

Davidson RJ (2003) Alterations in brain and immune function produced by mindfulness meditation. *Psychosom Med* 65(4): 564–70.

de Craen AJ et al (1996) Effect of colour of drugs: systematic review of perceived effect of drugs and of their effectiveness. *BMJ* 313(7072): 1624–6.

de Craen A et al (1999) Placebo effect in the treatment of duodenal ulcer. *Br J Clin Pharmacol* 48(6): 853–860.

de la Fuente-Fernandez R et al (2001) Expectation and dopamine release: mechanism of the placebo effect in Parkinson's disease. *Science* 293: 1164–1166.

Diamond EG et al (1958) Evaluation of internal mammary ligation and sham surgery in angina pectoris. *Circulation* 18: 712–713.

Di Blasi et al (2001) Influence of context effects on health outcomes: a systematic review. *Lancet* 10: 357(9258) 757–62.

Diener E (1984) Subjective well-being. *Psychol Bull* 95: 542–575.

Diener E, Chan MY (2011) Happy people live longer: subjective well-being contributes to health and longevity. Applied Psychology: *Health and Well-Being* 3(1): 1–43.

Diener E, Seligman MEP (2002) Very happy people. *Psych Sci.* 13: 81–84.

Dillon KM et al (1985) Positive emotional states and enhancement of the immune system. *Int J Psychiatry Med* 15: 13–18.

Dugdale DC (1999) Time and the patient–physician relationship. *J Gen Intern Med* 14(S1): S34–S40.

Ellis CN et al (2007) Placebo response in two long-term randomized psoriasis studies that were negative for rosiglitazone. *Am J Clin Dermatol* 8(2): 93–102.

ELSA (English Longitudinal Study for Aging) (n. d.) Online. Accessed 15 March 2015. Available: http://www. ifs. org. uk/ELSA.

Emmons Lab (2014) Online. Accessed June 2014. Available: http://psychology. ucdavis. edu/Labs/emmons/PWT/index. cfm?Section=4.

Emmons R, McCullough ME (2003) Counting blessings versus burdens: an experimental investigation of gratitude and subjective well-being in daily life. *Journal of Personality and Social Psychology* 84(2): 377–389, doi: 10. 1037/0022–3514. 84. 2. 377.

Eremin O et al (2009) Immuno-modulatory effects of relaxation training and guided imagery in women with locally advanced breast cancer undergoing multimodality therapy: a randomised controlled trial. *Breast* 18(1): 17–25.

Ernst E (2001) Towards a scientific understanding of placebo effects. In: Peters D (ed) Understanding the placebo effect in complementary medicine. *Theory, Practice and Research.* Churchill Livingstone, London, pp 17–30.

Evans D (2004) Placebo: mind over matter in modern medicine. London, HarperCollins.

Evans FJ (1974) The placebo response in pain reduction. *Adv Neurol* 4: 286–296.

Evans FJ (1985) Placebo: theory, research and mechanisms. New York, Guilford Press.

Ewald P (2000) Plague time. New York, The Free Press.

Feffer K et al (2011) Is it ethical not to prescribe placebo? The patient's perspective on the usage of placebo for the treatment of depression - a comparative study. *Eur Psychiatry* 26 (1): 1990.

Finding Joe (2011) Directed/written by Patrick Takaya. You Tube. Online. Accessed September 2014. Available: http://findingjoethemovie. com/.

Fisher S, Fisher RI (1963) Placebo response and acquiescence. *Psychopharmacologia* 4: 298–301.

Fisher S, Greenberg RP (1993) How sound is the double-blind design for evaluating psychotropic drugs? *J Nerv Ment Dis* 181(6): 345–50.

Fisher S, Greenberg RP (1997) The curse of the placebo: fanciful pursuit of pure biological therapy, in placebo to panacea: putting psychiatric drugs to the test. New York, Wiley.

Flammer E, Bongartz W (2003) On the efficacy of hypnosis: a meta-analytic study. *Contemp Hypn* 20 (4): 179–197.

Fordyce MW (1977) Development of a program to increase happiness. *J Couns Psychol* 24: 511–521.

Fordyce MW (1983) A program to increase happiness: further studies. *J Couns Psychol* 30: 483–498.

Frank JD, Frank JB (1991) Persuasion and healing (3rd edn). Baltimore and London, The Johns Hopkins University Press.

Frankel RM, Stein T (1999) Getting the most out of the clinical encounter: the four habits model. *Perm J* 3(3): 79–88.

Froh JJ, Sefick WJ, Emmons RA (2008) Counting blessings in early adolescents: an experimental study of gratitude and subjective well-being. J Sch Psychol 2008 Apr; 46(2): 213–33, doi: 10. 1016/j. jsp. 2007. 03. 005. *Epub* 2007 May 4.

Furlan AD et al (2010) Complementary and alternative therapies for back pain II. *Evid Rep Technol Assess (Full Rep)* (194): 1–764.

Furlan AD et al (2012) A systematic review and meta-analysis of efficacy, cost-effectiveness, and safety of selected complementary and alternative medicine for neck and low-back pain. *Evid Based Complement Alternat Med* 2012: 953139.

Garland EL (2007) The meaning of mindfulness: a second-order cybernetics of stress, metacognition, and coping. *Complement Health Pract Rev* 12(1): 15–30.

Gergen KJ, Gergen MM (1988) Narrative and the self as relationship. In: Berkowitz L (ed), *Advances in experimental social psychology*, vol 21. New York, Academic Press, pp 17–56.

Ghaly M, Teplitz D (2004) The biologic effects of grounding the human body during sleep as measured by cortisol levels and subjective reporting of sleep, pain, and stress. *J Altern Complement Med* 10(5): 767–76.

Gibbins J, Thomson AM (2001) Women's expectations and experiences of childbirth. *Midwifery* 17(4), 302–313.

Gibbs S, Harvey I (2006) Topical treatments for cutaneous warts. Cochrane Database Syst Rev Issue 3. Art. No. : CD001781.

Giles LC et al (2005) Effect of social networks on 10 year survival in very old Australians: the Australian longitudinal study of aging. *J Epidemiol Community Health* 59(7): 574–9.

Gracely RH et al (1985) Clinicians' expectations influence placebo analgesia. *Lancet* 5; 1 (8419): 43.

Green JM, Coupland VA, Kitzinger JV (1990) Expectations, experiences and psychological outcomes of childbirth: a prospective study of 825 women. *Birth* 17(1): 15–24.

Greenberg MA, Wortman CB, Stone AA (1996) Emotional expression and physical health: revising traumatic memories or fostering self-regulation? *Journ Pers Soc Psych* 71: 588–602.

Greenfield S et al (1985) Expanding patient involvement in care. *Ann Intern Med* 102(4): 520–8.

Greenfield S et al (1988) Patient participation in medical care: effect on blood sugar and quality of life in diabetes. *J Gen Intern Med.* 3: 448–57.

Greenhalgh T (2001) How to read a paper: the basics of evidence based medicine. London, BMJ Books, p ix.

Greenhalgh T, Hurwitz B (1999). Narrative based medicine: dialogue and discourse in clinical practice. London, BMJ Publishing Group.

Grenfell RF et al (1961) A double-blind study of the treatment of hypertension. *JAMA* 176 (2): 124–8.

Gruenewald TL et al (2009) Increased mortality risk in older adults with persistently low or declining feelings of usefulness to others. *J Aging Health* 21(2): 398–425.

Gryll SL, Katahn M (1978) Situational factors contributing to the placebos effect. *Psychopharmacology (Berl)* 31; 57(3): 253–61.

Hahn RA (1997) The nocebo phenomenon: scope and foundations. In: Harrington A (ed). *The placebo effect: an interdisciplinary exploration.* Cambridge, MA, Harvard University Press.

Hamer M, Chida Y (2008) Walking and primary prevention: a meta-analysis of prospective cohort studies. *Br J Sports Med* 42(4): 238–43.

Harker L, Keltner D (2001) Expressions of positive emotions in women's college yearbook pictures and their relationship to personality and life outcomes across adulthood. *J Pers Soc Psychol* 80: 112–124.

Harrington A (2000) The placebo effect: an interdisciplinary exploration. Cambridge, MA, Harvard University Press.

Hashish I et al (1986) Reduction of postoperative pain and swelling by ultrasound treatment: a placebo effect. Pain 33: 303–311.

Haskard-Zolnierek KB, DiMatteo MR (2009) Physician communication and patient adherence to treatment: a meta-analysis. *Med Care* 47(8): 826–834.

Häuser W, Hansen E, Enck P (2012) Nocebo phenomena in medicine: their relevance in everyday clinical practice. *Dtsch Arztebl Int* 109(26): 459–65.

Healy D (1997) The antidepressant era. MA and London, Harvard University Press, p. 90.

Hecimovich M et al (2014) Development and psychometric evaluation of scales to measure professional confidence in manual medicine: a Rasch measurement approach. *BMC Res Notes* 4; 7(1): 338.

Hillen MA et al (2011) Cancer patients' trust in their physician-a review. *Psychooncology* 20(3): 227–41.

Holwerda N et al (2013) Do patients trust their physician? The role of attachment style in the patient-physician relationship within one year after a cancer diagnosis. *Acta Oncol* 52(1): 110–7.

Hölzel BK et al (2008) Investigation of mindfulness meditation practitioners with voxel-based morphometry. *Soc Cogn Affect Neurosci* 3(1): 55–61.

Hunter P (2007) A question of faith. Exploiting the placebo effect depends on both the susceptibility of the patient to suggestion and the ability of the doctor to instil trust. *EMBO Rep* 8(2): 125–128.

Huskisson EC (1974) Simple analgesics for arthritis. *Br Med J* 26; 4 (5938): 196–200.

Hussain MZ, Ahad A (1970) Tablet colour in anxiety states. *Br Med J* 3(5720): 466.

Hrobjartsson A, Gotzsche PC (2001) Is the placebo powerless? An analysis of clinical trials comparing placebo with no treatment. *N Engl J Med* 344: 1594–1602.

Ikema Y, Nakagawa S (1962) A psychosomatic study of contagious dermatitis. *Kyoshu J Med Sci* 13: 335–350.

Ilnyckyj A et al (1997) Quantification of the placebo response in ulcerative colitis. *Gastroenterol* 112(6): 1854–8.

Ingraham P (2014) Your back is not out of alignment – debunking the obsession with alignment, posture, and other biomechanical bogeymen as major causes of pain. 9 July 2014. Online. Accessed Sept 2014. Available: http://saveyourself. ca/articles/structuralism. php.

Janssen I, Jolliffe CJ (2006) Influence of physical activity on mortality in elderly with coronary artery disease. *Med Sci Sports Exerc* 38(3): 418–7.

Jauk E et al (2012) Tackling creativity at its roots: evidence for different patterns of EEG alpha activity related to convergent and divergent modes of task processing. *Int J Psychophysiol* 84(2): 219–225.

Jenkinson CE et al (2013) Is volunteering a public health intervention? A systematic review and meta-analysis of the health and survival of volunteers. *BMC Public Health* 23; 13: 773.

Jensen MP, Karoly P (1991) Motivation and expectancy factors in symptom perception: a laboratory study of the placebo effect. *Psychosom Med* 53(2): 144–52.

Kabat-Zinn J et al (1985) The clinical use of mindfulness meditation for the self-regulation of chronic pain. *J Behav Med* 8 (2): 163–190.

Kaptchuk TJ et al (2000) Do medical devices have enhanced placebo effects? *J Clin Epidemiol* 53: 786–792.

Kaptchuk TJ et al (2008a) Do 'placebo responders' exist? *Contemp Clin Trials* 29: 587–595.

Kaptchuk TJ et al (2008b) Components of placebo effect: randomised controlled trial in patients with irritable bowel syndrome. *BMJ* 336(7651): 999–1003.

Kaptchuk TJ et al (2010) Placebos without deception: a randomized controlled trial in irritable bowel syndrome. *PLoS ONE* 5(12): e15591.

Karni A (1995) When practice makes perfect. *Lancet* 345: 395.

Keller VF, Carroll JG (1994) A new model for physician-patient communication. *Patient Educ Couns* 23: 131–40.

Kelley GA et al (2004) Walking, lipids, and lipoproteins: a meta-analysis of randomized controlled trials. *Prev Med* 38(5): 651–61.

Kelley JM (2009) Patient and practitioner influences on the placebo effect in irritable bowel syndrome. *Psychosom Med* 71(7): 789.

Kemmler W et al (2004) Benefits of 2 years of intense exercise on bone density, physical fitness, and blood lipids in early postmenopausal osteopenic women: results of the Erlangen Fitness Osteoporosis Prevention Study (EFOPS). *Arch Intern Med* 24; 164(10): 1084–91.

Kent S et al (1992) Sickness behaviour as a new target for drug development. *Trends Pharmacol Sci* 13: 24–28.

Khalsa DS, Stauth C (2002) Meditation as medicine: activate the power of your natural healing force. New York, Fireside Books.

Khan A, Redding N, Brown WA (2008) The persistence of the placebo response in antidepressant clinical trials. *J Psychiatr Res* 42(10): 791–6.

Kim YH et al (2013) Effects of meditation on anxiety, depression, fatigue, and quality of life of women undergoing radiation therapy for breast cancer. *Complement Ther Med* 21(4): 379–87.

King DE et al (2005) Dietary magnesium and C-reactive protein levels. *J Am Coll Nutr* 24(3): 166–71.

Kirsch I (2010). Emperor's new drugs: exploding the antidepressant myth. London, Random House Group, p. 111.

Kirsh I, Sapirstein G (1998) Listening to Prozac but hearing placebo: a meta-analysis of anti-depressant medication. Prevention and Treatment. 1 Article 0002a.

Kirschbaum C et al (1992) Conditioning of drug-induced immunomodulation in human volunteers: a European collaborative study. *Br J Clin Psychol* 31: 459–472.

Koivumaa-Honkanen H et al (2001) Life satisfaction and suicide: a 20-year follow-up study. *Am J Psych* 158: 433–439.

Kong J et al (2006) Brain activity associated with expectancy-enhanced placebo analgesia as measured by functional magnetic resonance imaging. *J Neurosci* 26(2): 381–388.

Krause N, Shaw BA (2003). Role-specific control, personal meaning, and health in late life. *Res Aging* 25: 559–58.

Lahmann C et al (2010) Effects of functional relaxation and guided imagery on IgE in dust-mite allergic adult asthmatics: a randomized, controlled clinical trial. *J Nerv Ment Dis* 198(2): 125–30.

Laine C et al (1996) Important elements of outpatient care: a comparison of patients' and physicians' opinions. *Ann Intern Med* 15; 125(8): 640–5.

Langs R (2004) Fundamentals of adaptive psychotherapy and counselling. Basingstoke, Palgrave Macmillan.

Lasagna L et al (1954) A study of the placebo response. *Am J Med* 16 (6): 770–779.

Lawler KA et al (2003) A change of heart: cardiovascular correlates of forgiveness in response to interpersonal conflict. *J Behav Med* 26(5): 373–93.

Lawler-Row KA (2008) Forgiveness, physiological reactivity and health: the role of anger. *Int J Psychophysio* 68: 1. 51–58.

Lazar SW et al (2005) Meditation experience is associated with increased cortical thickness. *Neuroreport* 28; 16(17): 1893–1897.

Lee CD et al (2003) Physical activity and stroke risk: a meta-analysis. *Stroke* 34(10): 2475–81.

Levine J et al (1978) The mechanism of placebo analgesia. *Lancet* 312 (8091): 654–657.

Levine JD et al (1979) Role of pain in placebo analgesia. *Proc Natl Acad Sci* USA 76(7): 3528–3531.

Levy BR et al (2002) Longevity increased by positive self-perceptions of aging. *J Pers Soc Psycho* 83(2): 261–270.

Liberman RP (1964) An experimental study of placebo response under three different situations of pain. *J Psychiatr Res* 2: 233–246.

Liberman BL (1978) The role of mastery in psychotherapy: maintenance of improvement and prescriptive change. In: Frank JD et al. *Effective ingredients in psychotherapy*. New York, Brunner Mazel.

Lichter S et al (1980) Increasing happiness through cognitive retraining. *New Zealand Psychologist* 9: 57–64.

Like R, Zyzanski SJ (1987) Patient satisfaction with the clinical encounter: social psychological determinants. *Soc Sci Med* 24(4): 351–7.

Linde C et al (1999). Placebo effect of pacemaker implantation in obstructive hypertrophic cardiomyopathy. PIC Study Group. Pacing in cardiomyopathy. *Am J Cardiol* 83(6): 903–907.

Lindström J et al (2003) Prevention of diabetes mellitus in subjects with impaired glucose tolerance in the Finnish Diabetes Prevention Study: results from a randomized clinical trial. *J Am Soc Nephrol* 14(7 Suppl 2): S108–13.

Livesey G, Taylor R (2008) Fructose consumption and consequences for glycation, plasma triacylglycerol, and body weight: meta-analyses and meta-regression models of intervention studies. *Am J ClinNutr* 88(5): 1419–37.

Longo DL et al (1999) Conditioned immune response to interferon-gamma in humans. *Clin Immunol* 90(2): 173–181.

Lowe NK (1989) Explaining the pain of active labor: the importance of maternal confidence. *Res Nurs Health* (4): 237–45.

Lowe NK (2003) Child-birth self-efficacy inventory. In: Redman BK (ed) *Measurement tools in patient education*, 2nd edn. New York, Springer.

Lucchelli PE et al (1978) Effect of capsule colour and order of administration of hypnotic treatments. *Eur J Clin Pharmacol* 17; 13(2): 153–5.

Luder E et al (2009) The underlying anatomical correlates of long-term meditation: larger hippocampal and frontal volumes of gray matter. *Neuroimage April* 15; 45(3): 672–678.

Luevano-Contreras C, Chapman-Novakofski K (2010) Dietary advanced glycation end products and aging. *Nutrients* 2(12) 1247–1265.

LuparelloTJ et al (1970) The interaction of physiologic stimuli and pharmacologic agents on airway reactivity in asthmas subjects. *Psychosom Med* 32: 509–513.

Luskin F (2002) Forgive for good – a proven prescription for health and happiness. New York, HarperCollins.

Lutz GK et al (1999) The relation between expectations and outcomes in surgery for sciatica. *J Gen Intern Med* 14(12): 740–744.

McQuay H et al (1995) Variations in the placebo effect in randomized controlled trials of analgesics; all is blind as it seems. *Pain* 64: 331–335.

Marks GN, Fleming N (1999) Influences and consequences of well-being among Australian young people: 1980–1995. *Social Indicators Research* 46: 301–323.

Martin P (1997) The sickening mind: brain, behaviour, immunity and disease. London, HarperCollins.

Meissner K (2011) The placebo effect and the autonomic nervous system: evidence for an intimate relationship. *Philos Trans R Soc Lond B Biol Sci* 366 (1572): 1808–17.

Merriam Webster Online: Dictionary and Thesaurus. Online. Accessed April 2013. Available: http://www. merriam-webster. com/.

Meyers S, Janowitz HD (1989). The 'natural history' of ulcerative colitis: an analysis of the placebo response. *J Clin Gastroenterol* 11(1): 33–7.

Miller FG, Kaptchuk TJ (2008) The power of context: reconceptualizing the placebo effect. *J R Soc Med* 1; 101(5): 222–225.

Miller MC (2010) Unconscious or subconscious? Blog. Mental Health Publishing, Harvard Health Publications. Online. Accessed June 2014. Available: http://www. health. harvard. edu/blog/unconscious-or-subconscious-20100801255.

Moerman DE (1983) General medical effectiveness and human biology. *Med Anthropol Q* 14(4): 3–16.

Moerman DE (2000) Cultural variations in the placebo effect: ulcers, anxiety and blood pressure. *Med Anthropol Q* 14: 1–22.

Moerman D (2002) Meaning, medicine and the placebo effect. Cambridge Studies in Medical Anthropology. Cambridge, Cambridge University Press.

Moerman DE (2006) Editorial: The meaning response: thinking about placebos. *Pain Practice* 6(4): 233–23. Online. Accessed June 2014. Available: http://www. academia. edu/4469275/EDITORIAL_The_Meaning_Response_Thinking_about_Placebos.

Montgomery GH, Kirsh I (1997) Classical conditioning and the placebo effect. *Pain* 72: 107–113.

Moseley JB et al (2002) A controlled trial of arthroscopic surgery for osteoarthritis of the knee. *NEJM* 11; 347(2): 81–8.

Nagao Y et al (1968) Effect of the color of analgesics on their therapeutic results. *Shikwa Gakuho* 68(4): 139–42 [Article in Japanese].

National Institutes Of Health (2013) We Can!' Community News Feature. Online. Accessed June 2014. Available: https://www. nhlbi. nih. gov/health/educational/wecan/news-events/matte1. htm.

Nickel JC et al (1996) Efficacy and safety of finasteride therapy for benign prostatic hyperplasia: results of a 2-year randomized controlled trial. *CMAJ* 155(9): 1251–9.

Nitzan U et al (2011) The informed consent not to be informed – a cross sectional survey on the use of placebo in clinical practice. *Eur Psych.* 26 (1): 756.

Ober C (n. d.) Clint Ober demonstrates earthing (Part 1/3). Online. Accessed: 16 March 2015. Available: http://www. youtube. com/watch?v=9OhYOsvJleA.

Ockene JK et al (2005) Symptom experience after discontinuing use of estrogen plus progestin. *JAMA* 294 (2): 183–93.

Okun MA et al (1984) The social activity/subjective well-being relation: a quantitative synthesis. *Research on Aging* 6: 45–65.

Ornish D et al (2008) Changes in prostate gene expression in men undergoing an intensive nutrition and lifestyle intervention. *Proc Natl Acad Sci USA* 105: 8369–8374.

Oschman JL (2007) Can electrons act as antioxidants? A review and commentary. *J Altern Complement Med* 13(9): 955–67.

Palermo TM et al (2010) Randomized controlled trials of psychological therapies for management of chronic pain in children and adolescents: An updated meta-analytic review. *Pain* 148(3): 387–97.

Park LC, Covi L (1965) Nonblind placebo trial. *Arch Gen Psychiatry* 12: 336–345.

Paul-Labrador M et al (2006) Effects of a randomized controlled trial of transcendental meditation on components of the metabolic syndrome in subjects with coronary heart disease. *Arch Intern Med* 166 (11).

Peabody FW (1984) Landmark article March 19, 1927: the care of the patient. By Francis W. Peabody. *JAMA* 252(6): 813–8.

Pennebaker JW (2004) Writing to heal: a guided journal for recovering from trauma and emotional upheaval. Oakland, CA, New Harbinger Publications.

Pennebaker JW, Seagal JD (1999) Forming a story: the health benefits of narrative. *Journ Clin Psych* 55(10): 1243–1254.

Pennebaker JW et al (1989) Disclosure of traumas and health among Holocaust survivors. *Psychosom Med* 1989 51(5): 577–89.

Petrovic P et al (2005) Placebo in emotional processing – induced expectations of anxiety relief activate a generalized modulatory network. *Neuron* 46: 957–969.

Pinto A et al (2006) Twenty-four hour ambulatory blood pressure monitoring to evaluate effects on blood pressure of physical activity in hypertensive patients. *Clin J Sport Med* 16(3): 238–43.

Platt FW (1992). Empathy: can it be taught? *An Intern Med.* 117(8): 700; author reply 701.

Platt FW, Keller VF (1994) Empathic communication: a teachable and learnable skill. *J Gen Intern Med* 9(4): 222–6.

Pluess M et al (2009) Muscle tension in generalized anxiety disorder: a critical review of the literature. *J Anxiety Disord* 23(1): 1–11.

Pogge R (1963) The toxic placebo. *Med Times* 91: 773–778.

Pollo A, Carlino E, Benedetti F (2011) Placebo mechanisms across different conditions: from the clinical setting to physical performance. *Philos Trans R Soc Lond B Biol Sci* 27; 366(1572): 1790–8.

Price D et al (1999) An analysis of factors that contribute to the magnitude of placebo analgesia in an experimental paradigm. *Pain* 83: 147–156.

Rabkin JG et al (1986) How blind is blind? Assessment of patient and doctor medication guesses in a placebo-controlled trial of imipramine and phenelzine. *Psychiatry Res* 19(1): 75–86.

Redhead S (2010) Keys to the laws of creation. Bloomington, IN, Xlibris.

Redman BK (2003) Measurement tools in patient education, New York, Springer.

Reynold T (2003) Researchers push for publication, registration of all clinical trials. *J Natl Cancer Inst* 95 (11): 772–774.

Roberts AH et al (1993) The power of non-specific effects in healing: implications for psychosocial and biological treatments. *Clin Psychol Rev* 13: 375–3.

Rodriguez-Laso A et al (2007) The effect of social relationships on survival in elderly residents of a Southern European community: a cohort study. *BMC Geriatrics* 1(7): 19.

Roscoe J et al (2004) Patient expectation is a strong predictor of severe nausea after chemotherapy. *Cancer* 101 (11): 2701–2708.

Rosengren A, Wilhelmsen L (1997) Physical activity protects against coronary death and deaths from all causes in middle-aged men. Evidence from a 20-year follow-up of the primary prevention study in Göteborg. *Ann Epidemiol* 7(1): 69–7.

Ross A, Thomas S (2010) The health benefits of yoga and exercise: a review of comparison studies. *J Altern Complement Med* 16(1): 3–12.

Rotter JB (1966) Generalized expectancies for internal versus external control of reinforcement. *Psychol Monogr* 80, Whole No. 609.

Rotter JB (1990). Internal versus external control of reinforcement. *Am Psychol.* 45 (4): 489–493.

Rubinstein SM et al (2013) Spinal manipulative therapy for acute low back pain: an update of the cochrane review. *Spine* (Phila Pa 1976) 38(3): E158–77.

Salkeld G et al (2004) A matter of trust – patient's views on decision-making in colorectal cancer. *Health Expect* 7: 104–114.

Samueli Institute (2013) Using placebo responses in clinical practice: is there a there, there? What do we need to know? Samueli Institute, January 20, 2012 p. 15 Online. Accessed June 2014. Available: http://www. samueliinstitute. org/File%20Library/Unassigned/RPT_Using-Placebo-In-Clinical-Practice-1-20-12. pdf.

Sandler A et al (2008) Children's and parent's perspectives on open-label use of placebos in the treatment of ADHD. *Child Care Health Dev* 34: 111–120.

Sarno J E (1998) The mindbody prescription. New York, Warner Books.

Sarsan A et al (2006) The effects of aerobic and resistance exercises in obese women. *Clin Rehabil* 20(9): 773–82.

Schedlowski M, Pacheco-López G (2010) The learned immune response: *Pavlov and beyond. Brain Behav Immun* 24(2): 176–85.

Schneider RH et al (2012) Stress reduction in the secondary prevention of cardiovascular disease: randomized, controlled trial of transcendental meditation and health education in blacks. *Circ Cardiovasc Qual Outcomes* 5(6): 750–8.

Schwartz C (1994) Introduction: old methodological challenges and new mind-body links in psychoneuroimmunology. *Advances* 10(4): 4–7.

Schweizer E, Rickels K (1997) Placebo response in generalized anxiety: its effect on the outcome of clinical trials. *J Clin Psychiatry* 58 Suppl 11: 30–8.

Schweitzer M et al (2004) Healing spaces: elements of environmental design that make an impact on health. *J Altern Complement Med* 10; Suppl 1: S71–83.

Scott DJ et al (2007) Individual differences in reward responding explain placebo-induced expectations and effects. *Neuron* 55 (2): 325–336.

Seaward B (2006) Managing stress: principles and strategies for health and well-being. Boston, Jones & Bartlett.

Seeman TE (1996) Social ties and health: the benefits of social integration. *Ann Epidemiol* 6(5): 442–51.

Shapiro AK (1959). The placebo effect in the history of medical treatment: implications for psychiatry. *Am J Psychiatry.* 116: 298–304.

Shapiro AK, Shapiro E (2000) The placebo: is it much ado about nothing? In: Harrington A (ed) The placebo effect: an interdisciplinary exploration. Cambridge, MA, Harvard University Press, pp 12–36.

Shapiro SL et al (2005) Mindfulness-based stress reduction and health care professionals. *Int J Stress Manag* 12 (2): 64–176.

Shapiro SL et al (2006) Mechanisms of mindfulness. *J Clin Psychol* 62(3): 373–386.

Silberman S (2009) Placebos are getting more effective. Drugmakers are desperate to know why. Wired Magazine 17. 09. Online. Accessed June 2014. Available: http://www. wired. com/medtech/drugs/magazine/17–09/ff_placebo_effect.

Simpson SH et al (2006) A meta-analysis of the association between adherence to drug therapy and mortality. *Br Med J.* 333: 15.

Smith M, Segal R (2014) HelpGuide. org. Stress management. Online. Accessed June 2014. Available: http://www. helpguide. org/mental/stress_management_relief_coping. htm.

Smucker DR et al (1998) Practitioner self-confidence and patient outcomes in acute low back pain. *Arch Fam Med* 7(3): 223–8.

Somerville M (2013) Ethical canary: science, society, and the human spirit. Georgetown, ON, McGill-Queens Press, pp 196–7.

Sox HC et al (1981) Psychologically mediated effects of diagnostic tests. *Ann Intern Med* 95(6): 680–5.

Spiro H (1992) What is empathy and can it be taught? *Ann Intern Med* 15; 116(10): 843–6.

Starfield B et al (1981) The influence of patient-practitioner agreement on outcome of care. *Am J Public Health* 71: 127–132.

Sternbach RA, Tursky B (1965) Ethnic differences in housewives in psychophysical and skin potential responses to electric shock. *Psychophysiology* 1: 241–46.

Stetter F, Kupper S (2002) Autogenic training: a meta-analysis of clinical outcome studies. *Appl Psychophysiol Biofeedback* 27 (1): 45–98.

Stewart SH et al. (2002). Relation between alcohol consumption and C-reactive protein levels in the adult US population. *J Am Board Fam Med* 15(6).

Strean WB (2009) Laughter prescription. *Can Fam Physician* 2009; 55(10): 965–967.

Su C et al (2006) A meta-analysis of the placebo rates of remission and response in clinical trials of active ulcerative colitis. *Gastroenterology* 132(2): 516–526.

Swinburn B et al (2009) Increased food energy supply is more than sufficient to explain the US epidemic of obesity. *Am J Clin Nutr* 90(6) 1453–1456.

Tamim H et al (2009) Tai Chi workplace program for improving musculoskeletal fitness among female computer users. *Work* 34(3): 331–8.

Tang YY et al (2009) Central and autonomic nervous system interaction is altered by short-term meditation. *Proceedings of the National Academy of Sciences* USA 106(22): 8865–70.

The Earthing Institute (2014) The Earthing Institute. Reconnecting people to the planet. Earthing research. Online. Accessed June 2014. Available: http://www. earthinginstitute. net/index. php/research.

Thom D et al (2004) Measuring patients' trust in physicians when assessing quality of care. *Health Aff (Millwood)* 23(4): 124–32.

Thomas KB (1987) General practice consultations: is there any point in being positive? *Br Med J (Clin Res Ed)* 294(6581): 1200–1202.

Thompson WG (2005) The placebo effect and health. Amherst, NY, Prometheus Books pp 40, 71–82.

Tilley BC et al (1995) Minocycline in rheumatoid arthritis: a 48-week double-blind placebo-controlled trial. *Ann Intern Med* 122: 81–89.

Toussaint LL et al (2012) Forgive to live: forgiveness, health, and longevity. *J Behav Med* 35(4): 375–86.

Tracey I (2010) Getting the pain you expect: mechanisms of placebo, nocebo and reappraisal effects in humans. *Nat Med* 16(11): 1277–83.

Turner J et al (1994) The importance of placebos in pain treatment and research. *JAMA* 271 (20): 1609–1614.

Tyrer P et al (2008) Risperidone, haloperidol, and placebo in the treatment of aggressive challenging behaviour in patients with intellectual disability: a randomised controlled trial. *Lancet* 371, 9606: 57–63.

University of Maryland Medical Center (2013). Health Information. Medical Reference Guide. Omega-3 fatty acids. Online. Accessed June 2014. Available: http://umm. edu/health/medical/altmed/supplement/omega3-fatty-acids#ixzz2s7tno8IB.

University of Pennsylvania Positive Psychology Center (2007) Online. Accessed June 2014. Available: http://www. ppc. sas. upenn. edu.

University of Southampton (2015) News release. 12 February 2015. Psychological factors play a part in acupuncture treatment of back pain. Ref: 15_27. Online. Accessed 13 March 2015. Available at: http://www. southampton. ac. uk/mediacentre/news/2015/Feb/15_27. shtml .

US National Library of Health, National Institutes of Health, MeSH term definition. Online. Accessed June 2014. Available: http://www. ncbi. nlm. nih. gov/mesh?Db=mesh&term=Placebo+Effect.

Vase L et al (2002) A comparison of placebo effects in clinical analgesic trials versus studies of placebo analgesia. *Pain*. 99: 443–452.

Vase L et al (2003) The contributions of suggestion, desire, and expectation to placebo effects in irritable bowel syndrome patients. *An empirical investigation Pain* 105(1–2): 17–25.

Verghese A (2011) Treat the patient, not the CT scan. New York Times Opinion Pages, Feb 26.

Voices of Beth Israel Deaconess Medical Centre Research at Harvard Medical School. Can a placebo pill help you feel better? Interview, 2012. Online. Accessed June 2014. Available: http://www. youtube. com/watch?v=2rt7WIK2OVE.

Volgyesi FA (1954). 'School for patients': hypnosis-therapy and psychoprophylaxis. *Brit J Med Hypn* 5: 8–17.

Voudouris NJ et al (1989) Conditioned response models of placebo phenomenon: further support. *Pain* 38: 109–116.

Waber RL et al (2008) Commercial features of placebo and therapeutic efficacy. *JAMA*. 299 (9): 1016–7.

Walters DD et al (1983) Spontaneous remission is a frequent outcome of variant angina. *J Am Coll Cardiol* 2(2): 195–9.

Webb JR et al (2013) Forgiveness and health: assessing the mediating effect of health behavior, social support, and interpersonal functioning. *J Psychol* 147(5): 391–414.

Weil A (1995) Spontaneous healing. New York. Fawcett, Columbine.

Whitfield TWA, Wiltshire TJ (1990) Color psychology: a critical review. *Genet Soc Gen Psych Monogr* 116(4): 387.

Wickramasekera I (1980) A conditioned response model of the placebo effect: predictions from the model. *Biofeedback Self Regul* 5: 5–18.

Wilmer HA (1968) The doctor-patient relationship and issues of pity, sympathy and empathy. *Br J Med Psychol* 41(3): 243–8.

Wilson A et al (1992) Health promotion in the general practice consultation: a minute makes a difference. *BMJ* 25; 304(6821): 227–230.

Wolf S (1950) Effects of suggestion and conditioning on the action of chemical agents in human subjects: the pharmacology of placebos. *J Clin Invest* 29: 100–109.

Wolf S, Pinsky RH (1954) Effects of placebo administration and occurrence of toxic reactions. *JAMA*. 155: 339–341.

Wolff B, Langley S (1968) Cultural factors and the response to pain: A review. *Am Anthropol* 70 (3): 494–501.

Wu CW et al (2007) Treadmill exercise counteracts the suppressive effects of peripheral lipopolysaccharide on hippocampal neurogenesis and learning and memory. *J Neurochem* 103(6): 2471–81.

Yin J et al (2013) Bounding the speed of 'spooky action at a distance'. Ar Xiv: 1303. 0614v1 [quant-ph] Online. Accessed June 2014. Available: http://arxiv. org/pdf/1303. 0614v1. pdf.

Young LR, Nestle M (2002) The contribution of expanding portion sizes to the US obesity epidemic. *Am J Public Health* 92(2): 246–249.

Zahl PH et al (2008) The natural history of invasive breast cancers detected by screening mammography. *Arch Intern Med*. 168(21): 2311–6.

Zborowsky T, Kreitzer MJ (2008) Creating optimal healing environments in a health care setting. *Minn Med* 91(3): 35–8.

Zhang W et al (2008) The placebo effect and its determinants in osteoarthritis: meta-analysis of randomised controlled trials. *Ann Rheum Dis* 67: 1716–1723.

Zubieta JK et al (2005) Placebo effects mediated by endogenous opioid activity on μ-opioid receptors. *J Neurosci* 25(34): 7754–7762.

Zunzunegui MV et al (2009) Longevity and relationships with children: the importance of the parental role. BMC Public Health. 18(9): 351. Online. Accessed June 2014. Available: http://www.biomedcentral.com/1471-2458/9/35100.

USEFUL WEBSITES

Forgiveness

http://theforgivenessproject.com/The Forgiveness Project
  Helpful resources for resolving forgiveness issues.
http://www.thepoweroforgiveness.com/
  The Power of Forgiveness contains excellent resources including a forgiveness quiz.
http://www.forgiving.org/
  Campaign for Forgiveness Research.
http://www.learningtoforgive.com/research.htm
  Stamford University Forgiveness Project.

Happiness

http://thehappinessshow.com
http://www. authentichappiness.sas.upenn.edu/
  Martin Seligman's website offers extensive happiness coaching.
http://www. psych.uiuc.edu/~ediener/
  Ed Denier's website.

Index